Neurodynamics of Personality

NEURODYNAMICS OF PERSONALITY

Jim Grigsby
David Stevens

THE GUILFORD PRESS
New York   London

#43051564

© 2000 The Guilford Press
A Division of Guilford Publications, Inc.
72 Spring Street, New York, NY 10012
www.guilford.com

Printed in the United States of America

This book is printed on acid-free paper.

Last digit is print number: 9 8 7 6 5 4 3 2 1

Library of Congress Cataloging-in-Publication Data
Grigsby, Jim.
  Neurodynamics of personality / Jim Grigsby, David Stevens.
    p. ; cm.
  Includes bibliographical references and index.
  ISBN 1-57230-547-9 (hard)
    1. Neuropsychology. 2. Personality. I. Stevens, David, 1954– II. Title.
    [DNLM: 1. Personality—physiology. 2. Brain—physiology. 3. Mental
Processes—physiology. 4. Neuropsychology. 5. Psychological Theory.
BF 698.2 G857n 2000]
QP360 .G745 2000
612.8—dc21
                                                              99-089082

A man can seldom—very, very seldom—fight a winning fight against his training; the odds are too heavy.

—MARK TWAIN, *As Regards Patriotism*

We do not initiate thought by an effort of self-consciousness. We find ourselves thinking, just as we find ourselves breathing and enjoying the sunset. There is a habit of daydreaming, and a habit of thoughtful elucidation. Thus the autonomy of thought is strictly limited, often negligible, generally beyond the threshold of consciousness.

—ALFRED NORTH WHITEHEAD, *Adventures of Ideas*

It is like learning to write. To acquire this art, one must practice much, however disagreeable or difficult it may be, however impossible it may seem. Practicing earnestly and often, one learns to write, acquires the art. To be sure, each letter must first be considered separately and accurately, reproduced over and over again; but once having acquired skill, one need not pay any attention to the reproduction [of the letters] or even think of them. He will write fluently and freely whether it be penmanship or some bold work, in which his art appears. It is sufficient for the writer to know that he is using his skill and since he does not always have to think of it, he does his work by means of it.

—MEISTER JOHANNES ECKHART, *The Talks of Instruction*

"It's a remarkable piece of apparatus."

—FRANZ KAFKA, *In the Penal Colony*

About the Authors

Jim Grigsby, PhD, is a research scientist at the University of Colorado Health Sciences Center, where he is Associate Professor in the Department of Medicine, Division of Geriatrics, and Senior Researcher at the Center for Health Services and Policy Research. He attended the University of Kansas and the University of Regina (formerly University of Saskatchewan), and obtained his doctorate at the University of Colorado. The primary focus of his research has been on the neuropsychological capacity to regulate purposeful behavior.

David Stevens, PhD, a practicing clinical psychologist and psychoanalyst, is Associate Clinical Professor in the Department of Psychiatry at the University of Colorado Health Sciences Center. He is on the faculties of the Denver Institute for Psychoanalysis and the Minnesota Psychoanalytic Institute, where he teaches classes in comparative psychoanalytic theory. He is also an adjunct faculty member of the University of Denver doctoral program in child clinical psychology. He lives in Denver with his wife, Jan, and their children, Alex and Abbey.

PREFACE

Speculation about the relationship between the brain and the mind began centuries ago, yet the details of that relationship have remained obscure. For centuries, damaged brains provided the primary window on the role of the brain in mediating personality and behavior. While this has been informative, the inferences that may be drawn from the study of pathology must be qualified, and they often cannot tell us how an intact, living brain works. In order to understand the brain we must study the neurophysiological and psychological processes characteristic of living organisms—something that has become possible only in recent decades. Despite significant progress, current knowledge remains relatively rudimentary. Nevertheless, enough is known that it is possible to formulate a number of reasonable hypotheses—a task we undertake in this book.

The scope of the model we present is broad, encompassing a number of scientific disciplines. In part, this is because a system as complex as the brain cannot be grasped without considering many kinds of information. Furthermore, we considered it important to establish a range of data and evidence with which, we believe, any general approach to personality theory must be consistent, and to attempt to shed light on psychological phenomena by establishing links between different fields of study. The result is a synthesis, a relatively comprehensive framework for thinking about personality functioning.

This book was written both for professionals (behavioral and neurobehavioral clinicians) and nonprofessionals who are interested in an evolving approach to the integration of biology and psychology. It is likely that we have not gone into sufficient depth in any given area to satisfy specialists in such matters as synaptic plasticity, functional neuroanatomy, or learning theory, but our intention was to produce a volume that would be of more general interest.

We are aware that most readers will already have a theory of the mind, and that they will perceive and critique the model we present through lenses shaped by the process of learning and repeatedly using that theory. Thus, each reader's theoretical perspective will serve as a kind of measuring stick, used not only to explain and predict psychological phenomena, but to assess the adequacy of other models (including our own).

From a psychological viewpoint, a theory is not only a systematic set of ideas and evidence; it is also a perceptual heuristic, a way of recognizing patterns—something people do automatically and nonconsciously. As one learns to navigate within a theoretical framework, developing habits of thinking and perceiving, it becomes a relatively effortless matter to find one's way around. At the same time, it may be more difficult to get one's bearings by means of a different theory, since the patterns one has already learned to recognize are easy to see, while those patterns that may become apparent through the medium of an unfamiliar model require deliberate consideration and somewhat effortful application if they are to be useful.

People think the way they habitually think, and to expect a book to change ingrained habits of thinking is a tall order. Whether this book is up to that task remains to be seen. It has taken many years for both of us to achieve the facility required to use this model relatively automatically. In any event, we believe the conceptual framework presented here is a useful one for understanding a number of important psychological phenomena, from the nature of the self to the basis of personality change. However, the reader will find it useful not as a collection of facts (i.e., declarative knowledge) but as a way of thinking (i.e., involving a kind of procedural knowledge as well).

—JIM GRIGSBY

As a practicing clinical psychologist and psychoanalyst I have had many opportunities to appreciate how profoundly difficult it can be for even highly motivated people to effect and maintain change in their behavior. It is common in clinical practice to encounter people who appear repeatedly to recreate life circumstances that engender one variety of predictable misery or another. As my appreciation for the difficulty associated with promoting useful change has deepened, my professional and scientific interests have increasingly focused on attempting to codify a set of clinical working principles that would sharpen clinical efficacy. A series of lively conversations with my friend Jim Grigsby, conducted over a period of 20 years, has fueled my conviction that findings from the neurosciences have riches to offer the mental health professional who perseveres in the effort to integrate neuroscience constructs into his or her conception of human beings and their behavior.

Although Jim speaks the language of neuroscience and physics while I am more immersed in psychoanalytic concepts, we have usually been successful at establishing a common ground in our conversations. On some occasions we might examine a piece of unfolding clinical material and/or some associated clinical or theoretical construct in light of ideas derived from Jim's study of clinical neuroscience. On other occasions we might more directly attempt to reconcile our perspectives on change. Gradually, across these conversations, it became increasingly clear to us that the neuroscientific perspective Jim articulated seemed to suggest a clinically useful and coherent set of organizing principles for conceptualizing the processes associated with change in the clinical situation.

Freud had originally hoped to establish an understanding of psychological phenomena that was grounded in neurology. In his *Project for a Scientific Psychology* he attempted to redescribe psychological events in terms derived from the neurophysiology of the day, but it turned out that the data and associated theoretical constructs available to Freud were too primitive and too blunt to provide him with the necessary scientific scaffolding for the metapsychology he had hoped to create. Although Freud abandoned his efforts to find a neuroscientifically based metapsychology, he remained hopeful throughout his career that psychoanalysis would eventually be grounded in findings from the scientific study of the brain.

Much has been learned about the organization and functioning of the brain since Freud's day and increasingly, journals read by psychologists and psychoanalysts interested in clinical applications contain papers dealing with constructs derived from the neurosciences. Yet for those of us whose intimate working knowledge of the brain may have been acquired in courses taken in graduate school many years ago, and subsequently added to in a piecemeal fashion, it can be difficult to make sense out of articles that attempt to bridge psychology and neuroscience. Many clinicians I know glaze over when confronted with an amygdala or prefrontal cortex. Furthermore, attempting to extrapolate or bootleg an understanding of brain functioning by reading articles in one's field that make use of neuroscientific constructs can lead to a fragmented understanding of how brains might work. Yet the prospect of acquiring the general grounding in neuroscience that would be required to be more informed about the applicability of neuroscientific ideas to psychology or psychoanalysis can make the non-neuroscientist faint-hearted.

I think this book's greatest value may lay in its synthesis of findings from many areas of science into a coherent, scientifically informed model of brain organization that is accessible to the non-neuroscientist. It is an exploration of how brains make minds, offering a systematic overview of diverse areas of science, and providing the clinician with a grounding in neural constructs that have immediate relevance to understanding personality processes.

—DAVID STEVENS

ACKNOWLEDGMENTS

This book, and the papers that preceded it, would not have been written without the collaboration of Jay L. Schneiders. Jay's contribution to the basic thinking outlined here was indispensable in the development of these ideas, and his comments on the manuscript were extremely helpful. Similarly, conversations with Kathryn Kaye over a number of years regarding a wide range of subjects (especially the significance of neural dynamics), and collaboration with her in research on the regulation of purposeful behavior, laid the groundwork for fundamental aspects of the model. George Hartlaub, a coauthor of an early paper on procedural learning and character, brought a number of insights to the clinical significance of multiple memory systems. Mary Sue Moore has been a strong supporter with a keen ability to apply the basic concepts of the model to clinical phenomena. From the beginning, she grasped where we were going with the model, and she has had a number of valuable ideas about it.

Other friends and colleagues have helped in a variety of ways, ranging from facilitating the development of our thinking, through critical review of the manuscript, and encouragement. Their individual contributions are too numerous to mention, but their assistance is very much appreciated. Among those we wish to thank are Stephen M. Allen, Susan D. Ayarbe, Patricia DeVore, Eugene S. Gollin, Dianne Sauder Jacobsen, Jerry Jacobson, Catherine L. Johnston, Zeke Kaye, John F. Kelly, Mike Kenny, Robert Kooken, Peter Levine, Jim Newman, Homer Olsen, Lisa Perry, Betsy Rubin, Robert Scaer, Allan Schore, and David Stephens (a different one).

It was always a pleasure to work with Kitty Moore, our editor at Guilford. We very much appreciate the direction and advice she provided throughout our work on the manuscript. We also want to express our thanks to Oliver Sharpe and the other staff at Guilford who made the final stages a tolerable process.

CONTENTS

	Introduction	1
1.	Overview	13
2.	Natural Selection and Adaptation	25
3.	Learning and Synaptic Plasticity	39
4.	Modularity of Brain and Psychological Functioning	54
5.	Modularity of Memory	83
6.	Dynamics	104
7.	Neurodynamics: Neurons and Neural Networks	131
8.	Normal and Pathological Dynamics	146
9.	The Physiological State and the Biology of Emotion and Motivation	164
10.	The Dynamics of Temperament	189
11.	Monkey Business: On the Nature of Cognition in Nonhuman Primates	203
12.	Conscious and Nonconscious Functioning	222
13.	Modularity, Dynamics, and Functional Systems	263
14.	Regulation of Behavior	279

15. *Development, Stability, and Change of Character*   305

16. *Biology of the Self*   327

17. *General Principles of Change*   355

References   377

Index   421

INTRODUCTION

In the fall of 1985, I (J. G.) was asked to examine Rodney, a 27-year-old man with 11 years of education. Rodney was unemployed, having been unable to work since sustaining his second significant head injury in 5 years. Drunk and driving at a high rate of speed, Rodney had rear-ended a tractor-trailer. The hood of his car slid under the rear of the trailer, and he came within a few inches of being decapitated. On arrival at the emergency department he was unconscious and unresponsive to painful stimulation. His body was rigidly positioned with his arms and legs extended and rotated inward, his back and neck arched, and his teeth clenched. This abnormal posture, referred to as *decerebrate rigidity,* is indicative of probable serious injury to the brainstem or thalamus. Radiographs showed a depressed skull fracture over his left parietal area—toward the top and rear of his head. There was considerable swelling of the brain, but the fracture was helpful in that it reduced the intracranial pressure that otherwise would have resulted. Rodney's condition was monitored closely, but the neurosurgeon elected not to perform surgery. By the eighth day after his injury, Rodney had regained consciousness, although he remained confused for several weeks. His disorientation and inability to recall recent events (posttraumatic amnesia) gradually cleared over a period of about 2½ months.

On examination 6 months later, it was clear that Rodney had not returned to his baseline level of cognitive functioning, which, judging from high school records, seemed to have been in the low average range, at about the 20th percentile. Rodney was less upset about his cognitive problems, however, than about the development of certain disturbing psychiatric symptoms. He said he had begun hearing "these two voices" in his head: "One is mean and the other is nice. The mean voice tells me to kick someone's ass, mess him up." The other voice, the "good one," would tell

1

him "Just behave, Rodney. Just mellow out, be cool." Rodney was unclear about when he first heard these voices, but he was aware of them only since his head injury, at a time before he became fully oriented and alert. They might have been present prior to the accident, but he was unable to remember anything for the 18 months or so that preceded his injury or the first few months afterward.

Rodney described the voices as being "male, but they're not human, and it's like they're in my head." He said he heard them "almost all the time." When I asked if he heard the voices at that moment, he nodded and said, "Yeah, it's like the mean one wants me to mess you up. The good one says, 'Hey, let's just sit down and see what this mother is saying.'" He didn't think the voices came from outside, and didn't think they were someone or something else really talking to him, yet they worried him quite a bit. Rodney had no obvious delusional system and was not exactly paranoid. Moreover, he seemed to have relatively good insight into the fact that what was going on in his mind was abnormal and not really happening.

Rodney was especially bothered by certain obsessive thoughts that he couldn't control. He said, for example, that he had "been saying sevens in my head for a long time now." He explained that he frequently counted either forward or backward by 7's, and demonstrated his prowess by subtracting serial 7's from 500 very quickly and accurately until I stopped him. He reported that he counted the number of steps it took him to walk to the store (usually just over 1,200), and said that counting, adding, and subtracting helped him distract himself from other thoughts, on which he refused to elaborate. Sometimes he would divide the total number of steps by 7, then subtract 7's from the answer until he reached a number less than 7. He claimed that none of this had gone on prior to his most recent injury.

Rodney discussed several specific phobias he had recently developed, and it seemed that even talking about them made him anxious. While discussing snakes and spiders, for example, he grew animated and agitated, and could barely sit still in his chair. He said he was afraid to walk on certain sides of certain streets, or specific blocks or sections of blocks. Sometimes one of the voices warned him to cross to the other side in order to prevent something "very bad" from happening. He wasn't sure he could say specifically what this might be, but he didn't really want to discuss it. On occasion, he looked as though he was ready to jump out of his skin, and I would recall the mean voice that was probably telling him that he should stomp my ass.

Another aspect of what Rodney referred to as his "mental disorder" was habitual, severe nail biting. I had noticed previously that his nails extended only perhaps one-quarter of the way from his cuticle to his finger tip. Several fingers had obviously been bleeding, and throughout the examination he picked and chewed on his fingernails, cuticles, and several scabs on his hands. He used to bite his nails, he said, but never as single-mindedly as he now seemed to do.

Rodney had been prescribed several different neuroleptic medications with little effect other than sedation with chlorpromazine, and a movement disorder with haloperidol. A psychiatrist had recently put him on carbamazepine—an antiepileptic drug—in an attempt to control his volatile mood. Rodney's mood could change quickly with little provocation, ranging from sadness through depression, anger, and euphoria. He found it nearly impossible to describe an event without rising from his chair and acting out the roles of the different participants, becoming more agitated in the process. He was very talkative and extremely preoccupied with insignificant details. He worried for several minutes, for example, about whether a trivial event had occurred at 7:00 P.M. or 7:30, or some time in between, although he was almost certain it had been at about that time, maybe 7:35, because he saw a clock at 7:15 but couldn't recall whether that was before, or after, or maybe during the event, but it could have been about 15 or 20 minutes later, and unfortunately he hadn't replaced the battery in his watch because he could have looked at it, because he always liked to check his watch, partly to see how many steps he had taken in a certain period of time (usually then dividing the number by 7), and partly because he liked to add to or subtract from the time in increments of 7 minutes, or 7 seconds, or 7 hours, or to subtract 7 days from the date, and 7 days from that, and so on. Needless to say, the examination was very time consuming.

The available history suggested that much of Rodney's symptomatology was, in fact, of posttraumatic onset. According to his parents and his ex-wife, he had been somewhat eccentric and mildly anxious before the most recent accident. Now, however, all shared his opinion that he was "just about ready for the loony bin." A series of neurologists, psychiatrists, and neuropsychologists had been unable to figure out just what was going on, and now it was my turn to be stumped. Even more frustrating for Rodney was the fact that none of the treatments that had been offered seemed to help, and he was certain he was rapidly getting worse.

In trying to understand what was happening with this unusual patient, I began to read the literature on head trauma and its effects on personality. There wasn't much to learn from the handful of studies that had been published. There was little well-designed research, and for the most part I ran across anecdotal papers and uncontrolled studies based on clinical data. I learned that head trauma frequently caused irritability and a low tolerance for frustration, and found a case report of obsessive–compulsive symptoms following one injury. Many of the behavioral effects of prefrontal cortex lesions had been described (e.g., Luria, 1966, 1980), but there was no objective evidence of injury to Rodney's frontal lobes, and moreover his pathology was not exactly characteristic of prefrontal injuries.

A paper that reported correlation coefficients between the scores of individual scales on the Minnesota Multiphasic Personality Inventory and individual tests on the Halstead–Reitan Neuropsychological Battery was typical of the research that had been done—not especially useful. A growing sense of frustration led me to the idea that a careful, scholarly review of the literature might be of some value, so I talked about my plan with Jay L. Schneiders, a friend and colleague at the Denver VA Medical Center, and we set out to write a literature review. Jay and I read a number of articles, and we had nearly completed a first draft when we began to think more carefully about the writings of A. R. Luria (1966, 1976, 1980) and Janos Szentágothai (1975, 1979, 1980, 1983).

Luria theorized that the brain was a hierarchically organized system characterized by both parallel and sequential processing. Szentágothai (e.g., 1975, 1979, 1980, 1983) had been investigating the hypothesis that the brain was a modular system—an architecture that had been suggested by the findings of M. E. Scheibel and A. B. Scheibel (1958), among others. I also found that Szentágothai had coauthored a paper with Michael A. Arbib (1974) in which they made the point that neuroanatomical structures and physiological functioning must be intimately related to organismic functioning—a point that might seem obvious but, if you stop to think about it, has some very interesting implications.

We were struck especially by the statement that "to understand anatomy, we must understand function—physics does not tell us what a beer can opener does!" (1974, p. 326). This idea, in conjunction with Luria's dictum that psychological *functions* really are *functional systems,* comprising many structural and functional subcomponents, led us to the realization (obvious in hindsight) that, if the brain has a modular architecture, and if function mirrors structure, and if perceptual, motor, and cognitive functions all seem to have a modular organization, then the same probably holds true for personality. Why should personality be any different?[1]

We began to lose interest in writing a literature review and embarked on an attempt to understand personality functioning starting from the premise that the brain (and hence personality) is a modular, distributed, hierarchically organized system. After several years and more than 50 drafts, we managed to get a couple of papers published (Grigsby & Schneiders, 1991; Grigsby, Schneiders, & Kaye, 1991), but the process of submission, rejection, revision, resubmission, and more rejection ad nauseam was frustrating. Moreover, it seemed that our thinking was always 3 or 4 years ahead of what we were writing about in the papers, so going over what felt like old ground was somewhat less interesting.

During the early development of our thinking, two colleagues in par-

---

[1]Not everyone has reached the same conclusion. Fodor (1983) argued that certain "central systems . . . are not plausibly viewed as modular."

ticular contributed significantly to various aspects of the model. Kathryn Kaye was especially helpful when it came to considering the *dynamics*—the processes—that were taking place in personality development and functioning. In addition, discussions with George Hartlaub starting in 1986 led to the evolution of our ideas about how multiple memory systems play a role in the development and manifestation of different aspects of personality, and in particular to the relationship between what is known as *procedural learning* and the habitual behavior sometimes referred to as *character*. A stripped-down version of our thinking on this subject was finally published by Grigsby and Hartlaub in 1994.

David Stevens and I have been hiking together for many years, at which time we frequently have discussions in which David raises and discusses some clinical phenomenon, then I cast it in a different light—usually biological—and we argue the matter until we reach some kind of resolution. Frequently we realize that despite apparent initial disagreement, our perspectives on the phenomenon are in many respects essentially similar, but that we have very different languages and conceptual schemes for explaining and understanding it. These conversations led ultimately to the writing of this book.

Although the reader will note that it has a heavily neurobiological and neuropsychological slant, this book is the result of a lot of thought by clinicians, and recovering clinicians, about what goes on in the clinical situation. It is rooted in an attempt to understand the things that people do, the ways in which people change, and why people tend to stay pretty much the same across time.

BRAIN INJURY AND THE PERSONALITY

Rodney obviously wasn't the first individual whose personality had undergone some kind of change, usually for the worse, as a result of a neurological disorder, but his pathology was at that time among the most puzzling and bizarre I had encountered. At least as far back as the case of Phineas Gage, it was known that certain central nervous system lesions could profoundly affect the personality. Mr. Gage was a construction foreman for a railroad in Vermont. In 1848, in a freak accident while preparing to blast some rock, an explosion propelled a meter-long tamping rod through the left side of Gage's face. The rod penetrated his head just under the cheekbone and exited through the top of his skull. Mr. Gage remained conscious during the wagon ride to a hotel where he was treated by a physician named John M. Harlow. Amazingly, Gage survived, and in a follow-up report of the case published some 20 years later Harlow (1868) described the profound change that had come over Gage. Once conscientious and a hard worker, he became "fitful, irreverent . . . manifesting but little deference for his fellows, impatient of restraint or advice when it conflict[ed] with his desires, at times pertinaciously obstinate, yet capricious and vacillating, devising many plans of future operation, which are no sooner arranged than they are abandoned in turn for others appearing more feasible" (p. 335).

NEUROSCIENCE AND THE MIND

Human personality is difficult to study, and scientific examination of the brain–personality relationship has been held up by historical factors and the lack of adequate technologies. Throughout much of the 20th century, behaviorists argued, with some justification, that all we could know about humans was learned by observing their behavior and the intricacies of its relationship to the environment. Many contended that it was unnecessary, and even counterproductive, to speculate about what goes on in the mind *or* the brain. Such phenomena were not even proper objects of study, since we could know nothing about them with any certainty. In part this philosophical position represented a reaction to psychoanalytic theorizing and the inferences that Sigmund Freud and his associates drew from their therapeutic work with patients.

While behaviorism may have been a useful corrective, one that eventually led theorists of other persuasions to adopt a more empirical approach to their subject matter, behaviorism also carried with it a lot of ideological excess baggage. For decades, the study of consciousness, unconsciousness, mind, and cognition became taboo, and even the objects of derision, for many academic psychologists. Although research into what goes on in the black boxes of the brain and mind never really went away, it became unfashionable, to say the least.

In the last quarter of the 20th century, new technologies facilitated a shift in the intellectual zeitgeist. Inexpensive high-speed computers and associated technology now permit the rapid and frequently real-time analysis of complex physiological processes, with a degree of spatial and temporal resolution undreamed of when Freud, Ivan P. Pavlov, J. B. Watson, and B. F. Skinner were at their zeniths. It is now possible to acquire images of the working brain, noninvasively, with spatial resolution of a few millimeters. By recording the activity of single neurons or groups of neurons, one can determine the timing of brain events on a scale of milliseconds. At the same time, the techniques of molecular neurobiology have allowed researchers to identify a host of neurotransmitters, neuromodulators, and receptors throughout different regions of the brain, as well as many of the genes that regulate them. As a consequence, we stand on the brink of a truly scientific understanding of human psychological functioning.

The various neurosciences—neuroanatomy, neurobiology, neurophysiology, neuropathology, neuropsychology, and neurodynamics—are not the only scientific disciplines contributing to this ferment. Cognitive psychology has matured as a science, as have other approaches to the study of behavior. Even advances in the understanding of the behavioral, emotional, and cognitive functioning of nonhuman animals have helped to illuminate this thing often referred to as "human nature," the attributes of which have been the subject of controversy for thousands of years.

PSYCHOLOGICAL THEORIZING BY THE LAY PUBLIC

One of the interesting things about people in general is that, as attribution theorists have demonstrated, we are all amateur psychologists. Nearly everyone has his or her own idiosyncratic understanding of why people do things and of the significance of the things they do. And as Nisbett and Ross wrote, "people's characterizations of themselves, like their characterizations of the objects and events that comprise their environment, are heavily based on prior theories and socially transmitted preconceptions" which "can survive seemingly potent empirical challenges" (1980, p. 197).

Some people, mental health professionals in particular, have been trained in a specific theoretical orientation—behavioral or psychoanalytic, for example. Many others have a perspective determined in large part by religious belief. In any case, most people have a theory, generally not very formally thought out, about what makes themselves and others tick.

The situation is like that described by John Stuart Mill in his articles on *Utilitarianism* (1861/1993). Writing on the subject of moral philosophy, he noted that "after more than two thousand years the same discussions continue, philosophers are still ranged under the same contending banners, and neither thinkers nor mankind at large seem nearer to being unanimous on the subject" (p. 1). We operate in a social world according to an implicit theory of personality. In fact, many investigators now think that all neurologically intact adult humans, and even adults among the great ape species, have a *theory of mind*, a conception of what goes on in the minds of other creatures. Scientists, philosophers, and poets have tried to express such theories in a more or less coherent fashion, while for most people these theories are rarely systematized. Scientific theories are models that attempt to provide ever more accurate approximate descriptions of reality. This is true as well of personality theories, but in some respects the latter are much more akin to literary metaphors than are the theories of more mathematically based sciences.

Philosophy and religion likewise have attempted to understand what is fundamentally true about human personality, and frequently the disagreements that arise represent a lack of consensus regarding the essential characteristics of human nature. For some Christians, human weaknesses are a consequence of original sin, potentially overcome by faith, good works, and divine intervention. For others, humans are completely depraved and only the elect have any hope of salvation. Western religion and philosophy has tended to emphasize the "ego," not necessarily the same as the ego about which Freud wrote, but reflecting a sense of individuality and identity. In contrast, Buddhism maintains that "our human nature is without ego. When we have no idea of ego, we have Buddha's view of life. Our egoistic ideas are delusion, covering our Buddha nature" (Suzuki, 1970, p. 100).

Such a wide range of ideas about the mind and human personality also may be seen in current theories of personality, of which there must be several dozen. Even among persons sharing a relatively uniform perspective, there is considerable variability, and idiosyncratic, individual, hairsplitting interpretations of theory probably are the rule rather than the exception.

READERS' OWN THEORIES

We assume that most people who read this book already have a personality theory of their own. Some may be favorably disposed to accept what we present, while others will no doubt find much that offends them. We acknowledge the possibility that we could be off base in our thinking, but we also are aware that a neuropsychological theory of personality may be hard for some to accept regardless of the degree to which it accurately models human functioning. Our model certainly may require a rather different way of thinking about the evidence than that to which many are accustomed.

We also are aware that "people often do not believe evidence that opposes some theory they hold. If the evidence cannot be discredited outright, it may nevertheless be given little weight and treated as if it were of little consequence. Thus, the theory often survives intact new data which ought, superficially, to force revision of confidence in the theory or perhaps even to reverse the theory" (Nisbett & Ross, 1980, p. 169). The brain has developed in such a way that it is exceptionally good at perceiving patterns of different kinds. At graduate school, say, with the acquisition of a particular personality theory, one learns to perceive only specific kinds of patterns. Eventually, it becomes habitual to see psychological phenomena through the lens of one's theory, yet—as Nisbett and Ross noted—it may be very difficult to observe that which is inconsistent with the theory.

DIFFERENT PSYCHOLOGICAL PERSPECTIVES ON PERSONALITY

There is no shortage of psychological theories of personality. Many aspects of these theories are reasonably well worked out and are of considerable practical value, so we wish to make it clear that the model we present is not intended to supplant them. Nevertheless, we anticipate that some readers will feel that we have attacked or challenged their beliefs, that we have called into question certain ideas of which they are convinced, ideas they believe have been empirically confirmed in some way. This is not our intent, and such reactions represent a misunderstanding of the relationship between our primarily biological model and models that are purely psychological in nature. That being the case, what *is* the logical relationship between our model and these other models?

As we see it, psychological phenomena represent a subset of the universe of biological phenomena. Therefore, because the model we present is grounded in a more basic level of analysis (i.e., biology), it is of a different *logical type* (Whitehead & Russell, 1910–1913) from that of purely psychological theories. Remember, we're only talking about theories here—abstract cognitive explanations about phenomena that actually occur in the world. In any event, a biologically based perspective of this sort logically should facilitate the explanation and understanding of a range of different psychological theories and should permit us to assess which of their precepts are more or less likely to pass scientific muster. It also should generate a large number of specific hypotheses that should enable us to put certain aspects of these psychological theories to the test.

What we propose is not an attempt to graft neuroscience onto a psychological theory. If one is thoroughly familiar with the concepts we outline here, the model may stand alone, directly serving as a means of understanding human functioning. On the other hand, it also may be used to complement more purely psychological theories—at least those that are well defined and amenable to some kind of empirical scrutiny. The model is not intended to replace those theories but to provide a context in which they may be understood and evaluated. In this sense, it may be a kind of metapsychological theoretical framework. Rather than giving license to wild eclecticism, our hope is that the model we propose may permit the integration of seemingly disparate approaches to understanding and changing personality functioning, and that it may do so within the context of an overarching empirically supported inductive framework. At the same time, this model is not intended to provide support for any particular theoretical orientation.

We believe this way of thinking may be of considerable utility for both clinicians and those who study personality and psychopathology. Although we rely heavily on others' work, many of the ideas here are new, and we believe we have managed to put the pieces together in a way that is novel.

FOR WHOM WAS THIS BOOK WRITTEN?

This book is intended primarily for clinicians—psychiatrists, psychologists, neuropsychologists, behavioral neurologists, and others who deal with the relationships between the mind and the brain—and for those who conduct research on the nature of personality. But despite the fact that there is much here of clinical significance, this is not really a clinical book per se.

We believe that our model may serve as the foundation for a comprehensive, scientifically based theory of personality and may facilitate the search for answers to a number of important clinical issues: What are the component parts of personality, for example? Of what is the "self" composed? What is it about personality that changes? What can and cannot change? What are the prerequisites for change? Why is change often so slow?

One obvious problem facing this way of thinking is that neuroscience is only just beginning to understand the connection between physiology and psychology. Nevertheless, data supporting the general idea have been accumulating rapidly. Rapidly enough, in fact, that we believe it is possible to learn a great deal about certain fundamental aspects of personality organization and function by studying data from the neurosciences even at this early stage. This book represents our attempt to undertake this task.

LANGUAGE

A basic aspect of professional and scientific education involves the acquisition of a specialized vocabulary for describing the phenomena in which one is interested. Advanced training in psychology, psychiatry, psychoanalysis, or related fields thus provides one with the ability to talk comfortably, efficiently, and intelligibly with persons possessing similar training. However, much confusion can result when specialized words lose their agreed-upon meaning or if no agreement can be reached on their meaning. While the cognitive neurosciences and psychology share many terms, they may mean very different things to those trained in the various disciplines. A *representation*, for example, means something different to cognitive neuroscientists than it does to psychoanalysts. We repeatedly discovered, in writing this book, that our own divergent biases and backgrounds, and our different vocabularies, could lead us into pseudocontroversies that reflected disagreements about jargon more than about basic concepts.

We therefore have tried to discuss things in functional terms throughout this volume, avoiding psychological terminology when possible and relying primarily on the language of neuroscience. It seemed only appropriate, in a neuropsychology-based theory, to adopt that course of action, and it permitted us to avoid making up any new words. However, the avoidance of many common psychological terms (e.g., *self, temperament*) would be so cumbersome as to make discussion difficult or impossible. We therefore use a number of these terms, but understand and define them in ways that we believe are consistent primarily with neuroscientific thinking.

Take the concept of *temperament,* for example. The word ordinarily is used to apply to certain *traits* that appear to be biologically based. Different authors have argued in favor of different numbers of specific fundamental traits such as shyness, extraversion, or neuroticism. We are concerned with the general concept of temperament but are not especially interested in the precise traits which it is thought to encompass. This does not reflect a failure to appreciate the accomplishments of the many psychologists who have studied traits. Instead, it reflects our emphasis on understanding the many dynamical subcomponent processes involved in those traits. As we see it, temperament is not something fixed and immutable, although clearly it tends to be stable throughout the lifespan. We believe, however, that this apparent stability is a *probabilistic* phenomenon and that, in a very real sense, an individual's temperament is never exactly the same from one moment to the next. Thus, a person who is shy is one who has a very high probability of engaging with others in a characteristically shy manner, and hence does so most of the time, but that does not preclude the capacity to behave at times in a more aggressive style. We are interested in the dynamics that influence these probabilities and in the modular distributed neural systems that lay behind them.

THE GOAL

Our goal is to synthesize material from neuroscience and from a number of other scientific disciplines into a single, comprehensive conceptual framework for understanding human personality. Ideally, such a model should be coherent, clinically useful, and empirically based. The model we develop here is not quite a personality theory, but it represents an intricate web of theory and evidence, spun from findings in a number of scientific disciplines, with which we believe any adequate theory of personality must be consistent. The various fields of study on which we have drawn may seem unexpectedly diverse, yet all of them—including contributions from physics, chemistry, dynamics, evolutionary biology, ethology, cognitive psychology, functional neuroanatomy, and cognitive neuroscience—have shed considerable light on who we are as human beings.

We have tried to develop this model from the ground up, rethinking and sometimes discarding concepts that have long been taken for granted— a task that in reality we can only approach as a limit. However, we believe that as a consequence there are two important differences between this way of thinking about personality and most others. The first is that this model is grounded in the findings and theories of several scientific disciplines, especially neuroscience, and what it asserts about personality functioning is consistent with neuroscientific models of mental processing. The second is that it is readily amenable to analysis from several levels, each of which is capable of illuminating familiar phenomena from a different perspective.

We have constructed a conceptual framework on the foundation laid by many other scientists, and therefore most of what follows is not new. William James, for example, anticipated many of our conclusions more than a century ago, and Ernest Hilgard, with his thinking about the hierarchical organization of the mind, also reached similar conclusions via a very different route, many years ahead of us. What *is* new, we believe, is the organization of this material into a more or less unified way of thinking about personality functioning, and a consideration of some of the implications of that model for clinical work.

1

OVERVIEW

PSYCHOLOGICAL PHENOMENA ARE EMERGENT PROPERTIES

Personality is an emergent property of brain processes. This means that specific psychological states are associated with specific states of the central nervous system, while psychological processes such as perception, thinking, emotion, and behavior reflect the activation of complex networks of neurons throughout the brain. This postulate has profound implications for how we think about human personality, suggesting that it is impossible to understand personality functioning fully until we know how personalities are created by brains.

PHILOSOPHICAL BASIS OF THE MODEL

We should be able to embed psychological *theories* within biological and chemical *theories*. As applied to psychology, this means that we try to understand how our biology affects our psychological state of mind. Biology *must* influence psychology. How else can we explain what happens when we have too much to drink, don't get enough sleep, smoke pot, watch a strobe light, take antidepressants, or sustain injuries to the brain? If the brain can influence our psychology in these matters, why would it not do so in others, and should we not be able to find some kind of systematic, orderly relationship between how the brain and mind work together? Establishing the nature of this relationship has the potential to enhance our understanding of the phenomena in question. As a bonus, it also provides further means of evaluating hypotheses about those phenomena.

13

We don't anticipate a precise one-to-one correspondence at the molecular level between physiological states and brain states. Nature doesn't work that way, and in any event things are messy in the natural world. Categories, labels, and theories are fundamentally arbitrary human inventions that will never completely fit the data. We do, however, believe strongly that there are lawful, probabilistic relationships between what takes place at the molecular and neural levels and associated psychological activity.

It seems probable and useful that psychological theories may be linked to biological theories, biological theories can be understood in terms of chemical concepts, and chemistry may be explained in terms of physics. Each level of analysis is itself valid, and study of each level may yield significant and important data. Yet it is essential to develop psychological theories which themselves may be understood in terms of more fundamental theories.

Collier (1988), for example, reasoned that "living systems are composed of chemicals. Although there may be laws governing very complex systems like organisms that are difficult or impossible to anticipate from our knowledge of simpler chemical systems, there is no good reason to suppose that biological systems violate the fundamental laws applying to chemical systems in general. The only open question about the relevance of physical and chemical theories to biology is whether they place useful constraints on biological theory" (p. 230). Similarly, there is every reason to suppose that psychological systems do not violate fundamental biological, physical, or chemical laws, and little reason to believe that psychological functioning is independent of those same laws. Might not more fundamental theories therefore place useful constraints on psychological theory? After all, humans are biological organisms that over the course of time have evolved to occupy certain ecological niches. Hence our psychological activity as humans is limited by, and simultaneously affects, our biological, evolutionary, and neurological status. Ideas about human psychological functioning require the constraints of biological thinking.

The model outlined in this volume draws from a variety of sources at many different levels of analysis. *Learning,* for example, is a *psychological* phenomenon. I might learn how to play the accordion or how to solve square roots, and subsequently demonstrate my learning through my behavior. In recent years it has become increasingly clear that learning is probably mediated by changes in the structure of the brain's neurons at the *synapse,* the junction between nerve cells, and hence learning has a biological aspect. The neurobiological processes that mediate our learning endow us with *synaptic plasticity*: when we learn something, it is not stored in any single neuron or any single area of the brain, but rather in the patterns of activation of a distributed array of neurons. Thus, learning is not only a psychological process but also a physiological process involving networks of neurons. Here we have at least two different levels of analysis, two different perspectives on what takes place when we learn something.

Theories of learning specify the cognitive and behavioral processes involved in acquiring a new skill or new information, whereas theories of synaptic plasticity concern themselves with what takes place in the brain while a person is learning. Learning (and the consolidation of memories) takes a certain finite amount of time. Why is this? Psychologists who have studied learning have come up with learning and forgetting curves—graphic means of showing how long it takes to learn something or to forget it. Yet curves of this sort only provide us with indirect information about the brain processes that mediate learning and about why they require the time they do. If one is interested in how habits are learned, psychology has experimental tools that are of considerable value in studying how an animal acquires habits. But by studying the neurobiology of learning, we can understand why learning takes a certain amount of time, why it is more or less permanent, and how we can obtain access to stored knowledge of different kinds. Psychologists, for example, have found that learning is consolidated by adequate amounts of subsequent deep sleep and rapid eye movement (REM) sleep. Neurobiologists seek the neural and chemical explanations for this phenomenon.

Both levels of analysis are valuable. If psychologists had not learned that something about sleep facilitates learning, no one would have thought to explore what goes on in the brain during sleep that is important in the consolidation of memories. On the other hand, without the biological or neurochemical explanation, the psychological phenomenon has an almost magical quality to it—explain things as a result of a vague concept such as instinct, for example, or simply state *that's just the way it is*. By bringing biology into the psychology of personality, we believe the two enrich one another. While a thorough causal reduction of psychological theories to more basic theories is impossible, perhaps even in principle, we believe that in order to fully understand personality functioning, biology, physics, and psychology all provide indispensable levels of analysis without which it is impossible to comprehend the activity of organisms as complex as human beings.

DUALISM AND EMERGENT MATERIALISM

Dualism, somewhat simplified, is the idea that reality is composed of two dissociable, immiscible parts: mind or spirit on the one hand, and body or matter on the other. René Descartes usually gets the credit (or the blame) for dualism, but this way of thinking about reality goes back at least to the pre-Socratic philosophers. Plato espoused a form of dualism, and Manichaeanism posited that there were separate kingdoms of good and evil. Descartes put a more modern spin on dualism, attempting to determine how the brain and mind are connected. The way he saw it, the mental and physical realms are separate but interact with one another. Hence his thinking is sometimes referred to as Cartesian interactionism.

Monism, the idea that there is only one fundamental substance, has taken a number of different forms. Among the so-called materialist philosophers, some strict reductionists believe mind can be explained away entirely. Others have adopted a kind of *emergent materialistic* viewpoint, and this, roughly speaking, is the position we espouse. We believe that mental states are in some sense identical to and emergent from specific processes (or states) of the brain. Mind is not some kind of substance, and neither is it distinct from brain in a dualistic sense. Consciousness and its associated properties are the manifestation of certain processes characteristic of a particular kind of self-organizing system.

THE ORGANISM AND ITS CONTEXT

One of the fundamental ideas underlying this model concerns the relationship between organisms and their environment. As Gollin (1966) has argued, all behavior is "a function of organism and environment," and therefore the proper way to study behavior is to "observe it in many organism–environment contexts" (p. 3; see also Gollin, 1984a, 1984b; P. A. Weiss, 1967, 1969, 1971). All species have evolved to occupy certain ecological niches, and thus their basic biological functioning has been shaped across time in interaction with the world in which they live. Moreover, each organism must survive in a specific context and thus must be able to respond flexibly to a variety of changing environmental demands. Given an organism's extreme sensitivity to contextual conditions, even trivial or momentary modifications of either external or internal environment may have striking effects on behavioral outcome. The relationship between brain and environment is especially clear in the development and adaptation of the mammalian central nervous system, in which experience has been shown to play a crucial role (Hubel & Wiesel, 1963; Kandel, 1984, 1991b; Wiesel & Hubel, 1963, 1965).

An animal must be adaptable if it is to survive in environments that may vary tremendously or that threaten it with predators, parasites, scarcity of resources, or harsh and unforgiving physical conditions (that pretty well covers the range of available environments on this planet). The brain must be continually responsive to the environment and must always be learning. Therefore neural plasticity is adaptive (Lynch, 1986; Matthies, 1982). Edelman (1987) even has argued that the brain itself develops (from both evolutionary and ontogenetic perspectives) and functions in response to selection pressures from an environment that demands adaptive behavior.

THE ORGANISM AND ITS ACTIVITY ARE PROCESSES

William James (1890) considered the mind to be a process rather than a thing. Some have argued more generally that life itself is most usefully thought of as a process or a set of processes. Jantsch, for example, maintained that any system, biological or otherwise, is "a set of coherent, evolving, interactive processes which temporarily manifest in globally stable structures that have nothing to do with the equilibrium and the solidity of technological structures. Caterpillar and butterfly, for example, are two temporarily stabilized structures in the coherent evolution of one and the same system" (1980, p. 6); thus the idea of a system "becomes dissolved into processes. In the domain of the living, there is little that is solid and rigid" (p. 7). In a sense, what we see as biological structures can be considered to be processes taking place on a timescale that makes them appear relatively unchanging. Yet viewed across the lifespan, an organ like the brain undergoes considerable change in structure and function from gestation to death. Strictly speaking, it is never the same from one instant to the next.

Similarly, personality is not a thing with a structure; rather, it is a set of *emergent properties* of complex biological systems behaving in a complex environment. Therefore, to understand personality within its context, it is necessary to think in terms of processes (Grigsby & Schneiders, 1991; Grigsby et al., 1991). Such an emphasis is not a new idea in psychology, having been espoused by William James and many others (e.g., Goldstein, 1939, 1942; Gollin, 1966; Goodglass & Kaplan, 1972; Kaplan, 1983; Schafer, 1976; Werner, 1937), but we consider it important to emphasize the point yet again. It is essential that an appropriate emphasis on process be applied systematically to the neuroscientific study of personality.

WHAT THIS BOOK IS NOT

It may be helpful if we explicitly state what this book is and what it is not. This book is not a psychoanalytic text (nor does it espouse *any* particular existing theoretical orientation), although one of us (D.S.) is a psychoanalyst, and many psychoanalysts have found certain of the ideas here interesting and useful. It likewise makes no attempt to discuss in depth any previous theory or research in personality theory. Such a discussion might, of course, be useful and interesting, but is not our objective. Similarly, the book is not a neuroscience text, nor a report of original findings in neuroscience, although in it we attempt to apply many of the findings of neuroscience to the understanding of personality. The emphasis of the book is on translating neuroscientific (and other) findings into a model that will be clinically and heuristically useful. In short, there is probably something missing from this volume that will disappoint and frustrate nearly everybody: not enough on trait theories, not enough on developmental psychoanalysis, too superficial a discussion of basic neuroscience, and so on.

Hence, the neuroscientist looking for new insights into the mechanisms of memory or for a discussion of the most current findings concerning long-term potentiation will be disappointed, unless he or she is curious about a different way of thinking of the role memory in the construction and treatment of personality. The psychoanalyst looking for a neuroscientific justification for psychoanalytic thinking, or who wonders what we have to say about Heinz Kohut's (or anyone else's) theory, likewise will go away feeling that something was missing. Behaviorists may complain that we provide inadequate coverage of reinforcement schedules or different paradigms of avoidance learning.

This is not a treatment manual or a how-to book for clinicians, although the clinician who reads the book carefully may come away with a rather different perspective on the assessment and treatment of persons with psychological or neurological disorders. Finally, our failure to review the work of everyone that every reader believes should have been reviewed reflects our twofold desire to begin predominantly from a biological perspective and to complete the manuscript in our current incarnations. We hope that we have not accumulated so much bad karma in this lifetime that we will be compelled to write a similar book in the next.

WHAT DOES THIS BOOK ATTEMPT TO DO?

So what is this book, anyway? It represents an attempt to approach the problem of the organization of personality from many different levels of analysis—biological, neuropsychological, cognitive, physical, dynamic— and to integrate these into a comprehensive model that is informed especially by cognitive neuroscience. The model is not only a theoretical exercise but also has a number of interesting clinical implications. For example, we propose that different memory systems contribute differentially to specific aspects of personality, suggesting the utility of specific clinical approaches for certain types of problems. Thus, that aspect of personality often referred to as *character*—the routine behaviors, gestures, mannerisms, and attitudes that make people knowable and predictable—can be understood as a manifestation of *procedural learning*. This hypothesis opens up many interesting research questions and allows us to think in a more systematic way about what kinds of interventions might be most effective in the treatment of character.

DEFINITION OF PERSONALITY

We understand personality as a set of emergent properties of the operation of various functional brain systems. These systems reflect the variable although relatively stable activity of many complex, interconnected neural networks, in transaction with the environment (Grigsby & Schneiders, 1991, p. 22). According to our model, personality *functions* (e.g., self, reality testing, control of behavior) are *functional systems* (Luria, 1980), subcomponents of larger systems. These functional systems themselves are composed of hierarchically ordered subsystems. *In short, personality reflects the emergent properties of a dynamic, hierarchically ordered, modular, distributed, self-organizing functional system, the primary objective of which is the successful adaptation of the individual to his or her physical and social environment.* The remainder of this volume will be spent unpacking and explaining this single sentence, and demonstrating the utility of a neuroscientific understanding of the phenomena of personality.

The definition of personality that guides our thinking is essentially similar to that proposed in our earlier work on the subject (Grigsby & Schneiders, 1991; Grigsby et al., 1991; Grigsby & Hartlaub, 1994). In a nutshell, this concept of personality includes (1) the typical behaviors, style, and attitudes that sometimes are referred to as an individual's *character;* (2) motivational and emotional states that are experienced and expressed by each individual in unique ways; and (3) the individual's relatively enduring representations of the self and the world. As we noted above, from our perspective there is no such thing as a personality structure per se. Instead, personality consists of a myriad of processes that are (despite their stability) exquisitely sensitive to environmental change. From what one observes when one examines an individual personality, one tends to infer certain enduring personal traits, although these are only *relatively* stable and actually represent the dynamic operation of numerous internal and external processes (Grigsby & Schneiders, 1991, p. 22).

OUTLINE OF THE BOOK

The book is roughly divided into two major parts. The first part (Chapters 2 through 8) deals with the biological and physical foundations of the model. In these chapters we present a body of research and theory from the fields of evolutionary biology, ethology, functional neuroanatomy, cognitive neuroscience, and the dynamics of biological systems. From these data, we believe it is possible to draw a number of important inferences about how the brain mediates personality. Of particular significance are the self-organizing processes that underlie brain functioning, the modular, massively parallel nature of brain structure and functioning, and the fact that the brain is modified as a result of experience. These three basic conceptual areas have profound implications for understanding how human beings function.

In order to establish a broad context for understanding human personality, in Chapter 2 we begin by discussing evolutionary biology. Natural selection operates to produce organisms that successfully adapt to their environments, and humans have evolved with the capacity to adapt to an incredibly wide range of environmental circumstances. Natural selection is driven by diversity and by the advantages some organisms obtain as a consequence of certain genetic variations. In this book we are less interested in specific behaviors that may have evolutionary significance and more concerned with such broad issues as randomness, self-organization, diversity, and conservation. Evolution and genetics establish the constraints within which we must operate, but one of the most important evolutionary achievements is the ability to refine one's adaptation through the capacity for learning from experience. Therefore, in Chapter 3 we deal with learning and synaptic plasticity—neurobiological processes of the utmost significance that work in conjunction with inheritance to shape personalities. The influence of evolution is manifested in the broad outlines of our cognitive and emotional capacities, which we share to some extent not only with the members of other species but with other humans as well. Postnatal modifications of the nervous system in association with experience serve further to refine our adaptation to specific niches and to create individual differences.

The problem of psychological development is extremely important, and we considered writing a separate chapter on the problem. It seemed, however, that a single chapter on development would fail to capture many of the essential features of these processes, so instead the reader will find that there are discussions of developmental issues throughout the book.

In Chapter 4 we take on the architecture of the brain, which is a hierarchically organized, modular, distributed system of extraordinary complexity. The brain functions as efficiently as it does by assigning tasks and subcomponents of tasks to a widely distributed array of highly specialized processors, which function in parallel to permit the automatic, efficient, and relatively nonconscious performance of most psychological activities. Chapter 4 goes into a moderate amount of detail concerning the visual system, in part because it is one of the most completely studied functional systems. Our discussion of the structure and function of the visual system is intended to illustrate the basic modular architecture that characterizes the brain. This architecture is manifested in the mind as well, a point that we discuss in Chapter 4 but go on to develop in more detail in Chapter 5, which deals with the modularity of memory. It has become apparent that what we call "memory" is not a unitary thing but a concatenation of different processes, having different neural substrates, operating on different timescales, all relatively independent of one another.

Chapters 6 through 8 deal primarily with the science of *dynamics*, which is the study of *processes*. Only by understanding neural and neuropsychological processes (as opposed simply to structures) can we begin to make the leap from neuroanatomy to psychology. Chapter 6, a general introduction to dynamics, covers the temporal organization of processes: some are periodic, some aperiodic, and others essentially appear to occur randomly. After dealing with background material that is important in the effort to study personality from different levels of analysis, we go on to consider such issues as self-organization in biological systems and the development of critical states. At a rather fundamental level, these principles are of considerable value in understanding the nature of stability and change in behavior and personality. We also deal briefly with biological rhythms that play an important role in regulating the individual's basic state.

The primary aim of Chapter 7 is to address the dynamics of neural networks and the brain. In particular, our focus is on the activity that occurs within and among neural networks, bearing in mind that while it is important to understand the structure of the brain, it is the processes that characterize that structure that give rise to the mind. In Chapter 8 we apply the material covered thus far to the understanding of normal dynamics and of dynamic disorders, many of which may be manifested as psychopathological syndromes. Over the course of an ordinary day, humans show significant and regular variability in their functioning. When disrupted, many of these regular processes may produce *dynamic disorders,* pathological conditions that may reflect disordered temporal dynamics. Among the many kinds of dynamic disorders we address are epilepsy (especially reflex epilepsy), jet lag, and depression, and we consider how anomalous sensory input (e.g., pain, overstimulation, sensory deprivation) and such influences as forced shifts in handedness may lead to changes in cognitive, emotional, and behavioral functioning. Our purpose is to demonstrate the sensitivity of the nervous system to environmental conditions, and to illustrate how the brain may be driven in ways that are manifested in experience and behavior.

In the second part of this book (Chapters 9 through 16) we develop the outline of a theory of mind based on inferences drawn from the material in the first eight chapters. In this part, we examine conscious and nonconscious functioning, the organization of personality functions, including the self and character, and the central organizing role of emotion and motivation in determining basic properties of one's state at any given time. In order to illustrate how the brain serves basic personality functions, we go into a detailed analysis of the regulation of behavior and of the organization of reality testing. Many of the clinical implications of the model are discussed in this section.

Chapter 9 addresses the concept of *instantaneous physiological state,* or what we refer to as *state* for short. This is the synthetic emergent property of a number of different systems influencing arousal, activity level, mood, short-term emotional status, motivational status, sleep–wake cycle, and other psychological phenomena. State, along with the environment, tunes the personality by establishing the probabilities that an individual will engage in a given behavior at a given time.

In Chapter 10 we deal with *temperament,* those basic, constitutional, behavioral and psychological characteristics such as predominant mood and activity level that are the result of genetic, intrauterine, and perinatal influences. We are especially interested in the dynamics of temperament and in the way the various neural components of temperament serve as a kind of template on which the different memory systems act.

In Chapter 11 our focus shifts from neurobiology and neuropsychology to a discussion of cognition in nonhuman primates. The great apes in particular seem to share certain cognitive abilities with humans: lying, tactical deception, self-awareness, the capacity to use symbolic language, and a theory of mind. The important similarities and differences among humans and closely related primate species help to illustrate the relative roles of genes, culture, and individual experience in the organization of our behavior. The acquisition of sign language by apes, for example, has produced behavioral changes both in individual animals and in their cultures. Sign language is so useful for chimpanzees that some of them have learned it spontaneously from other chimps, and animals familiar with the language have made deliberate efforts to teach it to those who are naive, including their children.

Conscious functioning and nonconscious functioning are the themes of Chapter 12. Cognitive neuroscience has shown that the vast bulk of the brain's processing occurs outside of awareness. Consciousness itself is a system with limited capacity, and without the brain's distributed, parallel architecture and automatic, nonconscious processing, even the simplest routine activities of daily life would require enormous effort. This chapter treats the relationship between conscious and nonconscious processing, and the respective strengths and weaknesses of the two systems—some data suggest that consciousness may be unnecessary for much of what we do, even rather complex behaviors. This chapter also considers the so-called split-brain studies, with particular emphasis on the issues of modularity and how we interpret our own behavior.

In Chapters 13 and 14 we analyze some specific personality "functions." In Chapter 13, we deal with the various systems involved in the representation and "testing" of reality, material that was first covered in a paper by Grigsby et al. (1991). In Chapter 14 our primary concern is with the regulation of behavior. Much of our activity is produced by nonconscious and automatic mechanisms that involve little deliberate conscious control, although the prefrontal cortex and medial frontal cortex contain regions that are part of a distributed network that permits us to engage in conscious, voluntary behavior. Because it may require considerable effort to engage in deliberate conscious behavior, and because the brain's dynamics favor automatic and nonconscious functioning, there is an innate tendency to acquire habits and to act predominantly out of habit.

Character is that aspect of personality involving the routine, typical things people do repetitively, and that make us knowable and predictable to others. Chapter 15 draws on material presented on the modularity of memory, the regulation of behavior, state, and dynamics, to present a theory of character that was previously outlined by Grigsby and Hartlaub (1994). We see character primarily as a dynamically regulated expression of processes that have become habitual through the operation of the procedural learning system. We suggest that many attempts to induce therapeutic character change have failed because they were not based on a clear understanding of this procedural learning system and of how it differs from other memory systems.

From our perspective the self, roughly speaking, is that system that involves one's representations of who one is. Although these representations may be explicit and verbalizable, they also have a constant, implicit quality that is associated with one's predominant state. Self-representations are all tangled up, psychologically and neurally, with representations of the world. In fact, injuries to the brain that impair some part of the capacity to represent the world may also leave the individual with a defective self-representation. We consider self-representations and self-awareness to represent two dissociable, modular systems that ordinarily operate in tandem, and argue that the modular, dynamic architecture of the self may be responsible for certain kinds of self psychopathology. These issues, discussed in Chapter 16, were first sketched out by Grigsby et al. (1991).

Chapter 17 focuses directly on the clinical implications of the model, although the reader will find that we have also attempted to address these issues throughout the first 16 chapters. This final chapter summarizes and integrates the implications of the model for understanding personality change, as we attempt to show how different aspects of personality change on different timescales as a result of different mechanisms. Our hope is to bring some sort of systematic way of thinking to discussions of change by grounding them in neurobiology and neuropsychology. We believe that this perspective has appreciable utility for the conceptualization of normal and pathological psychological functioning, for diagnostic assessment, and for therapeutic intervention.

THE UTILITY OF THIS BOOK
FOR MENTAL HEALTH PROFESSIONALS

We recognize that for many mental health professionals, especially those with little background in the natural sciences, some of the material in this book may seem too far removed from the clinical situation to be of interest. Our hope is that those readers willing to follow us as we work from biology through neurodynamics toward psychology will be rewarded by acquiring a model for understanding the brain that has many useful applications in clinical work. The intricacy of the transactions between persons and their environments is extremely complex and nonlinear. Our book offers the clinician a sort of metapsychology for conceptualizing how and in what ways the brain's organization and dynamics shape and delimit behavior. We believe that the implications of modularity and dynamics shed a new kind of light on human behavior that does justice to the complexity of the phenomena, while serving as a constant reminder of the unpredictability of human behavior.

The model we outline here provides a language of processes that can be useful for describing personality processes as well as the things that transpire in clinical situations. Many professionals of diverse theoretical perspectives are currently attempting to reconcile their theories with new ways of thinking that have influenced the natural sciences as well as other social sciences (e.g., complexity theory and social constructivist theory). In psychoanalysis, for example, a revolution is underway wherein theoretical language previously emphasizing mental "structures" (id, ego, and the like) is being discarded in favor of a theoretical language that emphasizes processes. It is because these dynamic activities are of such crucial importance that they are stressed here. The fact is that any individual brain, from gestation until death, is constantly reinventing itself in the here and now. Our hope is that clinicians from different theoretical backgrounds will find this way of thinking about people, their brains, and their contexts useful and consistent with emerging philosophical perspectives.

We also think this book offers clinicians a useful way of understanding the sorts of complex patterns of activity required for a brain to create an emergent mind. The chasm between neuroanatomy and psychology can appear vast, and for some clinicians the leap from the level of biochemical processes to that of human meaning may feel like one of dubious value. Our hope here is that the model provides an essential context for understanding the dynamic changes that characterize an emergent mind, a kind of a staircase between anatomy, physiology, and psychology.

Finally, we think a careful reading of this book will lead clinicians to a deeper appreciation of the degree to which most behavior is determined by nonconscious processes. Apparently one can never uncover enough evidence of the ubiquity of nonconscious processing to counteract the apparently hardwired experience of ourselves, first and foremost, as conscious agents and rational actors (which leads us to believe any number of wacky things, such as that we really do know why we do what we do, or that at least, after enough therapy or analysis, we will know). While we may in fact know some of the reasons for our behavior, it seems clear that our sense of intentionality itself is likely to have emerged from the complex, almost incomprehensible array of nonconscious distributed processes. A full appreciation of the role of these nonconscious processes as they are mediated by the brain is essential for formulating useful and accurate psychological theories.

2

NATURAL SELECTION
AND ADAPTATION

INTRODUCTION

This chapter involves a brief overview of evolutionary biology, presenting a larger framework for understanding the functioning of the brain and mind. Why stray off into evolution? According to evolutionary biologist Theodosius Dobzhansky, biology only makes sense in the context of evolution. Many would also argue the corollary that nothing in psychology makes sense except in the light of biology and hence of evolution.

We are not evolutionary theorists, and our aim is not to demonstrate the adaptive function served by various specific behavioral, emotional, and cognitive characteristics. We do not minimize the significance of evolutionary approaches to psychology, but we are more interested in understanding how the model we present fits into the theoretical framework of evolutionary biology.

Our goal in this chapter is to establish briefly the evolutionary context within which the human brain emerged. The advantages of the brain's modular architecture and its associated self-organizing capability can be properly understood and appreciated only when viewed within the context of the evolutionary pressures exerted by natural selection. Moreover, what evolutionary biology makes clear is that the development of the individual personality itself reflects an effort to adapt to a given set of circumstances with its many pressures and demands. Evolutionary adaptations, and learned behavioral adaptations, frequently are accompanied by characteristics or behaviors that are not adaptive, but that are associated with others that are adaptive. Superstitious behavior, although not itself adaptive, is an expression of pattern recognition, associative learning, and procedural learning, other facets of functioning that not only are adaptive but are found in both vertebrate and invertebrate animal species.

One of the most important evolutionary adaptations is the capacity of more complex individual organisms to adapt to their own unique circumstances in a way that goes beyond their genotypic programming. Thus the behavior of most complex animals is a function both of genotype and of learned adaptation to a social and cultural environment. The tremendous variation observed among both human and nonhuman cultures and the wide variability of individual behavioral repertoires are manifestations of this acquired adaptation in the context of certain biological constraints.

In this chapter we review certain basic ideas of evolutionary biology that are especially relevant to the model of mind we delineate in subsequent chapters. We first discuss natural selection and adaptation, with an emphasis on how biological diversity and genetic variability are the stuff upon which evolution exercises its influence. We then address the distinction between "adaptation" from the point of view of natural selection on the one hand, and what is referred to as "psychological adaptation" on the other. Highly maladaptive individuals from the point of view of psychology can be quite well adapted in terms of the pressures of their idiosyncratic environment. Finally, we briefly discuss the significance of the scientific literature on nonhuman primates in an effort to understand what can be learned by studying behaviors that appear to have been conserved across evolution. The fundamental organizing influence of genes on cognition and behavior can be appreciated by considering the similarities and differences within and among different primate species. The genotype imposes fixed limits on the psychological capacities of each species, but there is considerable diversity within these heritable constraints, reflecting genetic, environmental, and cultural influences.

EVOLUTION AND ADAPTATION TO CIRCUMSTANCES

Most people are familiar with the Darwinian phrase "survival of the fittest" but may not know precisely what is meant by "fit." It has nothing to do with late-night cable TV infomercials in which smiling models in spandex work out without breaking a sweat. Instead, the *fitness* of a particular animal "consists of its relative probability of survival from birth to adulthood" and consequent capacity to pass on its genes (Ridley, 1996, p. 113). Species evolve within specific ecological niches. While these niches may be very narrow, requiring extreme biological specialization (e.g., that of bacteria living around geothermal vents in ocean trenches), certain species have adapted to life in a wide variety of contexts (as is the case for both mosquitoes and humans). An animal's chances of survival—and hence its fitness—are maximized in the ecological niche to which it is best adapted. If the niche changes as a result of such factors as decreased precipitation, increased temperature, loss of forest cover or prey species, or the loss of a psychologically important caretaker, an individual animal's fitness may decrease concomitantly.

Because of the complexity of the natural environment, animals may be exposed to an essentially infinite variety of situations, many of which will demand rapid physiological or behavioral responses. Most specific situations cannot be foreseen, so it would not be possible to "hardwire" an animal genetically to be able to cope with every contingency that might arise. Moreover, such hardwiring might be maladaptive since, if the responses of organisms to most circumstances were determined a priori by their DNA, they likely would be physiologically and behaviorally rigid, and so unable to adapt flexibly to the demands of a changing environment.

It therefore is essential that animals have the capacity to respond adaptively to the environment, to maintain those adaptations if they are successful, and to try alternative behaviors if they are not. Hence, genes provide the basic blueprint for the structure and functioning of organisms, but ongoing experience within specific ecological niches is necessary to refine that master plan.

Humans have adapted to nearly every kind of habitat imaginable. While some physical characteristics are associated with evolution in a specific place (e.g., increased melanin production and the sickle cell trait among Africans, discussed below), much of the adaptation that occurs is experience dependent. As Gollin noted, "what we typically designate as environment is unique to each individual. This relationship may be stated in another way: The unique properties of each individual in a population will operate differently upon a given set of designated environmental conditions" (1981, p. 232). Thus there may be relatively few physiological impediments to a North American taking up a nomadic life in the Mauritanian Sahara, but such an individual would not have acquired, from earliest childhood, the learned repertoire of behaviors, knowledge, and attitudes that make life in the desert familiar, bearable, and meaningful.

It is important to note also that evolution is not a process of change *toward* something, as though there perhaps were some ideal state of the universe and evolution were a means of reaching that state. Instead, evolution operates more or less blindly: as circumstances change, so do species. Humans occupy no favored ecological niche and have a limited adaptive capacity; given the right kind of environmental change, we could follow the dinosaurs into oblivion, and in fact it's only a matter of time until that occurs.

NATURAL SELECTION AND VARIATION

Charles Darwin's major conceptual contribution to the theory of evolution (and that of his contemporary, Alfred Russel Wallace) was the concept of "Natural Selection, or the Survival of the Fittest," which Darwin defined as the "preservation of favourable individual differences and variations, and the destruction of those which are injurious" (1859/1958, p. 89). Because this concept has been misunderstood, misconstrued, and made to fit diverse ideological positions, it may be useful to discuss it briefly at this point. Natural selection, according to Ridley (1996), requires that four conditions be met. Two of these—that individual organisms must be capable of reproduction, and that the offspring of those organisms must inherit certain characteristics from the parent generation—are so obvious as to require little elaboration. The others have to do with the importance of diversity. There must be "variation in individual characters among the members of the population" (p. 72), and there must be variation in the fitness of organisms. Variation drives natural selection.

Consider the variability in body size observed among humans. There have been adults ranging in size from less than 3 feet to almost 8 feet tall, weighing anywhere from 40 pounds to nearly 1,000 pounds. Most people fall somewhere toward the middle of the distribution, while those at either end are outliers. Those individuals who have intermediate body sizes have greater fitness (in the evolutionary sense) than those at the extremes, and as a consequence body size remains relatively stable in the population. Body size could change, however, in response to a variety of influences. Although now extinct, at one time in the recent past there were small elephant-like creatures living on a number of islands, descendants of much larger elephantine ancestors.

Intelligence is another trait showing considerable variability and having a normal distribution. On most tests of intelligence (whatever it is they measure), by definition, approximately two-thirds of the population obtain IQ scores between 85 and 115. At the extremes, less than 1% of the population has IQ scores above 140 or below 60. This variability in intellectual functioning presumably reflects ordinary population-based, neuropsychological variation along a number of dimensions, in association with a number of genes and the vagaries of environmental influence.

In general, the heritability of intelligence is estimated at approximately 50% (i.e., about 50% of phenotypic variance is genetic in origin). Even among octogenarian identical twins, for whom one might expect life experience over the decades to have produced rather different patterns of functioning, one recent study estimated that more than 60% of the contribution to general cognitive ability is genetic (McClearn et al., 1997). The figure of 60% means, however, that approximately 40% of this ability may be a result of environmental influence.

Variation exists not only at the level of body morphology, intelligence, and other global psychological abilities. In fact, the key to understanding the whole process is to realize that what is expressed at the cellular, physiological, and behavioral levels is the result of processes that occur at the biochemical level. The occurrence of molecular mutations and recombination in the process of reproduction constantly produces new variations on old themes. A few of these changes are adaptive, but most are likely either to have no effect or to be detrimental to the individual organism.

THE EFFECTS OF GENETIC MUTATIONS

Evolution takes a good deal of time—about 400,000 generations to produce an efficient eye, for example, according to one computer simulation (Nilsson & Pelger, 1994). Complex adaptations must wait for the right combination of genetic mutations and environmental conditions. Hence, existing species are the products of millions of years of adaptation to their respective environments and as such have developed extremely successful mechanisms of survival. It is difficult to improve on this record, and new mutations (if they have any effect) are most likely to produce undesirable changes or none at all. As long as there is considerable variation in the gene pool, improved adaptations will be favored by natural selection, but such increases in fitness tend to occur infrequently and take considerable time (Maynard Smith, 1978).

Some mutations confer both advantages and disadvantages, or may have little effect on fitness. For example, many Africans and their descendants have a gene responsible for producing unusually shaped red blood cells. Individuals who are *heterozygous*[1] for this trait (i.e., from one parent they received a normal gene, while from the other parent they received a gene that produces altered blood cells) are protected to some extent against the malaria parasite. However, they also have what is known as the *sickle cell trait*. On the other hand, persons who are *homozygous* for this trait (i.e., they received the sickle cell gene from both parents) are affected by the blood disorder known as sickle cell anemia. If we were to assume that a trend toward global warming could lead to the proliferation of drug-resistant malaria in North America, the 10% of African Americans with the sickle cell trait (i.e., heterozygotes) would have an advantage over persons without the trait. Given the problems associated with sickle cell anemia, however, homozygotes would have no advantage.

A different situation is observed with regard to the thalassemias, genet-

---

[1]A heterozygote has inherited one gene that codes for a specific trait and one gene that codes for a different trait. A homozygote has inherited two identical genes (e.g., either both code for sickle cell or neither do).

ically transmitted blood disorders leading to defective synthesis of hemo-globin and associated anemia. The thalassemias appear to confer no adaptive advantages. If genetic conditions such as these do not kill or severely disable those who have them by the time they reach childbearing years, the conditions are likely to persist in the population. This persistence of a genetic disease in the gene pool is the case with Huntington's disease (also called Huntington's chorea), a disorder with autosomal dominant transmission (meaning that the offspring of an affected individual have a 50% chance of inheriting the trait). Huntington's disease is a rapidly progressive neurodegenerative disorder that tends to have its onset after the age of about 40 years, so the condition can be transmitted to one's children before one knows whether one is affected.

Some conditions considered disorders in our society actually may reflect ordinary heritable variability in the population. This may be the case for many people with attention-deficit disorders (ADD) and learning disabilities. For example, just as height, weight, head circumference, and intelligence are roughly normally distributed, so it is likely that the capacity to attend to the task at hand and to inhibit responses to extraneous stimuli also are normally distributed. Hence, a small percentage of people at one end of the distribution are likely to have exceptional powers of attention and concentration, just as a minority at the other end are likely to be extremely distractible. In recent years, the number of people diagnosed as having an ADD—both adults and children—has grown significantly. This probably reflects the fact that not only those individuals at the tail of the distribution but those who are somewhat more toward the center report improvement in their functioning when they take stimulant medication.[2] While some unknown percentage of the population may have an ADD resulting from such cerebral insults as perinatal hypoxia, for many people it is likely that their ADD is a normal variant rather than the result of a neuropathological process.

Likewise, it seems plausible that a certain percentage of so-called learning disabilities are cases of developmental *dyscalculia* (a difficulty with arithmetic) or developmental *dyslexia* (a difficulty with reading) that do not reflect a neurological problem per se, but rather indicate normal variation that has come recently to be socially defined as a medical or psychological problem and which may be of little or no consequence to the process of natural selection. Modern humans (*Homo sapiens*) have been around for about 100,000 years, and over that time nature did not select people for their ability to read or to perform calculations. Natural selection doesn't care whether you can read until such time that the ability to read improves your fitness (i.e., your capacity to reproduce). If you were illiter-

---

[2]Not to mention diagnostic fads and economic considerations.

ate as recently as 100 years ago, you had a lot of company (and still would today in much of the world) and it didn't matter if your brain was organized somewhat differently than were the brains of most other people. If our society did not place considerable value on the ability to calculate and to read, most developmentally dyscalculic or dyslexic persons never would be aware of their "deficit." Such genetic variants may affect functioning in society and the type of occupation a person might have, but because they don't influence fitness in the evolutionary sense (i.e., reproductive success) they remain in the gene pool.

MUTATION AND EVOLUTION

Mutation involves the substitution of one nucleotide for another, the inappropriate insertion or deletion of a pair of nucleotides (a base pair), or a translocation.[3] The other major mechanism by which changes occur in the DNA of a gamete is *crossover,* in which a segment of the DNA from one parent is inserted into the strand of DNA from the other parent, and vice versa. These processes occur randomly, uninfluenced by the kind of changes in form or function that might result, although at the molecular level certain mutations are more likely to occur than others. (A nucleotide that contains a *pyrimidine*—either cytosine or thymine—is more likely to be replaced by a nucleotide containing another pyrimidine than by a nucleotide containing a *purine*—adenine or guanine; a purine-containing nucleotide is more likely to be replaced by a nucleotide containing another purine than by a nucleotide containing a pyrimidine.)

One of the major mechanisms by which evolutionary change occurs is alteration in the timing of certain developmental processes; that is, genes may code for the same proteins in different species, but the timing of production of those proteins in fetal development differs. The face of an infant chimpanzee, for example, is closer in structure to that of a human than is the face of an adult chimp; the mouth and jaw protrude further in the adult chimpanzee. One genetic difference between chimpanzees and humans, then, may be that homologous genes responsible for the protruding mouth and jaw in chimps are "turned off" early in human development but remain active for a longer time in the chimpanzee (thus causing the lower face to protrude farther in chimps than humans).

---

[3]These nucleotides are chemical subunits of DNA. Their sequence on a DNA molecule encodes and transmits information essential to development. Four nucleotides, each containing one of the following bases, make up the genetic code: adenine, cytosine, guanine, and thymine; these each are covalently bonded to a five-carbon sugar (deoxyribose) linked to a phosphate group. In the two DNA strands, nucleotides containing adenine are paired with those containing thymine; those containing cytosine are paired with those containing guanine.

EVOLUTIONARY ADAPTATIONS ARE NOT NECESSARILY THE MOST EFFICIENT DESIGNS

Although natural selection works exceptionally well, it has a tendency at times to produce some seemingly bizarre or perhaps less-than-optimal organisms and parts of organisms. Consider the striking diversity of organisms that exist today—the leech, octopus, platypus, tapeworm, dung beetle, sea anemone, slime mold, guinea worm, career politician, and vampire bat, for example. Consider also that, as different species evolve, they are not designed by engineers starting with a clean slate. Instead, natural selection must work with what is already there, so that whales' fins still contain the vestigial bones characteristic of their terrestrial ancestors' legs, for instance. In a similar fashion, brains are bound to their evolutionary history.

ADAPTATION IN TERMS OF EVOLUTION DIFFERS FROM PSYCHOLOGICAL ADAPTATION

In a thoughtful article that clarifies a number of issues, D. M. Buss et al. (1998) noted the conceptual confusion that has characterized the emerging field of evolutionary psychology as a result of failure to distinguish clearly between "adaptation" as an evolutionary concept and "adaptation" as a psychological construct. They argued that many discrete expressions of "personality" are properly conceptualized as "noise" from the evolutionary point of view, representing the essentially random effects associated with the processes of evolution. What evolution shaped in the case of human beings is a species that possesses a brain with a modular architecture capable of supporting self-organizing activity. The individual expressions of this self-organizing activity (i.e., the diverse expressions of personality) are for the most part the work of what are referred to as *spandrels*: the unintended, specific consequences of possessing a brain with a self-organizing capability interacting with the infinite varieties of circumstance.

Although psychological adaptation is a matter of considerable importance to individual human beings, it probably is of little consequence to evolution. Where psychological adaptation and Darwinian adaptation intersect, from an evolutionary point of view, is that for human beings "adaptation to a specific environmental niche" is to a great extent tantamount to adjustment to a specific set of psychosocial circumstances. A brain such as humans possess is especially well suited to supporting the emergent cognitive processes required for adaptation to a unique set of psychosocial circumstances. Thus, when we speak of adaptation in subsequent chapters we are referring to adaptation from the evolutionary perspective. If we discuss "psychological adaptation," we will explicitly refer to it as such.

CONSERVATION OF TRAITS ACROSS EVOLUTION

Certain traits are conserved across evolution (i.e., they are found in many different species, orders, or phyla) because they serve essential purposes for the organisms that possess them. Other adaptations so obviously contribute to fitness that it should be no surprise that they have evolved independently several times. For example, eyes are so complex it is almost hard to believe that they could have resulted from natural selection alone. Nevertheless, it has been estimated that light-sensing organs of varying degrees of complexity have evolved between 40 and 60 times among different invertebrates alone (Ridley, 1996).

THE ORDER PRIMATES

The importance of genotype in determining both similarities and differences in behavior within and among species can be appreciated by discussing some of the primate species, with special attention to the conservation of certain traits across those species. The order Primates is one of several major subdivisions of the taxonomic class of mammals (Mammalia). For a species to be classified by biologists as a primate, it must possess several characteristics, including five fingers and five toes on each hand and foot. These digits must be capable of grasping, and must have flattened nails rather than claws. Primates also have a shortened muzzle, overlapping visual fields for the two eyes, a specific pattern of teeth, considerable development of the brain (especially the cerebral cortex), and long gestation with birth of a single infant at a time (W. E. Le Gros Clark, cited in Bramblett, 1994).

There are two suborders of primates. One suborder, the Prosimii (prosimians), tend to be small, with small brains, heavy reliance on the senses of touch and smell, and *vibrissae* (specialized facial "whiskers" that convey tactile information, also found on cats, rodents, and many other animals). Prosimians, including lemurs and tarsiers, generally are nocturnal and live primarily in the trees. The other suborder, the Anthropoidea (anthropoids), is divided into three *superfamilies:* New World monkeys, Old World monkeys, and hominoids (apes and humans). The brains of anthropoids are larger than those of prosimians in proportion to overall body size. Their eyes are shifted farther forward, and they have much more precise control of individual fingers. Finally, their offspring experience a very lengthy period of physical dependency and social immaturity (Bramblett, 1994). Old World monkeys and the hominoids are the most closely related of these superfamilies and appear to have shared a common ancestor approximately 30 million years ago (Bramblett, 1994). Old World monkeys include macaques, baboons, and a number of other species. Some of these species (e.g., the macaque) are related closely enough to humans that study of their brains has proven quite helpful in enhancing our understanding of human functioning, especially vision.

Hominoids typically are divided into three families: gibbons (Hylobatidae), great apes (Pongidae), and humans (Hominidae). Gibbons, apes, and humans are thought to have descended separately from a common ancestor beginning about 22 million years ago. The great apes include the orangutan (*Pongo pygmaeus*), gorilla (*Gorilla gorilla*), chimpanzee (*Pan troglodytes*), and the bonobo (*Pan paniscus*, sometimes referred to as the pygmy chimpanzee); see Figure 2.1. Orangutans diverged from the other hominoids about 16 million years ago, and gorillas about 7 million years ago. Based on immunological evidence, it is thought that humans shared a common ancestor with chimps and bonobos as recently as about 5–6 million years ago (Sarich & Wilson, 1967). According to Sibley and Ahlquist (1987), who used DNA hybridization to study the similarity in genetic material between humans and several other primate species, the DNA of humans, bonobos, and chimpanzees is approximately 98.5% similar.

CONSERVATION OF COGNITIVE ABILITIES ACROSS THE ORDER PRIMATES

Certain cognitive and behavioral traits appear to be conserved across evolution, suggesting that they increase the fitness of members of different species. For example, there are data suggesting that even pigeons may be able to learn to make at least simple abstract categorizations (Herrnstein & Loveland, 1964; Herrnstein, 1979, 1985). Findings such as this has led some scientists who study animal cognition to argue that basic cognitive functions may be more similar than they are different, at least for mammals, and only the possession of speech and a complex natural language may set humans apart from other species. According to Bramblett (1994), for example, "we have little evidence that the nature of cognitive processes of anthropoids, if not mammals, differs in any fundamental ways from those of humans" (p. 62).

CHIMPANZEE CULTURES

Culture is not a strictly human phenomenon; it is an important aspect of life for many species (Bonner, 1980). A powerful shaper of individual behavior, culture itself is a product of evolution. Primatologists have observed that there is considerable variation in the cultures of geographically disparate groups of members of the same species. Such differences in culture demonstrate the importance of learning, and especially of social learning, in the acquisition of adaptive behavior.

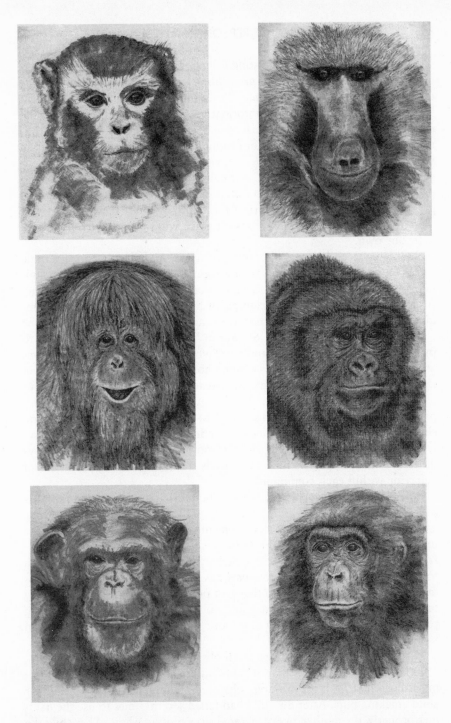

FIGURE 2.1. Clockwise from top left: Female rhesus macaque (*macaca mulatta*); male baboon (*papio hamadryas*); male gorilla (*gorilla gorilla*); female bonobo (*pan paniscus*); male chimpanzee (*pan troglodytes*); female orangutan (*pongo pygmaeus*). Drawings by Kathryn Kaye.

The social practices that distinguish one culture from another are mediated to a large extent by the *procedural learning* system, which will be discussed at length in later chapters. Procedural learning involves the learning of *processes* rather than information, and is characterized by the nonconscious and automatic performance of these processes. Among humans, such things as greetings, for example, are so overlearned and routine within a culture that it is possible to greet a friend or acquaintance and engage only in habitual behavior. Other cultural phenomena—such as kinship patterns, work, child care, and entertainment—are more complex than greetings but become such a part of the fabric of life that we seldom give them a second thought until we visit a place with a very different culture than our own.

Chimpanzees have cultures of their own, and there is considerable variation among these cultures with respect to a number of issues, including tool acquisition and use, the ingestion of medicinal plants, hunting strategies, and grooming. For example, it has been found that not all communities of wild chimpanzees use tools, and not all groups use the same tools. Chimpanzees at Gombe Stream in Tanzania use grass or sticks to probe and "fish" for termites and ants, whereas chimps at other locations use neither. Chimps at Lopé in Gabon ignore termites entirely; at Kibale in Uganda chimpanzees use their hands instead of tools to dig for termites but use chewed leaves as sponges to absorb water. Near Taï, Ivory Coast, chimpanzees use a stone hammer and anvil to crack nuts, whereas in Gabon chimpanzees seem to consider these same nuts inedible and therefore don't bother trying to crack them at all (McGrew, 1992, 1994). The differences described above appear to reflect culturally transmitted, learned patterns of behavior within each community.

Tool use, among chimpanzees or humans, is an acquired skill. As Matsuzawa (1994) points out, learning to use tools takes considerable time and practice, and proceeds in developmental steps. Matsuzawa stresses the importance of social learning in the acquisition of this skill, noting that infant chimpanzees often observe closely while adult animals work with tools. In some cases, an adult tool user has been observed handing the tools over to her young observers so they can practice the skill. (It is interesting to note that humans also require a fair amount of practice before becoming proficient in the manufacture and use of chimpanzee tools, not to mention human tools.)

Young chimpanzees learn to use tools by emulating others (Tomasello, 1994), but it also appears that at times adults actively instruct young animals. Boesch (1991), for example, observed a chimpanzee mother and her child cracking nuts. After the child had failed several times to use the hammer properly, the mother, in exaggerated slow motion, showed her child the way to use the stone hammer. Following this demonstration, the young chimp's performance with the hammer and anvil improved.

A particularly interesting aspect of chimpanzee culture is that chimps use medicinal plants and that each culture seems to have its own distinct formulary (Huffman & Wrangham, 1994). For example, in areas where they are at high risk for parasitic infections, chimpanzees have been observed consuming a number of plant species that ordinarily are not a part of their diet. Chimpanzees tend to eat these plants during the rainy season, when they are most susceptible to parasitic infestation. The plants, which have demonstrated a variety of medicinal properties (such as treating parasitic worms, amoebas, and bacteria), tend to have a bitter taste and chimps ordinarily avoid them.

Chimpanzees are not the only animals with an interest in some of these natural medicines. The pith of one such plant reportedly also was used by many African people to treat gastrointestinal problems and intestinal parasites (Huffman & Wrangham, 1994). The leaves of a second plant, often swallowed by chimpanzees, are commonly used by Ecuadorian Indians as a treatment for headaches (Russo, 1992). At Kibale, Uganda, the berries of yet another plant are eaten by chimpanzees; compounds derived from these same berries have been studied for the control of schistosomiasis, a serious parasitic disorder to which both chimpanzees and humans living in Africa are susceptible.

How chimpanzees initially acquired their knowledge of medicinal plants is unknown, but transmission of the behavior appears to be culture bound. Some chimp communities use plants that other groups ignore, or use in different ways (Huffman & Wrangham, 1994). Moreover, the use of many plants crosses species. Some leaf-swallowing behavior, apparently for medicinal purposes, has been observed among chimpanzees, bonobos, gorillas, and humans.

SUMMARY AND CONCLUSION

Although evolution has produced a wide range of organisms that occupy nearly every conceivable ecological niche, the environment is always in flux and successful species must be able to exploit their environs in ways that ensure their survival. Over many generations, changes in form and function occur in response to different environmental demands, but new evolutionary developments do not produce entirely novel organs or organisms de novo. Instead, they build on extant designs, modifying existing structures to perform new tasks.

Genetics imposes specific constraints on the psychological capacities of each species, but diversity also reflects environmental influences, mediated by a considerable capacity for adaptive learning. This capacity of individual organisms to adjust to their own unique circumstances by learning is one of the most crucial evolutionary adaptations. It is simply impossible for genes to provide us with all we need to know in every conceivable situation. Therefore, because acquisition of the ability to learn must have produced a significant increase in fitness, nearly all animals have a well-developed potential to profit from experience.

To a large extent, the temperaments and behavioral repertoires of the different primate species are determined by genetic influences. Each species has what might be considered a kind of modal temperament; in this respect, the more gregarious chimpanzees are quite different from the more reticent gorillas or from orangutans (who seem to prefer solitude). Yet primate behavior is very complex, and there is tremendous variability in the personalities observed within each species. Individual animals are different from one another, and groups of individuals differ from other groups in the same species. Careful observation reveals that primate behavior is a function both of genotype and of adaptation to a social and cultural environment.

The significance of learning is demonstrated by the fact that individual primate communities have distinct cultures. Different groups of chimpanzees display habits that vary across groups, including different ways of making and using tools, settling dominance disputes, and learning from one another. Chimpanzees use medicinal plants when they are ill; the plants used and the typical ways in which they are used differ from one group to another even when the same plants are widely available.

In short, natural selection leads to change in populations and species over many generations. Although learning produces change in individual animals within a generation, it cannot change the genotype, thereby affecting future generations directly. Learning can, however, influence subsequent generations via the medium of learning and social or cultural change.

As we discuss next in Chapter 3, for both humans and nonhuman primates learning is a manifestation of the malleability of the central nervous system. The wide variability observed among and within cultures and the variability of individual behavioral repertoires (also among and within cultures) are manifestations of this learned adaptation in the context of certain biological constraints. To understand the processes involved in psychological change, it is essential that we examine the biological bases of such change. Therefore, we now turn our attention to learning and its neurobiological substrate—synaptic plasticity—the mechanism by means of which the individual organism responds adaptively to its environment.

3

LEARNING AND SYNAPTIC PLASTICITY

INTRODUCTION

Personality is shaped by the interaction of constitutional processes and the experiences of individuals in unique environments. In other words, we are, at least in part, who we learn to be. As a result of these experiences, learning drives the acquisition and refinement of a wide repertoire of enduring perceptions, attitudes, thoughts, and behaviors. The relative permanence of learning and memory reflects the operation of processes that modify the microscopic structure of the brain, yielding changes in different aspects of functioning over time as a result of the individual's interactions with the world. These experience-dependent changes in brain structure and functioning are known by the general term *synaptic plasticity*.

In this chapter, we are especially concerned with the following themes. First, memory and learning are mediated by processes involving structural changes at the junction between nerve cells (i.e., the synapse). Learning involves the concerted activity of large numbers of neurons, sometimes referred to as cell assemblies, neural ensembles, or neural networks. While the synaptic changes that undergird learning occur between individual neurons, they must occur across many individual synapses to produce learned, complex behavior. The functional manifestation of such changes is an altered *probability* of activation of those neural networks mediating specific kinds of activity as a result of experience. Therefore, to understand behavior it is necessary to understand the role probability plays in the activation of various neural networks (and behaviors), since the activity of the brain, though not strictly predictable, is predictable in a statistical sense.

Among mammals, learning probably occurs continuously, but there is a kind of learning that occurs in association with sensitive periods in development. These sensitive periods play a crucial role in shaping the central nervous system (CNS) and behavior, continuing the processes of cellular differentiation that begin *in utero*. For example, there is considerable research on experience-dependent development of the visual system, and Spitz's work on sensitive periods in interpersonal attachment (1945, 1946) demonstrated the significance of appropriate experience for healthy emotional development.

NEURAL AND PSYCHOLOGICAL DEVELOPMENT

A human infant enters the world with an incompletely developed CNS, which subsequently must undergo considerable change in the way of myelination of axons and branching of dendrites, synapse formation, and programmed cell death (K. W. Fischer & Rose, 1994). Different regions of the brain reach adult developmental configurations over a period of many years and as a consequence of several neuronal growth spurts. Certain aspects of brain maturation (e.g., full development of the prefrontal cortex) may not be complete until the mid-20s (Yakovlev & Lecours, 1967). Psychological development in periods such as adolescence, during which an increased breadth of experience occurs, thus take place against the background of a developing nervous system.

As many as 12 cycles or spurts of brain development occur between birth and the end of the second decade of life (Fischer & Rose, 1994). These periods of brain development are associated with behavioral and cognitive maturation, and are influenced by the child's transactions with the environment. For example, development of the prefrontal cortex is an essential precursor to the acquisition of the ability to understand another person's perspective. Yet, even while the brain is developing on its own time line, learning from experience involves other kinds of structural change in the brain; the psychological phenomena we refer to as learning are the emergent properties of experience-dependent change, whereas maturation is a function of both brain development and learning.

SUMMARY OF NEURONAL STRUCTURE AND FUNCTION

In this section, we provide a brief review of neuronal structure and function as preface to a discussion of synaptic plasticity. The basic work of communication in the nervous system is the function of the neuron, of which there are perhaps 50 billion in the fully developed human brain. The neuron is one of two major classes of cells in the brain; the other consists of *glia* (the three primary types of glial cells being *astrocytes, oligodendroglia,* and *microglia*). Glia have been overshadowed by their flashier companions, the neurons (Travis, 1994); many of the functions of glial cells are only now beginning to be understood. While they serve a number of important supportive roles, we will not discuss them here.

Our discussion of neurons will be somewhat cursory and oversimplified. Figure 3.1 shows a schematic drawing of a neuron. Most neurons consist of a cell body (or *soma*), which contains the nucleus and other cellular subcomponents, as well as two types of *processes,* or extensions: *dendrites,* which transmit incoming neural stimulation toward the cell body, and an *axon,* which transmits nerve impulses away from the cell body. Dendrites have a number of knobby structures on their surfaces called *dendritic spines.* The purpose of the spines appears to be to increase the surface area available for formation of connections with other neurons. Axons roughly approximate the shape of a branching tree, with multiple branches leading to smaller and smaller branches. Because of this resemblance, the branches of the axon are referred to as *arborizations.* The terminal arborizations,

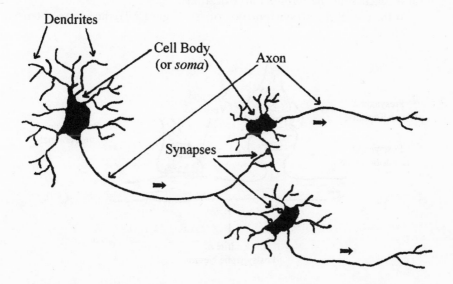

FIGURE 3.1. Schematic drawing of one type of neuron. The dendrites conduct excitatory and inhibitory postsynaptic potentials toward the cell body. If there is a sufficient amount of excitatory input in a short enough interval, an action potential is initiated. The short bold arrows show the direction of the propagation of the action potential along the axon. At the axon terminal, a *synapse* is formed with the postsynaptic neuron(s). In this case, the synapse is located at a dendrite for the top postsynaptic neuron (an *axodendritic* synapse) and at the cell body for the lower postsynaptic neuron (an *axosomatic* synapse).

sometimes called terminal *boutons,* form connections (also known as *synapses*) with other neurons or other receptor sites (e.g., in glandular and muscle tissues).

The entire neuron is surrounded by a *plasma membrane* which, through the operation of both passive and active chemical processes, maintains a somewhat skewed balance between negative and positive ions, so that the inside of the cell is electrically negative relative to the outside. The electrical potential difference across the membrane fluctuates continually at around –70 millivolts (actually, different types of neurons have different resting potentials). Excitatory stimulation received from other neurons tends to *depolarize* a neuron, making the electrical potential somewhat less negative. Inhibitory stimulation received from other neurons tends to *hyperpolarize* the cell, making the potential even more negative. When the total input of excitatory and inhibitory neurons over a very brief period of time (a few milliseconds) is sufficient to *depolarize* the neuron to a certain threshold level (somewhere in the vicinity of –40 to –50 millivolts, depending on a number of different factors), the neuron fires (or, in more technical terms, it initiates an *action potential* or *nerve impulse*). The action potential is propagated along the length of the neuron, without any loss in strength, until it reaches all the terminal arborizations.

At the end of the presynaptic neuron (see Figure 3.2), the action poten-

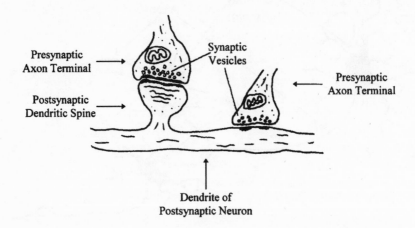

Presynaptic Axon Terminal

Synaptic Vesicles

Postsynaptic Dendritic Spine

Presynaptic Axon Terminal

Dendrite of Postsynaptic Neuron

FIGURE 3.2. Schematic drawing of a chemical synapse. In this case, one axon terminal makes contact with a dendritic spine, the other with the body of a dendrite. When a presynaptic action potential reaches the axon terminal, electrical changes in the membrane increase the permeability of the presynaptic terminal to calcium ions (Ca^{++}), which then enter the neuron through Ca^{++} channels. This leads to fusion of the synaptic neuronal membranes). The vesicles contain a neurotransmitter substance, which then is released into the cleft. The neurotransmitter binds to postsynaptic receptors, leading to excitatory or inhibitory postsynaptic potentials.

tial causes release of a relatively fixed amount of a chemical neurotransmitter into the synapse, which is a junction between the presynaptic and postsynaptic neurons. The neurotransmitter then forms a transient molecular bond to proteins on the surface of the membrane of the postsynaptic neuron (known as *receptors*), producing one of three kinds of effects. If the neurotransmitter is excitatory, it causes a partial depolarization of the postsynaptic neuron (an *excitatory postsynaptic potential*, or EPSP). If it is inhibitory, it results in a partial hyperpolarization of the postsynaptic neuron (an *inhibitory postsynaptic potential*, or IPSP). Finally, a neuron can have a neuromodulatory influence, changing the membrane properties of the postsynaptic neuron and possibly altering the threshold of presynaptic stimulation necessary to produce an action potential. The postsynaptic neuron sums and integrates all the IPSPs and EPSPs that stimulate it, and when there is sufficient excitatory stimulation within a sufficiently brief period of time to depolarize the neuron to its threshold, an action potential is produced.

Neurons can be classified in many different ways—excitatory, inhibitory, and neuromodulatory (as above), for example. They also may be categorized by the distance they cover and the cells with which they form synapses. *Projection neurons* have relatively long axons that convey action impulses to other areas of the nervous system. Some projection neurons, for example, travel from the motor cortex downward into the spinal cord. *Interneurons* have relatively short axons, and in some cases no axon at all (e.g., *granule* or *amacrine* cells). Interneurons sometimes form connections between neurons in restricted areas, often making inhibitory links between neighboring excitatory cortical neurons.

SYNAPTIC STRUCTURE AND FUNCTION

The pattern of neuronal connections (and hence the organization of synapses) accounts for the emergent properties of neural networks. There are many different types of synapses; however, in order to keep things simple we'll limit our discussion to a kind of caricature of the *chemical* synapse. Figure 3.2 shows a small space, or *synaptic cleft*, between the pre- and postsynaptic neurons; around this cleft the membranes are fused. Inside the presynaptic neuron at the synapse itself are many *synaptic vesicles*, which are spherically shaped containers made of plasma membrane and holding a more or less uniform amount of a neurotransmitter. When an action potential reaches the synapse, the change in the electrical potential of the presynaptic membrane causes calcium ions to enter the terminal bouton from the space surrounding the cell. This calcium influx in turn causes the synaptic vesicles to fuse with the cell membrane at the synapse and to release their contents of neurotransmitter into the cleft.

The neurotransmitter substance crosses the cleft and binds to receptor proteins on the surface of the postsynaptic membrane, producing an EPSP or IPSP, or modulating the functioning of the postsynaptic neuron. Depending on the type of postsynaptic cell involved, the neurotransmitter has either a direct or indirect effect on the postsynaptic membrane. If sufficient excitatory stimulation reaches the postsynaptic neuron in a sufficiently short period of time from a number of neurons, the postsynaptic neuron will depolarize and propagate an action potential. If the sum of EPSPs and IPSPs produces a depolarization insufficient to bring the neuron to its threshold, there is no action potential and the membrane will continue its fluctuation around the resting potential.

Most neurons form synapses with thousands of other neurons, both receiving and sending action potentials. There thus is a constant background of spontaneous synaptic activity, in addition to synaptic potentials resulting from organized incoming information. Much of this synaptic activity, because it is below the threshold for generating an action potential, produces no nerve impulses, although it generates the brain electrical activity recorded by electroencephalography (EEG).

Immediately after a nerve impulse has been conducted, a neuron enters what is referred to as its *absolute refractory period*. During this time, the membrane's resting electrical potential is being restored and the temporary state of the neuron makes a new action potential impossible. This refractory period, which is of very brief duration, is followed by a *relative refractory period*, during which the neuron is able to generate an action potential, but only in response to a greater than usual amount of excitatory stimulation.

SYNAPTIC EFFICACY

Synapses vary with respect to their *efficacy*, or the strength of the connection between two neurons. An action potential transmitted by neuron *A* at a synapse with neuron *B* has a certain probability of depolarizing neuron *B* and producing an action potential in neuron *B*. In many cases, that probability is zero or near zero, although it may range as high as 0.20 for some cortical synapses. That is, there is a 20% chance that a discharge by neuron *A* will cause neuron *B* to fire. It has been estimated that the average synaptic strength in the cortex is close to 0.003 (Abeles, 1991). These probabilities vary as a function of the state of both pre- and post-synaptic neurons, which is determined by the overall physiological state of the organism, by such local factors as recent neuronal activity (e.g., the presynaptic neurotransmitters may have been depleted by a sustained high-frequency volley of firing, or the postsynaptic neuron may be in a relative refractory state), or by neuromodulatory influences. Many of these influences on synaptic strength are transient, in some cases lasting only a few milliseconds, in other cases lasting minutes or hours; others may persist for months, years, or an entire lifetime.

HEBB'S MODEL OF SYNAPTIC MODIFICATION

Fifty years ago, D. O. Hebb proposed a hypothesis for the neural basis of learning that in many respects remains current today. According to Hebb, "the persistence or repetition of a reverberatory activity (or 'trace') tends to induce lasting cellular changes that add to its stability. The assumption can be precisely stated as follows: *When an axon of cell A is near enough to excite a cell B and repeatedly or persistently takes part in firing it, some growth process or metabolic change takes place in one or both cells such that A's efficiency, as one of the cells firing B, is increased*" (1949, p. 62; emphasis in original). Hebb supposed that this might occur through the development of new synapses between the two neurons, although at that time he had no evidence to support this hypothesis.

In the process of modification of synapses by experience, as in so many others, timing is everything (e.g., Markram et al., 1997). Assume that two neurons, A and C, are presynaptic neurons, both of which form synapses with neuron B. The strength of synapse A–B is strong, while that of C–B is weak. If neurons A and C fire at different times, A may produce a depolarization in neuron B, the postsynaptic cell, while neuron C is unlikely to do so; over time, C's connection with neuron B may even weaken. If neurons A and C repeatedly fire simultaneously, however, the connection between neurons B and C is likely to strengthen over time.

Whether Hebb's hypothesis is precisely correct is uncertain (Cruikshank & Weinberger, 1996). Much experimental work remains to be done before the details are fully understood. Importantly, however, there is wide agreement that structural changes of some kind occur at the synapse in response to experience and that the effect of these changes is to alter the probability that an action potential from a presynaptic neuron will lead to a discharge in a postsynaptic neuron.

CRITICAL PERIODS AND NEURAL PLASTICITY

In general terms, plasticity refers to the modifiability of the CNS in response to experience. This plasticity is manifested in different ways. For example, Hubel and Wiesel (1962, 1963; also Hubel, Wiesel, & LeVay, 1977; Wiesel & Hubel, 1963) demonstrated that appropriate experience may be necessary for the survival or normal functioning of certain populations of neurons in the visual system (see also Greenough, 1986). That is, they found that specific kinds of stimuli must occur during *critical* or *sensitive periods* of development for associated functional–structural adaptations to result.[1]

Early in human life, as already noted, the CNS is not fully developed. Many neurons are immature, and neuronal connections supporting various functions have not yet been fully established. A considerable amount of brain development must take place after birth for several reasons. First, if the brain were fully developed, the head would be so large as to make even more difficult its passage through the birth canal without a high rate of infant and maternal mortality. Second, the computational complexity of the human brain is so great that detailed specification of precise neuronal connections would complicate the process of development and potentially limit the individual's capacity for flexible responses to the environment; thus, learning is essential. Finally, because certain aspects of brain development are left up to brain–environment interaction, better adaptation to the infant's specific biological, family, and social niche is facilitated.

The timing of critical and sensitive periods may be a function of several different factors. One is the occurrence of *apoptosis,* or programmed cell death. A normal part of development, apoptosis follows the "exuberant" proliferation of neurons that occurs during uterine development. In some areas of the brain, more than half of all neurons that develop in utero may be eliminated in this manner. A second factor is the myelinization of neurons (the formation of a myelin sheath around certain kinds of nerve cells, which appears to increase the speed at which an action potential is conducted), a process that can continue for many years after birth. A third factor is the presence of neurotrophic factors—substances that promote growth and development of neurons—in various regions of the brain during sensitive periods. A fourth is the growth of dendrites and dendritic spines, and formation of new synapses. There is evidence that different areas of the brain develop in "waves" over time, beginning with the primary motor and sensory cortex, proceeding to the posterior association areas, and finally to the prefrontal cortex (Chugani, Phelps, & Mazziotta, 1987; Harwerth et al., 1986; Shrager & Johnson, 1995).

CRITICAL PERIODS AND THE DEVELOPMENT OF PERCEPTUAL ABILITY

Von Senden (1932/1960) reported that children born with cataracts who had their lenses replaced after several years never developed normal vision. Congenitally blind individuals who underwent this surgery in late child-

---

[1]A critical period is a window of time during which experience *must* occur or a developmental failure will result. A sensitive period is an interval during which, if experience occurs, the effects will be more robust than if the experience occurs at a later time.

hood, adolescence, or adulthood often had a poor postoperative course. Blind since birth, these individuals frequently had learned to navigate without vision and may have adapted well to blindness. When the cataracts were removed, instead of finding a new and exciting visual world, some experienced their situation as worsened. They had difficulty seeing things in detail and interpreting what they saw; depth perception was especially problematic. These people in effect had to deal with visual stimulation that could not be integrated properly with their other, more familiar senses. They commonly reported particular problems in negotiating stairs, thresholds, and such transitions as from hardwood to carpet or dirt to pavement, and usually experienced no significant improvement in their condition as time passed. The problem was that they had failed to experience normal visual stimulation during a critical period of development, and the same kind of stimulation occurring after that developmental period had passed was ineffective in properly tuning their brains.

Hubel and Wiesel studied this phenomenon of critical periods in vision with a series of experiments using kittens and infant monkeys (Hubel & Wiesel, 1963; also Hubel et al., 1977; Wiesel & Hubel, 1963). In one such experiment, they sutured shut one of a kitten's eyes shortly after birth and found on follow-up that only about one cell in six preferred the sutured eye, rather than the usual 50%. Similar findings were reported for monkeys. Most of the cortical cells failed to respond that ordinarily would have been responsive to the eye if unsutured. Those that did respond were abnormal in their functioning (Hubel, 1988, p. 195).

Subsequent studies determined that the problem was with a lack of exposure to shapes, rather than to light itself. Other researchers (Blakemore & Cooper, 1970) observed that kittens reared most of the time in darkness, except when exposed for a few hours each day to visual stimuli consisting only of vertical black and white stripes, demonstrated cortical cells that responded to vertical lines but not to lines oriented at other angles. Similar findings were reported by Hirsch and Spinelli (1971). Cyander, Berman, and Hein (1973) raised kittens in darkness punctuated by stroboscopic flashes of light. If you think about how things look when a strobe light is flashing, it makes sense that in such an environment the animals could perceive form but not movement. The result was a paucity of cortical cells responsive to motion. Pettigrew and Garey (1974) took this finding one step further and restricted the visual environment to movement that could be observed in only one direction, with analogous results.

Experimental manipulations such as those just described have no effect on the organism unless they are performed during specific critical periods. Among kittens, that period is from the fourth postnatal week until the fourth month, but it is most prominent during the first few weeks. In monkeys, the sensitive period begins at birth and ends at about 1 year of age, although the first 2 weeks of life are most important. In part, this difference between species is because infant monkeys have a visual system that is functional at birth whereas kittens do not. If one or the other eye of an adult animal is sutured shut, no such effects are observed. Only if the animal is deprived of visual stimulation during the first few weeks and months of life are deficits produced. These deficits are irreversible.

CRITICAL PERIODS AND EMOTIONAL ATTACHMENT

Critical periods associated with emotional development among infant monkeys were demonstrated by Harry F. Harlow's well-known studies of animals raised either with their mothers or with cloth or wire surrogates (Harlow, 1958; also Harlow & Harlow, 1973). The monkeys with wire mother surrogates, although fed appropriately, showed severe emotional disorders. Those with cloth mother surrogates showed pathology that was less severe than that of the monkeys raised with wire "mothers." Relative to the normally reared monkeys, they nevertheless showed significant pathology and impaired social functioning. Although the anatomical substrate for these effects is unclear, many studies of early separation of primates from their mothers have shown similar lifelong effects on psychological functioning.

The same kind of finding holds true for humans, of course. Goldfarb (1943) and Spitz (1945, 1946; see also Bowlby, 1969) showed that severe emotional disturbances develop among children raised without the presence of any mother figure during a critical period of infancy and early childhood. Spitz (1945, 1946; Spitz & Wolf, 1946) demonstrated the presence of a critical period for attachment in his study of two groups of infants. The first was composed of babies living in a nursery; their mothers were incarcerated in a women's prison to which the nursery was attached, and they had regular (but limited) daily contact with their mothers as well as other people. The second group of infants was composed of babies raised in a foundling home; they had minimal contact with nursing staff each day, and their contact with other people was very limited.

After the first year it was found that the motor and cognitive development of the children of the prison inmates was superior to that of the children in the foundling home, who appeared depressed and socially withdrawn. With longer follow-up, language development also was shown to be impaired among the children in the foundling home. Schore (1994, p. 97) has concluded that while signs of attachment are evident earlier in infancy, a "critical period of socialization for the formation of enduring attachment bonds to the early primary caregiver" occurs between about 10 and 18 months of age.

SHORT-TERM SYNAPTIC ENHANCEMENT

A somewhat different kind of plasticity, not necessarily linked to sensitive developmental periods, occurs in association with learning and memory. If you recall any of the ideas in this book, or even if you recall having read the book, the structure of your brain has changed in order to maintain that memory. A similar process occurs when you learn any kind of skill—typing, knitting, playing the accordion, or juggling machetes—your brain is modified by experience. These long-term memories are mediated by structural change.

Short-term (or working) memory also must involve some kind of temporary synaptic modification, but rather than producing structural change, these memory processes are likely to involve transient alterations in the concentration, binding, or uptake of various neurotransmitter substances. The process known as *short-term synaptic enhancement* (STE; see S. A. Fisher, Fischer, & Carew, 1997) may be the best-developed model of certain short-term memory processes, and whether or not it applies to short-term memory across the board, it suggests a way in which neurochemical activity might maintain memories by modifying the synapse for brief periods of time.

STE consists of at least four components: fast-decaying facilitation (lasting 10s of milliseconds), slow-decaying facilitation (lasting 100s of milliseconds), augmentation (lasting for fewer than 10 seconds), and post-tetanic potentiation (lasting for periods of more than 10 seconds). The evidence to date suggests that the mechanisms subserving STE occur primarily in the presynaptic neuron, possibly involving an increase in the number of synaptic vesicles releasing neurotransmitter substance into the cleft in response to an action potential (S. A. Fisher et al., 1997).

NEURAL PLASTICITY IN THE ADULT:
LONG-TERM MEMORY

Long-term memory appears to alter the structure of the synapse permanently. These synaptic changes probably involve some kind of learning-induced gene expression (Rose, 1993). They are likely to occur at the synapse, and not elsewhere in the neuron, because as Lynch observed (1986, p. 3), "since individual neurons receive and generate thousands of connections and hence participate in what must be a vast array of potential circuits, most theorists have postulated a central role for synaptic modifications in memory storage. To do otherwise (e.g., to assume that whole cell changes are involved) would impose severe limits on both the capacity and the selectivity of the memory system."

The current prevailing models of synaptic plasticity for long-term memory are referred to as *long-term potentiation* (LTP) and *long-term depression* (LTD). Although they are not universally accepted, there is a reasonably large body of evidence supporting them as models of synaptic plasticity. According to Linden and Connor (1995), LTP has come to refer to a persistent increase in synaptic efficacy resulting from any of a number of neural mechanisms, but it is clear that LTP (initially reported by Bliss & Lømo, 1973) is not a one-size-fits-all process underlying all types of long-term memory. Long-term depression involves persistent experience-dependent *decreases* in synaptic efficacy. Multiple forms of both LTP and LTD apparently exist (Artola & Singer, 1993; Bear & Abraham, 1996; Linden & Connor, 1995). Their precise relationship to specific memory mechanisms is as yet unclear, but Murphy and Glanzman (1997) may have reported the first persuasive evidence of a direct link between LTP and classical conditioning.

LTP may involve several processes, including an increase in the number of synapses between axons and dendrites, changes in neurotransmitter release, and modification of the shape of dendritic spines. These modifications of the synapse and spine may occur "within minutes of a stimulation train that lasts for a fraction of a second" (Lynch, 1986, p. 7). According to Lynch (1986), even very brief periods (less than 1 second) of high-frequency neuronal stimulation in the hippocampus may produce alterations in the strength of synaptic responses that last for periods of up to several months or more. The details of this process have yet to be determined, though we are not concerned with the specific nature of the pre- and postsynaptic changes that mediate memory. For our purposes, the significant points are that changes in synaptic structure as a result of experience have been documented by a number of investigators (Kauer, Malenka, & Nicoll, 1988; Lynch, 1986; Morris, Davis, & Butcher, 1990; Muller, Joly, & Lynch, 1988, Siegelbaum & Kandel, 1991; Thompson, 1986) and that synaptic plasticity alters the probability that a neuron will be activated by incoming stimulation.

FUNCTIONAL IMPLICATIONS
OF SYNAPTIC PLASTICITY: NEURAL NETWORKS

As we will discuss later, among complex organisms and for all but very simple types of learning, most changes in neural structure and function associated with learning involve networks of many neurons rather than pairs of neurons or very small linear neuronal groups. Of particular importance is the *pattern* of activity across populations of neurons, or neural networks. A *neural network* is an array of neurons, arranged both in parallel and in series, often distributed throughout many regions of the brain, that work in concert to effect particular emergent properties. Both active and silent neurons participate in these networks to transmit information in the brain.

The *functional* outcome of the neural plasticity involved in long-term memory is a change in the probability that a set of postsynaptic neurons will respond with action potentials to a given level of stimulation by presynaptic neurons. From a behavioral perspective, this means that with practice (i.e., in association with the repeated use of a particular neural network), the probability of the future activation of that network (i.e., the occurrence of a given behavior) changes. In other words, learning leads to either an increased or decreased likelihood that an animal will engage in a particular cognitive, perceptual, or motor activity.

The occurrence of a learned behavior is a *probabilistic* phenomenon. A given behavior may have a high probability of occurring, but whether it actually takes place depends on several variables. Outcomes other than the expected one may ensue, and what actually happens is a function of the specific neural pathways involved and of the constantly changing status of the internal and external environment of the organism (G. G. Globus, 1992). The emergent behavior shows a *sensitive dependence on initial conditions* (Lorenz, 1963; Mandelbrot, 1982). Even an apparently trivial change in circumstances may produce a profoundly different behavioral outcome.

In practical terms, when an organism's activity is effective, that activity is likely to recur in the future. This facilitation of specific behaviors is generally nonconscious and does not necessarily occur because an animal knows that it should behave in a particular manner. Instead, an activity that previously has been adaptive is likely to recur because the brain functions automatically, but probabilistically, to produce that behavior in similar circumstances. To a certain extent, each repetition of a response has the effect of making the same response more likely to occur in the future.

PLASTICITY OF SOMATOSENSORY CORTEX

Between the transient neurochemical synaptic modifications associated with short-term memory, on the one hand, and the relatively permanent structural synaptic changes that accompany long-term memory on the other, there exists a kind of plasticity that shows flexible reorganization of neural tissue in response to varying kinds of experience. Much of the research in this area has been carried out on primate somatosensory cortex, which integrates and interprets information arriving at the brain from somesthetic or bodily sense receptors (e.g., touch, pain, heat/cold, position sense, sensitivity to pressure), although there also is evidence that the auditory cortex may reorganize itself in adults following hearing loss (King & Moore, 1991).

The somatosensory cortex is topographically organized. This means that the surface of the body is mapped out on the surface of the cortex in an organized manner, so that cells in one region receive impulses coming from the index finger, for example, while cells in another region receive impulses from the palm of the hand. For many years it was thought that these cortical maps were relatively fixed and that little plasticity was possible. Over the past 10 years, however, several investigators have demonstrated that in fact the topographic representation of the body on the cortex is quite malleable.

For example, Merzenich and his associates (see Jenkins, Merzenich, Ochs, Allard, & Guic-Robles, 1990; Jenkins, Merzenich, & Recanzone, 1990; Kaas, 1991; Merzenich et al., 1983a, 1983b, 1990) performed a number of experiments on monkeys in which the investigators first recorded the responses of neurons in the somatosensory cortex to stimulation of the individual fingers of the hand, thereby mapping out the representation of the hand and fingers on the cortex. Subsequently, they performed one of several different manipulations and observed the response of the same neurons over time.

In one experiment, the above investigators amputated either one or two fingers. A few months after surgery, they determined that the neurons formerly receiving input from the amputated fingers had become responsive to stimulation of the remaining adjacent fingers and the palm of the hand. The cortical map had reorganized itself, and neurons now served a different function than previously had been the case. In a second experiment, these investigators sutured the skin of adjacent fingers together, forcing the animals to use the two fingers as though they were a single digit. In this case, after several months the receptive fields of the "fused" fingers—once independent—now overlapped. When the surgical fusion was reversed, after a period of time the original receptive fields again were observed. Finally, these investigators trained their monkey subjects to obtain a reward (food) by using a device that made contact with the tip of one or two fingers. Over nearly 4 months of daily stimulation, for about 90 minutes a day, the representations of the fingers used by the monkeys increased significantly (Jenkins, Merzenich, Ochs, et al., 1990).

Pons and his collaborators (1991) observed findings suggesting considerable plasticity of the somatosensory cortex in a monkey with a completely deafferented arm. While recording neuronal responses from the area of cortex normally dedicated to that extremity, stimulation of the arm or hand produces no neural activity, but light touch applied to the face produced reactions throughout the area of cortex one would expect to be associated with the arm. It is thought that this plasticity is modulated by the basal nucleus, a forebrain structure. Lesions of the basal nucleus prevent such changes in cortical sensory maps from occurring (Kilgard & Merzenich, 1998).

SUMMARY AND CONCLUSION

Evolution demands the adaptation of species to hostile and changing conditions, and individual organisms must have the capacity to adapt their behavior to unique ecological niches. Among organisms with nervous systems, the mechanism by which this experience-dependent modification of structure occurs is synaptic plasticity, a process that seems to be an inherent property of neural tissue.

Synaptic modifications take place on a wide range of timescales, lasting anywhere from a few milliseconds through several decades. Some of these alterations are transient, mediated by neurochemical processes of only brief duration. Other changes involve permanent alterations in the structure of the junction between neurons. Between the two extremes are dynamic processes that produce flexible patterns of cortical organization.

A good deal of experience-dependent modification of the CNS takes place during critical (or sensitive) periods of development. Unless an individual has the right kind of experience during those periods, neural and psychological functioning go awry, sometimes with serious and enduring consequences. The visual system is the best studied site of such experience-dependent maturation, but critical periods also have been demonstrated for attachment and the acquisition of language. Sensitive periods probably also exist for the development of basic self-representations and for character, both of which are discussed in later chapters.

On a functional level, the effect of synaptic plasticity is a change in probabilities. Learning induces structural changes that make it either more or less likely that stimulation of a given neuron or (more accurately) a population of neurons will cause the stimulated neurons to fire. This point cannot be overemphasized, and we will return to it repeatedly in this book. The probabilities are determined to a large extent by the overall state of the individual at any given time (we refer to this as the *physiological state* and discuss it in Chapter 9). Changing one's state can reset the probabilities for almost all kinds of behavioral, perceptual, cognitive, and mnestic activity.

4

MODULARITY OF BRAIN AND PSYCHOLOGICAL FUNCTIONING

INTRODUCTION

This chapter deals with the way the brain is organized and with the implications of that organization for psychological functioning. Because the architecture of the brain is of great importance for our understanding of personality, we will discuss it in considerable detail. In short, the brain is a modular distributed, self-organizing system of neural networks. Cognitive, emotional, and behavioral functioning are mediated by the parallel and sequential processing patterns of neural networks originating in different structures and distributed throughout the brain. Even within specific cortical or subcortical regions, functional abilities are mapped on the brain in a modular distributed manner. This chapter addresses the meaning and general implications of this architecture, examining in particular the following issues.

The visual system provides a compelling example of the modular distributed architecture of the brain, and it demonstrates some of the implications of modularity for neural and psychological activity. The visual system synthesizes information that is simultaneously processed by a large number of different modules, at many different levels of neural and perceptual complexity, with discrete processing areas for such basic phenomena as color, contour, and direction of movement. Separate visual subsystems have such basic functions as the detection of motion and sensing of the position of objects in space, the conscious awareness and representation of visual information, control of ocular reflexes, and regulation of the body's circadian

pacemaker. The effects of focal neurological syndromes affecting subcomponents of the visual system illustrate the fundamental parallel capacities necessary for normal visual processing.

Vision is not the only neuropsychological process organized in a modular fashion. Rather, it seems likely that psychological functioning in general is characterized by a modular distributed architecture. To further illustrate the concept of modularity, we will examine the modular basis of
motor functioning. As with vision, many regions of the brain are involved
in movement, and our discussion of the varied nature of specific movement
disorders below serves to illustrate the modularity of the motor system.

The performance of various tasks—even ones that appear superficially
to be relatively simple in their nature—involves rather complex patterns of
parallel and sequential processing that could be accomplished only by a
massively parallel modular system. Thus, specific psychological functions—
for example, language, reasoning, impulse control, or reality testing—are
more accurately thought of as *functional systems,* processes comprising
varying numbers of functional subcomponents.

One of the major theoretical problems facing neuroscientists is to determine the mechanisms by which widely separated modular arrays of neurons can function coherently to produce an organized representation of the
world, a representation that permits purposeful behavior and the precisely
timed integration of perception, cognition, and activity. Referred to as the
binding problem, there is evidence that this integration of neuronal activity
appears to involve the synchronous and oscillatory firing of large, distributed populations of neurons.

The phenomenon of modularity underscores the central importance of
the brain's capacity to integrate (i.e., to bind) vast amounts of processing in
the service of adaptive activity. It seems logical, then, that some kinds of
psychopathology may best be understood as reflecting failures or anomalies
of integration. A modular architecture provides a basis for understanding
certain aspects of such disorders as dissociation and borderline personality
disorder. Moreover, various psychological functions (e.g., impulse control)
can be explained more convincingly by examining the neural basis of their
various subcomponents. The modularity of memory, discussed in Chapter
5, has significant implications for understanding how psychotherapy produces or fails to produce change.

HIERARCHICAL ORGANIZATION
OF BIOLOGICAL SYSTEMS

Organisms differ from simpler physicochemical systems in that they possess
highly complex, nonlinear, self-organizing structures. Such structures yield
the sort of emergent properties—behavior, cognition and the like—that

characterize living things. How this happens is not yet well understood, but as a general rule those biological systems that show a greater degree of differentiation and development show a correspondingly more complex organization.

It has become apparent that the brain is a hierarchically organized system that is capable of massively parallel (simultaneous) processing across large numbers of interconnected regions, with exquisitely timed sequential operations. Hierarchical structure as a general organizing principle in biology was of great interest to biologist Paul A. Weiss (1971, p. 23). He studied the ways in which hierarchy contributes to "the orderliness of the living state" (p. 26) and applied his ideas to neuroscience (1967). Weiss (1971) considered organisms to be "units composed of smaller units subordinated to the system as parts or components" (p. 24). In this way, according to Weiss, nature "reveals itself to be ordered 'hierarchically' in descending steps from supersystems through systems to subsystems, and so on down through different orders of magnitude and levels of systemic stability" (1971, p. 24).

A comprehensive hierarchical theory of brain functioning was proposed by A. R. Luria (1973, 1980), who suggested that the brain was composed of three principal "functional units" (1973): one regulating arousal and cortical activation; one encompassing perception, cognition, and memory; and one concerned with the regulation and monitoring of purposeful activity. According to Luria's scheme, the second and third units are composed of a large number of different subsystems, each of which functions at a primary level of organization (the receipt of basic sensory data in a single modality, such as vision), a secondary level (the integration and interpretation of basic perceptual data within each modality), and a tertiary level (the integration of perceptual data from multiple sensory modalities and functional systems, such as the combination of visual and auditory images with words that describe or attribute meaning to those images).

CURRENT THEORIES OF BRAIN FUNCTIONING

The structural–functional organization of the central nervous system (CNS) has become somewhat more clear over the past 20–25 years as a result of the work of many neuroscientists (e.g., Eccles, 1984; Edelman, 1979; Gazzaniga & LeDoux, 1978; A. Globus & Scheibel, 1967; G. G. Globus, 1992; Goldman-Rakic, 1984; Hubel & Wiesel, 1963; Kaas, 1987, 1989; Mountcastle, 1979; Rumelhart & McClelland, 1986; Szentágothai, 1975, 1979, 1980; Szentágothai & Arbib, 1974), and it appears that in fact the brain defies description by simple hierarchical models. As Kaas noted, "the true complexity of the system should be remembered. Processing has both parallel and hierarchical components, but 'later' stations receive inputs from both 'intermediate' and 'early' stations, confounding simple hierarchical schemes" (1987, p. 144). Some areas of the brain, for example, are considered to be "networks," involving functionally related regions that "are interconnected in a manner that is not obviously hierarchical, or at least in a manner where hierarchical processing across areas is not the dominant feature" (Kaas, 1989, p. 129).

Current models depict the brain as a modular distributed system—a complex nonlinear hierarchy, perhaps better described by McCulloch's term *heterarchy* (1945). Such a hierarchy has a number of advantages over other architectures—but for the brain, efficiency of processing is one of the most important (Szenthágothai & Arbib, 1974). The lowest levels of the hierarchy are specialized for the quick and automatic handling of routine tasks (e.g., reflexes, eye movements, and basic perception) that do not require deliberate processing. The higher stages in the hierarchy then are relieved of the burden of such processing and are freed to perform tasks at a more complex level of integration (e.g., planning). Simple tasks like talking, walking, and understanding speech would be absurdly difficult if they did not become automatic early in childhood. Consider the difficulty, and the demand for attentional resources, that one encounters in trying to speak or understand a foreign language with which one is barely familiar, or in learning a demanding motor skill like juggling or playing the organ. When behaviors of this kind can be performed unconsciously, effortlessly, and automatically, an individual has the capacity to devote his or her limited processing capacity to higher-level activities like planning, self-monitoring, and organizing one's activity.

The "computational" aspect of neural processing may provide the incentive for neural systems to evolve toward modularity. Shallice (1988), for example, noted that computers controlling complex engineering or manufacturing processes require very elaborate programs to direct the executive functions that manage lower-level subcomponents of the process in real time. These executive programs, which can account for as much as 30–40% of the programming code, reduce the flexibility of the system and significantly increase response time. When engineers break such problems into many decentralized subsystems, parceling them out to nonexecutive parallel processors, the demand for central executive control is greatly diminished and the efficiency of these systems improves significantly. In the case of brains, which must create all of an individual's perceptual, cognitive, and motor phenomena, the demand on executive resources would be prohibitive were the CNS designed in any way other than a massively parallel, widely distributed, hierarchical system in which the vast bulk of functioning takes place entirely outside the purview of the upper levels of the hierarchy.

Higher levels of the hierarchy may have only limited direct control over lower levels, but they do receive constant feedback about the status of the organism's overall functioning and they may effect changes in functioning at relatively complex levels of integration (e.g., change in the meaning of a percept, but not in the fundamental sensory properties of the percept itself). Heterarchies, while possessing many of the basic characteristics of hierarchies, are even more complex. The different subcomponents of heterarchies may be relatively independent, yet they also interact with, influence, and are informed by one another at different levels of integration.

THE RELATIONSHIP BETWEEN STRUCTURE AND FUNCTION

In biology, structure and function are intimately related. Although there is no strict one-to-one correspondence, the structure and function of biological systems and subsystems have evolved in tandem, with various biological structures developing in ways that serve the successful functioning of the organism. Functioning (behavior, cognition, perception, and so on), insofar as it *reflects* structure, must be organized in a similar manner to structure. The significance of this point cannot be overemphasized and should not be interpreted metaphorically. Human functioning, like the architecture of the brain, is heterarchically organized.

THE MODULE IS A STRUCTURAL AND FUNCTIONAL UNIT

Although the individual neuron is in some respects the fundamental building block of the brain, the basic functional unit is the *module* (A. Globus & Scheibel, 1967; Manger et al., 1998; Mountcastle, 1979, 1997; M. E. Scheibel & A. B. Scheibel, 1958; Szentágothai, 1967, 1975, 1980). The module is an array of developmentally related neurons that is difficult to define precisely (Shallice, 1988) and that varies across brain structures and levels of organization.

In the brain, each of a multitude of modules contains a systematically arranged collection of excitatory and inhibitory neurons. There may be as few as a handful of nerve cells or as many as several billion. The basic *cortical* module is a column or cylinder of radially oriented neurons (i.e., they are oriented so they are perpendicular to the surface of the cortex) whose processes extend across all six layers of the cortex, making horizontal connections with other modules in the immediate vicinity, as well as with structures located some distance away. Each module thus is capable of influencing and being influenced by modules in many cortical and subcortical areas, a phenomenon referred to as *reentrance* or *reentry* (Edelman, 1979; Goldman & Nauta, 1977; Goldman-Rakic & Schwartz, 1982).

Szentágothai (1983) estimated that 90% of all cortical connections may serve a reentrant function by which already processed signals from various subsystems may "reenter" other systems "so that they may be correlated at later times with succeeding input signals" (Edelman, 1987, p. 60). Thus, while there are myriad quasi-independent modules operating throughout the brain, each is closely integrated with various other neuronal groups. As a consequence, brain (and psychological) functioning, despite its modular character, emerges as a synthetic, coherent whole.

Modules exist at different levels of organization, so that each module mediates either a specific function, a component of a function, or a complex of functions. Although each module operates somewhat independently, each also is woven into the structural–functional fabric of the whole brain. According to Mountcastle (1979, p. 22), these "closely linked and multiple interconnected subsets of modules in different and often widely separated entities thus form precisely connected but distributed systems." Excitatory and inhibitory neurons connect modules within any given subsystem, and also connect systems and subsystems with one another at various levels of integration. A functional system such as language is mediated not by a single localized brain region (e.g., Broca's area), or even two regions (e.g., Broca's area *and* Wernicke's area), but by a number of areas that are distributed throughout both cortical and subcortical structures.

The absolute size of modules varies widely depending on the level of organization one wishes to consider. Some authors reserve the term *module* for the basic functional unit of the nervous system, but the concept of module may be used to describe relatively independent neuronal systems at different levels of complexity as well. For example, one might argue that individual neurons represent the modular subcomponents of the cell columns which Szentágothai (1975) has identified as modules. Larger structures, or sets of structures, also may be considered to be more complex modules. For example, the cerebellum as a whole could be considered a module, as could the cerebellum's dentate nucleus, or groups of cells within the dentate nucleus. Thus modules at one level may comprise subcomponent modules at several other different levels and may themselves be subcomponents of higher-level modules.

At the most basic level of anatomy, these modules may be quite small, and because of their variability, their exact topographic limits have been difficult to specify (A. B. Scheibel, 1979). Some are composed of vertically oriented cell columns, whereas others are characterized more by horizontally oriented neurons ("tangential modularity"; Manger et al., 1998). At the lower limit of size, Szentágothai (1975) has proposed the existence of one system of inhibitory modules in cortical layer II containing fewer than

10 pyramidal cells. Yet interactions among these and other modules take place, for example, in cortical layer I, where cells may form connections with neurons from deeper cell layers as well as from places distant in the cortex. Basic modular neuronal units have been identified across species (Krubitzer, 1995; Manger et al., 1998), suggesting that they are a fundamental building block of brains (Kaas, 1995; Krubitzer, 1995; W. Singer et al., 1997). In a simple organism such as *Aplysia californica*, the sea hare, a marine invertebrate used extensively in research on synaptic plasticity, the module involved in the gill and snout withdrawal reflex may involve only a few dozen neurons (Castellucci, Carew, & Kandel, 1978), whereas the human right cerebral hemisphere is a higher-level module composed of billions of neurons. Simpler cortical modules are organized into large fields of neurons, the degree of complexity of which appears to increase with the complexity of the organism (Kaas, 1987).

There are considerable data to support the idea of a modular cortical architecture, a type of organization described as "almost a logical necessity" by Szentágothai (1979, p. 407). In his assessment, so many aspects of this concept are supported by experimental data that "it seems almost trivial to try further to elaborate upon them" (Szentágothai, 1987, p. 330). Not everyone agrees that the brain is fundamentally and thoroughly modular, however; some authors (e.g., Fodor, 1983) have maintained that only input systems are modular, whereas others have argued that only and motor systems are modular. Central processing is thought to be organized in a more diffuse, equipotential manner. Nevertheless, the evidence for modularity is compelling, and the concept is widely accepted (see also Shallice, 1988).

MODULAR ORGANIZATION OF THE VISUAL SYSTEM

In this section, we discuss the organization of the visual system. Our intention is to demonstrate the complex manner in which a large number of functional subsystems are interwoven to yield a complete picture of the world. A similar pattern of organization underlies all personality functions.

Analysis of the visual system of primates reveals an unmistakably modular organization. There are, for example, at least four major visual systems—one cortical, and three subcortical. These mediate control of the ocular reflexes, the detection of movement and location in space, regulation of the body's biological rhythms, and conscious awareness of visual stimuli. We now discuss each of these briefly, addressing in particular the organization of the system for conscious visual processing.

Neurons travel from the retina to several areas of the brain via the optic nerve. One of these regions, located on the superior and dorsal (back) surface of the midbrain (see Figures 4.1 and 4.2), is called the *pretectal area*. There is a *pretectum* on both the right and left sides, located a short distance from the midline. Each pretectum receives input from retinal neurons that respond to changes in level of illumination. A bright light shined in the right pupil sends impulses to the right pretectum, which in turn transmits nerve impulses that cause a symmetrical constriction of the pupils in both the left and right eyes. This reflexive process is automatic, occurring unconsciously and requiring the action of the retina, optic nerve, brainstem, and third cranial nerve only. It is not under direct conscious control and cannot be deliberately inhibited.

In mammals, a second visual pathway (the *retinohypothalamic tract*) runs from the retina to the suprachiasmatic nucleus (SCN) of the hypothalamus, an area that appears to contain a circadian pacemaker (Meijer & Rietveld, 1989) responsible for driving certain periodic and quasi-periodic processes such as cycles of activity and the sleep–wake cycle (Czeisler et al., 1989; Ralph et al., 1990). Specialized retinal receptors are stimulated by light, and activity in this circuit during certain regular hours of each day serves to entrain the circadian pacemaker; in other words, exposure to light on a regular schedule presumably leads to the expression of certain genes on a regular daily basis. The proteins produced by a gene or genes, synthesized as a result of exposure to light, regulate the activity of the SCN (Takahashi, 1991).

A third visual pathway involves nerve fibers running from the retina to the *superior colliculus,* a small, bilaterally symmetrical set of structures on either side of the dorsal midbrain tectum, near the pretectal area. The superior colliculus is composed of several layers containing precisely aligned sensory maps, so that sensory stimuli of various kinds are represented in an organized way and distributed across a layer of cells. A cellular map of the visual world is the most superior of these, and it provides the basic template for the other sensory maps. Immediately beneath this is a map of the body (a *somesthetic* map), and under that is a map of auditory space. Visual information also is reentrant into the lower levels of the colliculus. Beneath these various sensory maps is a motor map—that is, a systematic representation of the body as it moves in space. These maps are precisely aligned in order to integrate information regarding the location of stimuli in three-dimensional space. The superior colliculus is involved in the control of head, neck, and eye movements (Schiller, True, & Conway, 1980) and also appears to be essential for accurate perception of the movement of objects in space.

The fourth visual pathway contains neurons that project from the retina through the optic nerve and optic tract to the *lateral geniculate nucleus* (LGN), a cluster of cell bodies in the thalamus. Like the superior colliculi, the LGN is a layered structure. Neurons carrying information regarding movement terminate in layers of the LGN different from those carrying in-

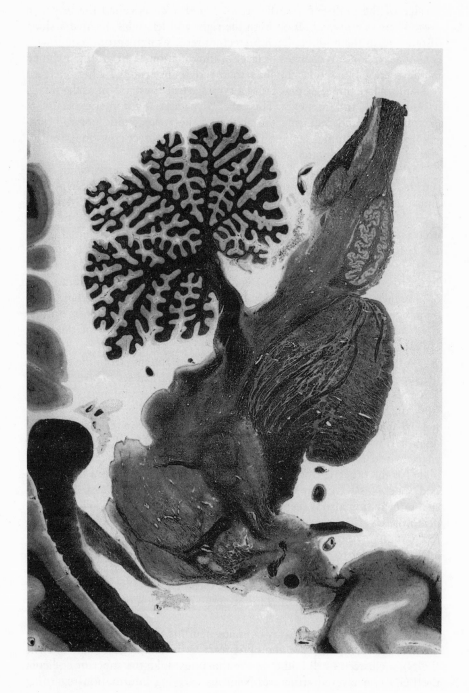

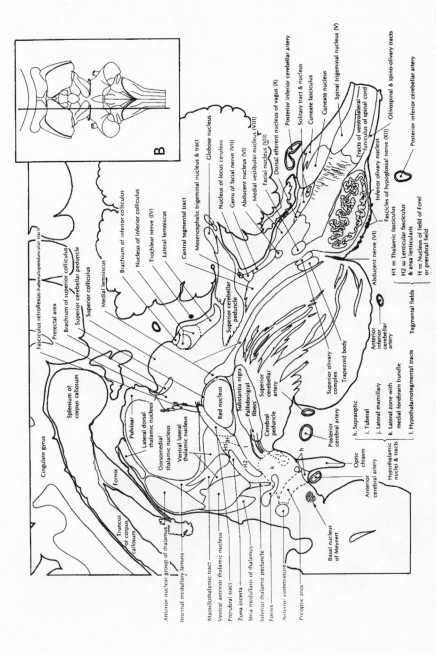

FIGURE 4.1. Parasagittal (parallel to the midline) section of the human brainstem, cerebellum, and thalamus. Part A shows a section through the brain while Part B shows the angle of the cut through the brain. Part C shows the locations of a number of structures in this region. From DeArmond, Fusco, and Dewey. (1989, pp. 154–155). Copyright © 1974, 1976, 1989 by Oxford University Press, Inc. Used by permission of Oxford University Press, Inc.

63

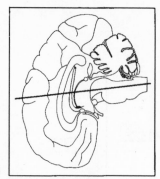

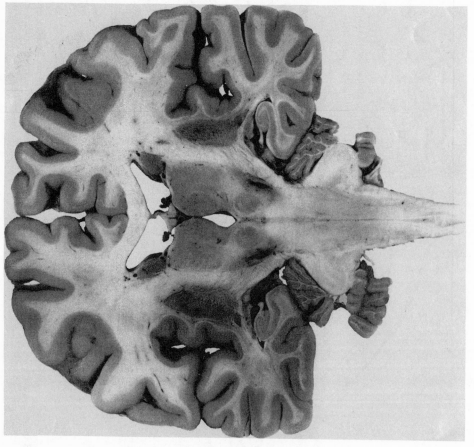

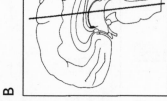

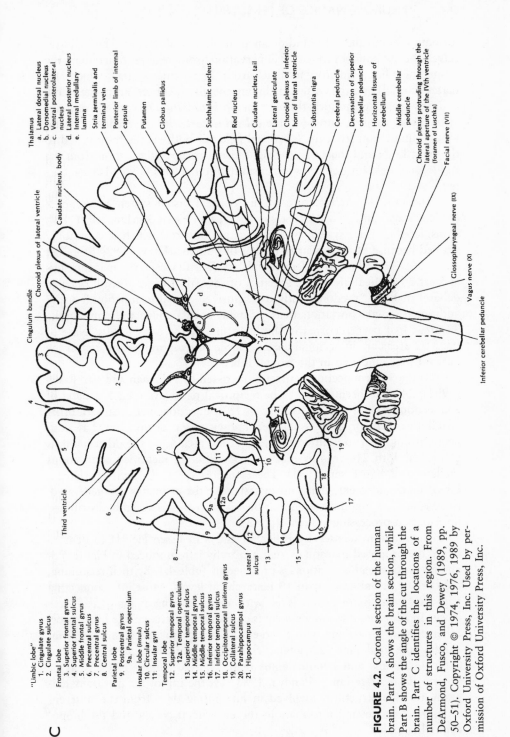

"Limbic lobe"
1. Cingulate gyrus
2. Cingulate sulcus

Frontal lobe
3. Superior frontal gyrus
4. Superior frontal sulcus
5. Middle frontal gyrus
6. Precentral sulcus
7. Precentral gyrus
8. Central sulcus

Parietal lobe
9. Postcentral gyrus
9a. Parietal operculum

Insular lobe (insula)
10. Circular sulcus
11. Insular gyri

Temporal lobe
12. Superior temporal gyrus
12a. Temporal operculum
13. Superior temporal sulcus
14. Middle temporal gyrus
15. Middle temporal sulcus
16. Inferior temporal gyrus
17. Inferior temporal sulcus
18. Occipitotemporal (fusiform) gyrus
19. Collateral sulcus
20. Parahippocampal gyrus
21. Hippocampus

FIGURE 4.2. Coronal section of the human brain. Part A shows the brain section, while Part B shows the angle of the cut through the brain. Part C identifies the locations of a number of structures in this region. From DeArmond, Fusco, and Dewey (1989, pp. 50–51). Copyright © 1974, 1976, 1989 by Oxford University Press, Inc. Used by permission of Oxford University Press, Inc.

Thalamus
a. Lateral dorsal nucleus
b. Dorsomedial nucleus
c. Ventral posterolateral nucleus
d. Lateral posterior nucleus
e. Internal medullary lamina

Stria terminalis and terminal vein

Posterior limb of internal capsule

Putamen

Globus pallidus

Subthalamic nucleus

Red nucleus

Caudate nucleus, tail

Lateral geniculate

Choroid plexus of inferior horn of lateral ventricle

Substantia nigra

Cerebral peduncle

Decussation of superior cerebellar peduncle

Horizontal fissure of cerebellum

Middle cerebellar peduncle

Choroid plexus protruding through the lateral aperture of the IVth ventricle (foramen of Luschka)

Facial nerve (VII)

Glossopharyngeal nerve (IX)

Vagus nerve (X)

Inferior cerebellar peduncle

Cingulum bundle

Choroid plexus of lateral ventricle

Caudate nucleus, body

Third ventricle

Lateral sulcus

C

65

formation about the color and detailed resolution of images. The LGN receives the preponderance of its innervation from regions other than the retina, including regulatory feedback from the reticular system (which regulates arousal) and the cortex, including the visual cortex. From the LGN, neurons project posteriorly through the *optic radiation* toward the primary visual area, a region known as the *calcarine cortex* of the medial occipital lobes. Stimulation from the *left* visual field for both eyes is transmitted to the right LGN and thence to the right visual cortex. Stimulation from the *right* visual field for both eyes is transmitted to the left LGN and visual cortex.

The modular architecture of the cortical visual system is complex (Felleman & Van Essen, 1991; Kaas, 1987; Van Essen & Maunsell, 1983). Consider the visual system of the macaque monkey, which is commonly studied because of its similarity to that of humans (Kaas, 1992; Tootell et al., 1996). According to Felleman and Van Essen (1991), the macaque has at least 25 cortical areas (the specifics of several of these are still open to debate) that are "predominantly or exclusively visual in function," and 7 additional visual association areas. As many as 305 connections among the 32 areas had been reported in the literature by the early 1990s. Nine of these 32 areas are in occipital cortex, eleven in temporal cortex, ten in the parietal lobe, and two in the frontal lobe.

Of the 305 connecting pathways discussed by Felleman and Van Essen (1991), 242 had been shown to be reciprocal pathways (i.e., 121 pairs of connections). There was an average of 19 connections per area with other visual areas. The primary visual area, known as V1, demonstrated 16 connections linking it to 9 different areas. Visual area 4, on the other hand, is connected with 21 areas by means of 39 different identified connections (Felleman & Van Essen, 1991). These authors concluded, with perhaps a bit of understatement, that "no matter how the estimates are generated, there is no escaping the notion that the visual cortex is a highly distributed information-processing system" (p. 13).

The diagram devised by Felleman and Van Essen (1991) to demonstrate the proposed macaque visual hierarchy is reproduced in Figure 4.3, and a key for the abbreviations is provided in Table 4.1. By their reckoning, the cortical visual areas span 10 hierarchical levels. Most interconnecting pathways cross more than 1 level, with some crossing as many as 7 or 8 levels. In addition, the visual system is extensively interconnected with most other cortical areas, and with a large number of subcortical structures including the thalamus, amygdala, claustrum, caudate nucleus, superior colliculus, pons, and hypothalamus (e.g., Iwai & Yukie, 1987; Kaas & Huerta, 1988; Yeterian & Pandya, 1985). At the top of the hierarchy diagram are two structures involved in integrating data from the different senses and processing information: the entorhinal cortex and the hippocampal complex.

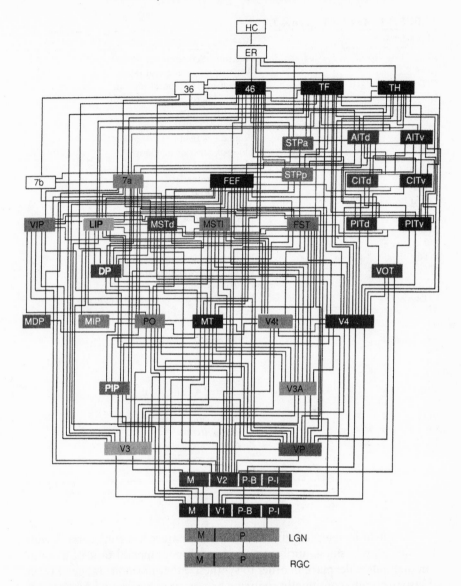

FIGURE 4.3. Hierarchy of visual areas as proposed by Felleman and Van Essen (1991). There is a total of 32 visual cortical ares and 2 subcortical areas (retinal ganglion cell layer [RGC] and lateral geniculate nucleus [LGN]) shown. Several nonvisual areas also are included to demonstrate links with other sensory modalities or processing areas (e.g., area 7b of somatosensory cortex; hippocampus). The proposed cortical visual hierarchy spans 10 levels. Most interconnecting pathways traverse more than 1 level, although some cross as many as 7 or even 8 levels. At the top of the hierarchy diagram are 2 structures that are essential for information processing and the integration of data from different senses: the hippocampal complex (HC) and the entrohinal cortex (ER). From Felleman and Van Essen (1991, p. 36). Copyright © 1991 by Oxford University Press. Reprinted by permission of Oxford University Press.

TABLE 4.1. Key for Figure 4.3

Abbreviation	Area
AITd	Anterior inferotemporal (dorsal)
AITv	Anterior inferotemporal (ventral)
CITd	Central inferotemporal (dorsal)
CITv	Central inferotemporal (ventral)
DP	Dorsal prelunate
ER	Entorhinal cortex
FEF	Frontal eye field
FST	Floor of superior temporal
HC	Hippocampal complex
LIP	Lateral intraparietal
MDP	Medial dorsal parietal
MSTd	Medical superior temporal (dorsal)
MSTl	Medial superior temporal lateral
MT	Middle temporal
PIP	Posterior intraparietal
PITd	Posterior inferotemporal (dorsal)
PITv	Posterior inferotemporal (ventral)
PO	Parieto-occipital
STPa	Superior temporal polysensory (anterior)
STPp	Superior temporal polysensory (posterior)
V1	Visual area 1
V2	Visual area 2
V3	Visual area 3
V3a	Visual area V3a
V4	Visual area 4
V4t	Visual area 4 transitional
VIP	Ventral intraparietal
VOT	Ventral occipitotemporal
VP	Ventral posterior
7a	Brodmann area 7a
36	Brodmann area 36
46t	Brodmann area 46

We might be tempted to wonder whether nature has gone berserk with this hierarchy business until we consider the monumental task of integration that must take place in order to synthesize the enormous range of types of visual stimuli, continually changing as our eyes, heads, and bodies constantly move, so that different images are projected accurately to the visual cortex. At the most basic level of the hierarchy—individual cell columns in area V1—there is considerable specificity in the nature of the stimuli to which cells respond. *Simple cells,* for example, may respond only to precisely oriented lines. This was demonstrated by Hubel and Wiesel (1959, 1962), who placed microelectrodes within simple cells and found that these neurons were maximally responsive (i.e., showed the greatest frequency of firing) when they were stimulated by lines projected onto a particular spot on the retina at specific angles. Rotation of a line by as little as 10° from the preferred orientation led to a decrease in firing of the cells, while cells in adjacent columns might show a simultaneous increase in their frequency of discharge.

Hubel and Wiesel (1962) also identified what they called *complex cells*. Like simple cells, these are most responsive to stimuli with a specific axis of orientation, but an image does not have to fall on a precise spot on the retina to lead to a discharge. Instead, movement of an image across the retina at a particular angle will produce an increase in the rate of firing in complex cells. Hubel and Wiesel concluded that complex cells receive input from groups of simple cells having the same responsivity to stimuli oriented at a specific angle but having different receptive fields on the retina. Through the combined functioning of simple and complex cells, every possible stimulus angle at every point on the retina can be represented. The integration of these basic stimuli is a daunting integrative task, one that requires a complex hierarchy for synthesis of these elemental components of perception.

In addition to the simple and complex cells in the primary visual cortex, there are cell columns referred to as *blobs* (Ts'o, Gilbert, & Wiesel, 1986), which are responsive to color rather than line orientation. At the next-higher level of organization, there also are *ocular dominance columns* in primary visual cortex. These juxtaposed columns of cells receiving similar input for the same visual field from either the left or right eye play a role in binocular vision. Also at a higher level of integration in area V1, Hubel and Wiesel (1962) identified what they called *hypercolumns,* modules composed of groups of columns of simple and complex cells (as well as blobs) receiving stimuli from both eyes, at all angles of rotation, over a limited spatial extent.

THE EFFECTS OF INJURY TO SPECIFIC REGIONS OF THE VISUAL SYSTEM

Injury to specific regions of the visual system tends to produce consistent, relatively predictable region-specific effects, providing additional evidence that the brain has a modular distributed architecture. We first examine the manifestations of lesions affecting the four major visual systems described at the beginning of the section on vision: the pretectum, SCN, superior colliculus, and visual cortex.

Injury to the brainstem may disrupt circuits involved in the pupillary reflexes mediated by the pretectum. If this occurs, an individual is liable to be unconscious, since neural networks in the core of the brainstem also are necessary for arousal. In any case, if a light is directed into the pupil of each eye, one at a time, an asymmetrical response might be observed, or there may be a failure of the pupil to constrict in response to the light. If the lesion were sufficiently circumscribed (as might be the case in an injury to the oculomotor nerve), the visual system otherwise might well be unaffected. Injury to the superior colliculus alone may impair both quick responses to moving stimuli, and the individual's judgment of the location of stimuli—especially moving objects—in space. Lesions of the SCN, retinohypothalamic tract, or any injury involving bilateral destruction of the retinas or loss of the eyes will abolish the stimulation of the SCN by light, with a resulting tendency for the individual to develop disturbances of circadian rhythms, showing physiological deviation from the normal patterns entrained by the light–dark cycle.

A lesion at any point along the visual system between the retina and the occipital cortex may produce unique patterns of visual disturbance that can be useful in localizing the lesion. For example, complete transection of either optic nerve produces blindness for the eye transmitting stimulation through that nerve, while vision remains normal in both right and left visual fields for the other eye. Complete destruction of either primary visual cortex (area V1) produces conscious blindness for the visual field on the side opposite the damaged hemisphere, a condition referred to as *homonymous hemianopia*. If neurons in the left superior optic radiation (the part of the visual tract between the LGN of the thalamus and the occipital cortex that passes through the lower parietal lobe) are damaged, *right inferior quadrantanopia* results: defective vision in the right lower quadrant of space.

In contrast, relatively diffuse lesions of cortical regions serving higher levels of the visual hierarchy do not produce blindness (M. P. Alexander & Albert, 1983; Campion & Latto, 1985). Instead, they yield a class of complex phenomena known as *agnosias*. A visual agnosia is an impaired ability to interpret visual information correctly in spite of the fact that the individual's primary visual system is intact. There are a number of these agnosias, each of which involves a unique deficit in higher-level visual processing. For example, the term *apperceptive agnosia* refers to a class of disorders involving an inability to recognize objects visually as a result of impaired perception. Farah (1990) suggested that these apperceptive disturbances could be classified into three categories: apperceptive agnosia narrowly defined, and two variants of a syndrome called *simultanagnosia*.

Apperceptive agnosia per se is an inability to recognize objects by means of vision, associated with a seriously compromised ability to perceive and copy even very simple shapes, in the presence of intact basic visual functions such as color discrimination and acuity. There is a loss of the ability "to recognize differences that distinguish two similar objects" (Hécaen & Albert, 1978; Lissauer, 1890). In severe apperceptive agnosia, an individual may be unable to name objects, pictures of objects, letters, or other visual stimuli without the assistance of other senses. The fundamental problem in this disorder is one of visual recognition, not of naming. The visual system is impaired; the language system (and probably its connections with the visual system) is not. When presented with the same objects and asked to touch or manipulate them, the patient is likely to know immediately what they are.

In simultanagnosia, despite the fact that the visual fields and elementary visual functions are intact, patients frequently cannot see more than one object, or one small region of visual space, at a time. If two objects are held out in front of a simultanagnosic person, he or she will see only one of them unless the objects are both quite small and located next to each other at a distance from the patient. For example, one of Luria's patients (see Luria, Pravdina-Vinarskaya, & Yarbuss, 1963), when looking at a face could recognize it as a face, but would become caught up in the details of the face and then lose sight of the rest of the face—an extreme case of failing to see the forest for the trees. According to Farah (1990), individuals with one type of simultanagnosia (*dorsal simultanagnosia*, presumably resulting from bilateral lesions of parieto-occipital cortex) can see only one object at a time even though they have no visual field defects. Those persons with the other version of this disorder (*ventral simultanagnosia*, presumably a consequence of lesions of left inferior occipitotemporal cortex) are able to see more than one object at a time but cannot recognize them. Luria thought simultanagnosia reflected a "loss of the ability to convert successively presented stimuli into simultaneously perceived structures" (1966, p. 89), however the precise nature of the deficit is unclear.

There are several disorders that might be classified as associative agnosias, or what McCarthy and Warrington (1990, p. 34) call "disorders of object 'meaning'." We will consider only one of them here: *associative agnosia,* as narrowly defined by Farah (1990). She proposes the following criteria for diagnosing associative agnosia: (1) difficulty identifying visually presented objects; (2) normal object recognition through other sensory modalities; and (3) adequate perception of forms and intact basic visual functioning. Individuals with associative agnosia are able to tell objects apart on the basis of their form, but they cannot identify them, nor can they explain the use of an object without handling it or obtaining other sensory data about it.

Hécaen and Albert (1978, p. 195) discussed such a patient who "called a hat a 'little pot'; a ball was misidentified as 'a round block of wood'; a bicycle was called 'a pole with two wheels, one in front, one in back.' " Presented with a pen and a cigar, he called them "cylindrical sticks of variable length." Luria (1980, p. 161) had a similar patient who called a picture of a pair of glasses a bicycle because it had two circles connected by "some sort of crossbar . . . it must be a bicycle." Characteristic of persons with visual associative agnosias is the fact that they attempt to deduce the nature of the object with which they are presented using whatever features of the object they are able to recognize. When basic perception of form is preserved, as in associative agnosia, this may lead to responses such as the bicycle seen by (or, more accurately, inferred by) Luria's patient. Persons with apperceptive agnosia, on the other hand, have even greater difficulty because they may not adequately perceive form. Thus, a patient of Landis et al. (1982) who based inferences on the color of objects came to the conclusion that scrambled eggs were vanilla ice cream.

MODULARITY OF THE VISUAL SYSTEM: SUMMARY

We have discussed the modularity of the visual system in detail to provide a relatively comprehensive perspective on the architecture of both structure and function in the CNS. In reality, however, the system is more complex than we have described. As we noted earlier, the cortical visual system in macaques may have as many as 35 visual areas, with more than 300 connecting pathways, and 10 or more hierarchical levels. These areas are interconnected with other, nonvisual cortical areas and with a large number of subcortical structures as well.

We also have discussed some of the wide variety of visual disorders resulting from injury to different regions of the visual network. When the brain is injured, it undergoes a spontaneous reorganization of its functional systems, and the resulting syndromes are like a net with holes in it—it will still catch some fish, but depending on where they are in the net, some will escape. The point we wish to underscore is that vision itself, and not merely the neurons and cell populations composing the visual system, is modular in character.

MOVEMENT AND MODULARITY

Because the concept of modularity is so fundamental to our model of personality functioning, we will briefly examine the architecture of a second functional system. Although in principle any system would serve our purpose, we have chosen motor functioning. The hierarchical organization of motor and sensorimotor activity has been studied extensively (Bernstein, 1967; Felleman & Van Essen, 1991; Szentágothai & Arbib, 1974); as is true for vision, the capacity to move and to control one's movement is an emergent property of a widely distributed, massively parallel brain network. A sense of the complexity of the hierarchical organization of the motor system can be gained from even a rather superficial analysis of the various motor deficits that follow lesions in a number of areas of the brain.

First we will consider the primary motor cortex, the most posterior area of the frontal lobe (Figure 4.4). This area contains pyramidal neurons

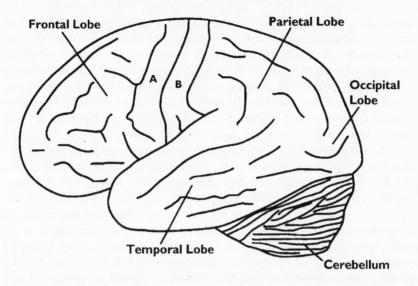

Frontal Lobe

Parietal Lobe

A B

Occipital Lobe

Temporal Lobe

Cerebellum

FIGURE 4.4. Lateral view of the left human cortex. The primary motor area is in the precentral gyrus (A), while the primary somatosensory area is in the postcentral gyrus (B). From Walsh, Brown, Kaye, and Grigsby (1994, p. 45). Reprinted by permission of The West Group.

that descend into the spinal cord, where they form synapses with motor neurons. These "lower" motor neurons exit the anterior part of the cord and form synapses with muscle fibers. The activation of muscle fibers by lower motor neurons causes them to contract. If lower motor neurons are injured, the result is weakness in the affected muscles; in severe cases, the outcome is paralysis. Moreover, without constant innervation by motor neurons, the denervated muscles atrophy.

Modularity is seen as well in the distribution of neurons in the primary motor cortex, which is *somatotopically* mapped onto the cortex. This means that specific regions of the motor cortex are dedicated to the activation of groups of muscles in specific parts of the body. As a consequence of the somatotopic mapping of the primary motor cortex, electrical stimulation of the medial surface of the cortex produces movement of the feet and legs, while stimulation of the superior surface of the brain causes movement of muscles in the trunk. As an electric probe is moved down the lateral surface of the cortex, stimulation produces movement in the hands and arms, face, tongue, and muscles involved in swallowing. Injuries to the primary cortex are likely to result in focal areas of weakness on the opposite (contralateral) side of the body. The severity of impairment may range from minor circumscribed weakness of certain muscles through complete paralysis of one entire side of the body (hemiplegia). Such disorders usually are associated with abnormalities of muscle tone; spasticity (inconsistently increased tone) is common, but flaccidity (reduced tone) is not unusual. Primitive reflexes—normally elicited only in young infants—may be observed. In many animals, ablation of the primary motor cortex may not interfere with the performance of stereotyped activities such as walking or feeding, which seem to be mediated by the brainstem, although the precision and efficiency of movement may be affected (Passingham, 1993). Humans with such lesions show more severe motor deficits, however.

Another region that is important for movement, just adjacent and posterior to the primary motor cortex, is the primary somatosensory cortex, the most anterior portion of the parietal lobe. This region, like the motor cortex, is also somatotopically mapped in a way that resembles the representation of the body on the motor cortex. The somatosensory (or *somesthetic*) area is concerned primarily with physical sensation on the contralateral side of the body. Touch, pressure, and the sensation of the position of one's limbs in space (the *kinesthetic* sense) all are mediated by the primary somatosensory cortex. Stimulation of a small percentage of neurons also may cause movement of the sort observed when the primary motor area is stimulated. Lesions of the postcentral gyrus thus may affect movement directly, though not profoundly, by damaging these motor neurons. More importantly, such lesions may impair kinesthetic or other somesthetic sensation. Hence, without precise information on the exact location of one's limbs, an individual's movements become less precise and somewhat clumsy.

Among the subcortical structures involved in movement are the *basal ganglia,* a bilateral set of nuclei that lie roughly to the outside of the thalamus and upper brainstem deep within each cerebral hemisphere (see Figure 4.2). They include the *caudate nucleus, putamen, globus pallidus, substantia nigra,* and *subthalamic nucleus.* Various parts of the basal ganglia operate as subcomponents of several parallel circuits involving the thalamus and frontal cortex (G. E. Alexander & Crutcher, 1990). Most input to the basal ganglia enters the putamen and caudate nucleus from the thalamus and the entire cortex, with cortical input topographically organized. Although the specific roles of different regions of the basal ganglia are not fully understood, damage to different structures may result in tremor or other involuntary movement, hypoactivity, hyperactivity, and perseveration. The signs of Parkinson's and Huntington's diseases, quite different in their manifestations, are in large part the result of degeneration of neurons in the substantia nigra and caudate nucleus, respectively. Chevalier and Deniau (1990) proposed that the unique contribution of the basal ganglia to the initiation of movement is the disinhibitory arousal of executive motor areas that regulate the performance of voluntary motor activity.

Another subcortical motor area is the *red nucleus,* a structure located in the midbrain that is somewhat less important for apes and humans than for other species. A major portion of the red nucleus (the *magnocellular* division) is involved in the control of independent movements of the limbs (Houk, 1991), and Houk suggested that the normal function of the red nucleus is to control the use of the digits and limbs in the performance of skilled tasks. When electrically stimulated, the red nucleus may produce flexion of the extremities. Studies of laboratory animals suggest that the effects of lesions of the red nucleus on motor functioning typically are transient. Injury to this nucleus may, however, cause a coarse contralateral tremor somewhat similar to the so-called *intention tremor* observed in cerebellar disease.

The *cerebellum* traditionally has been considered important primarily for movement, and while a few investigators continue to maintain this viewpoint (e.g., Glickstein, 1993), recent research has demonstrated the structure's probable significance for cognitive functions as well (Appollonio et al., 1993; Leiner, Leiner, & Dow, 1986, 1989; Middleton & Strick, 1994). Leiner and associates suggested that "the cerebellum functions, in effect, as a general-purpose computer whose special purpose applications can differ in each species, depending on the input–output connections that evolved between the cerebellum and the other parts of the brain" (1986, p. 450). Ivry and Keele (1989) reported research suggesting that the cerebellum is essential for timing of disparate brain activities, and it has been shown to be important in the acquisition of certain conditioned behaviors (Yeo, Hardiman, & Glickstein, 1984).

However the cerebellum functions, it appears to be much involved in feedforward and feedback activity necessary for the proper temporal integration of perception and movement. (Feedforward and feedback are discussed in Chapter 7 on neural dynamics.) The cerebellum receives considerable sensory input (most of which is processed nonconsciously) and is extensively interconnected with a number of cortical and subcortical structures. Input comes especially from the brainstem, including the *pons, inferior olive* (a nucleus in the upper *medulla oblongata*), the *spinocortical tract* (a sensory nerve tract running through the brainstem from the spinal cord to the cortex), and the *vestibular nucleus*. The cerebellum in turn projects fibers back to the vestibular nucleus, the cortex (via the thalamus), and the red nucleus.

Lesions of the *vermis*, the area of the cerebellum nearest the midline, disturb movements of the trunk and proximal musculature (hips and shoulders), whereas lesions of the *cerebellar hemispheres* affect movement of the limbs. Changes in posture, balance, muscle tone, and coordination follow cerebellar injury. The precision of movement may be impaired, as it becomes difficult to control the speed and trajectory of movements of the limbs. Both smooth pursuit movements and rapidly alternating movement may be defective following lesions of the cerebellum (Gilman, Bloedel, & Lechtenberg, 1981).

The *prefrontal* cortex plays what has been described as an "executive" role in movement. When the prefrontal cortex is damaged, the basic capacity for movement remains intact. Depending on the exact locus of a lesion in the prefrontal cortex, however, one may observe failure to initiate purposeful motor activity (*adynamia*) or failure to inhibit irrelevant or inappropriate actions (*disinhibition*). Thus the voluntary regulation of behavior goes awry. Somewhat similar syndromes may be observed following lesions of the dorsomedial thalamus, since the prefrontal area receives a large number of neurons from this area (Fuster, 1997), and as a result of injury to parts of the basal ganglia, especially the caudate nucleus and putamen. In severe bilateral or left-hemisphere lesions of the prefrontal cortex (Luria, 1966, 1980), an individual may be entirely unable to engage appropriately in purposeful activity. Lesions of the *medial premotor area* (also known as the *supplementary motor area*) and the *anterior cingulate gyrus* produce deficits in the initiation of purposeful, voluntary movement (A. R. Damasio & Van Hoesen, 1983; Passingham, 1993).

The interdependence of perception and action requires that the motor system be integrated with the various sensory systems at different levels. The vestibulo-oculomotor reflex, for example, stabilizes the direction of gaze during changes in head position. Without this reflex, visual perception would be extremely unstable during any kind of movement. Although the reflex involves vision, it is initiated by signals arising in the labyrinths (organs of the inner ear involved in maintaining equilibrium) and occurs entirely outside awareness. The eyes themselves are in constant movement in order to prevent the stabilization of images on the retina (saccades), to track moving objects (optokinetic movement), to pursue moving objects smoothly, and to converge accurately on specific positions in visual space. In each case the motor, visual, and other systems operate by means of reentrant signaling to integrate activity at a very basic unconscious level.

Felleman and Van Essen (1991) proposed a hierarchical architecture for the integration of 3 motor and 10 sensorimotor cortical areas, using 62 known connections among these areas. Their proposed hierarchy contains 10 levels but does not include the prefrontal cortex. It also does not include connections with the different subcortical structures addressed here, such as the cerebellum, basal ganglia, and red nucleus. Inclusion of these would make the wiring diagram considerably more complex.

Some of the implications of the distributed heterarchical organization of motor functioning were discussed by Szentágothai and Arbib (1974). In their analysis, two points in particular are noteworthy. First, the motor system uses both feedforward and feedback mechanisms. Feedforward systems respond quickly and can be used to control movement in a general sense, producing movements that are more or less accurate. Slight inaccuracies in the trajectory or force of movement then can be corrected using feedback systems that integrate perceptual and possibly cognitive processing into the network. Feedforward permits a quick and efficient but somewhat inaccurate response. Feedback permits more accurate movement, but by its nature requires more time for the initiation and coordination of activity. The second point has to do with the fact that basic movements tend to be organized into functional groups that operate as *synergies*. Even a simple movement such as flexion of the arm requires contraction of the biceps and simultaneous relaxation of the opposing triceps muscle. Stimulation of the primary motor cortex tends to produce movements of groups of muscles but not of individual muscles themselves. By organizing movement in this way, the organism loses some control over the details of movement, but the trade-off is that higher-level "executive" systems are freed of the necessity to choose these fine details of each motor act. This decrease in the degrees of freedom enhances the organism's capacity for a wider range of purposeful activity, since the same basic act may be performed in a variety of ways with a minimal expenditure of deliberate effort. The executive system formulates a general objective and strategy, and lower-level systems carry out the program.

Examination of different disorders of movement, as well as of the role played by the different parts of the sensorimotor hierarchy, reveals a high degree of modular order in the motor system. The motor behavior of most neurologically intact persons (even klutzes) has an apparently seamless quality; that is, its functional fractionation—its modular character—is not at all obvious. It seems likely, however, that a careful study of the motor activity of ostensibly normal individuals would yield evidence of significant individual differences in all of these various subcomponents of the motor system.

THE BINDING PROBLEM

If the brain is essentially modular, why is its activity not fragmented and temporally disorganized? How does the brain produce coherent patterns of perception, cognition, and movement? Since the brain operates in a massively parallel manner, with simultaneous information processing in several sensory modalities occurring in conjunction with language, recollection, formulation of intentions, planning, and movement, it is essential that these processes occur in a precise, temporally organized manner. As W. Singer and Gray (1995) describe the problem for vision, "any given image consists of a collection of features, consisting of local contrast borders of luminance and wavelength, distributed across the visual field. For one to detect and recognize an object within a scene, the features comprising the object must be identified and segregated from those comprising other objects. This problem is inherently difficult to solve because of the combinatorial nature of visual images" (p. 555).

The problem becomes even more difficult when we consider that a single neuron or a population of neurons may participate in divergent processes but may not always generate an impulse even in situations that appear to be very similar to one another. For example, a single neuron might fire in response to images of different kinds of deciduous trees but not to images of conifers. Moreover, that same neuron may be silent much of the time when the retina is exposed to images of deciduous trees. How are neurons grouped together? The answer is quite complex, since the processing of information involves many populations of neurons, widely distributed over the entire brain. How is the functioning of these neurons integrated? What process ensures that everything happens when it is supposed to happen? This is known as the *binding problem,* and its solution is one of the major issues with which neurophysiologists must contend.

The prevailing and best-articulated (albeit somewhat controversial) viewpoint is that the neuronal signaling occurring in populations mediating a specific activity is *time locked.* That is, it happens synchronously or nearly synchronously (Llinás & Paré, 1996; P. M. Milner, 1974; W. Singer, 1996; W. Singer & Gray, 1995; von der Malsburg, 1981, 1996; von der Malsburg & Schneider, 1986). Kelso (1995) put it simply when he said that, for vision, the key idea is "that spatially separated cell groups should synchronize their responses when activated by a single object" (p. 252). The problem of binding and neuronal synchronization has been studied most thoroughly in the visual system, but data have been obtained that suggest that the kind of synchronous oscillatory activity that would be expected of such time-locked dynamic processes is characteristic of other subsystems, including olfaction (Freeman, 1995) and physical sensation such as touch (Bouyer et al., 1987).

According to W. Singer (1996, p. 104), when a specific pattern of input has led neurons to begin responding, "a self-organizing process is initiated by which subsets of responses are bound together according to the joint probabilities imposed by the specific input pattern, the functional architecture of the coupling network, and the signals arriving through reentry loops from higher processing stages. The essential advantage of such a dynamic, self-organizing binding process is that individual cells can bind at different times, for example, when input constellations change, with different partners." Such self-organized, correlated firing is associated with both regional and large-scale patterns of oscillatory neurophysiological activity. Llinás and Paré (1996, p. 12) suggest that stimuli arriving at the brain within what they call one "perceptual quantum" (a period of 12—15 milliseconds) are "bound into one cognitive event rather than perceived as separate entities" (an idea that we return to later in Chapter 12 on consciousness).

Much work remains to be done to solve the binding problem, but the evidence accumulated thus far regarding synchrony and oscillatory activity is suggestive. Llinás and Paré (1996), for example, note that this explanation for binding could explain how "the activity of cells coding for different aspects of a given object would form a coherent, synchronized group, leading to the transient formation of functional cell assemblies" (p. 9). Thelen and Smith (1994, pp. 140–141) argue also that the theory helps us to understand how different neural networks may overlap. As they noted, it is "a mechanism whereby both flexibility and uniqueness can coexist. Although cell groups coexist and overlap, their activity can be recognized as distinct because of a unique temporal code. At the same time, the same cell or group of cells may participate in different assemblies by changing their temporal relationships, providing a mechanism for both the extreme context sensitivity of perceptual responses and their gestalt character."

WHAT DOES THE MODULAR HYPOTHESIS CONTRIBUTE TO THE UNDERSTANDING OF NORMAL PERSONALITY?

The clinician reading this book may not yet have a clear sense of the significance of this modular line of thinking for the everyday clinical problems of assessment, diagnosis, therapy, and patient management. Nevertheless, the modular theory of personality has a number of important implications for clinicians. They are best understood in the light of other material yet to be discussed on memory and dynamic processes, but we will address some of the distinguishing features of our model briefly here.

Psychological phenomena can be understood in modular terms. In this sense, *personality* itself is not unitary, but, rather consists of a complex array of systems and subsystems, characterized by consistent patterns of behavior, thinking, perceiving, and feeling. For example, (later in Chapter 16) we examine the concept of the self in considerable detail, but for now we note that there is considerable evidence that "the self" actually is a set of different, transiently stable representations and that it is never exactly the same from one moment to the next. A neuropsychological theory of the self might help us to determine more precisely what the self is and how it functions. The data we discuss later in this book suggest that even among healthy individuals there are many self-representations, overlapping in greater or lesser degree depending on the individuals, their state, and the circumstances. Some representations may be more accurate depictions of reality than others, but all are only approximations, models of who one believes oneself to be.

WHAT DOES THE MODULAR HYPOTHESIS CONTRIBUTE TO THE UNDERSTANDING OF PSYCHOPATHOLOGY?

Certain psychopathological phenomena might be usefully conceptualized in this framework. For example, if the self is a modular system, this modularity of self-representations could provides a partial explanation for such disorders as borderline personality organization and the spectrum of dissociative disturbances. While we are unable fully to discuss this subject without going into some detail regarding neural dynamics, we can address here the nature of self-representations, the manner in which they shift across time, and the dynamics of the memory systems that mediate self representations. We also address the relative independence of different personality systems (e.g., self-representations and the system that mediates habitual behavior). This dissociability provides important insights into a number of interesting phenomena. It provides a clear explanation for disorders in which there is a marked difference between how people view themselves and what they actually do (as in passive–aggressive personality), and it suggests a clear rationale for the use of various therapeutic approaches that involve dealing with different memory systems in unique ways.

WHAT DOES THE MODULAR HYPOTHESIS CONTRIBUTE TO ASSESSMENT AND DIAGNOSIS?

The model we propose is a *functional* theory rather than a *trait* theory of personality. The study of traits has been an important aspect of psychological research, but the identification of specific traits may fail to do justice to individual differences in the subcomponent processes contributing to those traits. We view personality itself as a complex emergent process, and hence we are more interested in the processes that contribute to the development and stability of traits than in the traits themselves. For this reason, this modular model is somewhat consistent with an approach like that of Bellak, Hurvich, and Gediman (1973), who attempted to specify a number of "ego functions" that they considered important aspects of personality (e.g., reality sense, reality testing, judgment, impulse control, and affect regulation) and devised a method of assessing the subcomponents of each in different clinical populations.

The diagnostic category of schizophrenia, for example, includes people with widely varying symptoms, functional capacities, and adaptive abilities. We believe that in many ways it is more useful to study individual variation in discrete functional abilities within diagnostic groups than to collapse, for either research or clinical purposes, all individuals into a single category (e.g., paranoid schizophrenia). Certainly, if we are to understand the neuropsychological and neurological basis of schizophrenia, it is important that a much more fine-grained approach be taken to understanding the functioning of people with this disorder.

In contrast, while it may have nosological value, a system like DSM-IV (the *Diagnostic and Statistical Manual of Mental Disorders,* 4th ed.; American Psychiatric Association, 1994) inadequately deals with the individual differences that may make members of certain diagnostic groups (e.g., conduct disorder or antisocial personality disorder) rather different from one another. Similarly, the Minnesota Multiphasic Personality Inventory (MMPI) may provide somewhat useful descriptions of personality styles but provides no information on the underlying processes that contribute to those styles. In the long run, we believe that a modular theory that emphasizes functions over traits and diagnostic categories may be of significant utility in the rational choice of treatment approaches.

Finally, in evaluating personality it is essential to bear in mind that psychological *functions* in fact are *functional systems,* having a modular architecture. When we attempt to assess the integrity of such functional systems as impulse control, we must consider the contributions of a number of different processes to an individual's ability to regulate his or her behavior. These processes, themselves relatively complex modular systems comprising still other subcomponents, include attachment, moral judgment, the ability to inhibit inappropriate behavior, the ability to see things from another's perspective, and guilt sense, for example. Each of these has its own unique neural foundation, and mechanisms of change and stability may vary significantly from one of these processes to another. There undoubtedly are many routes to poor behavioral self-control, and the modular hypothesis will allow us to explore these systematically on different levels of analysis.

By itself, modularity is of somewhat limited heuristic value. The reader will find, however, that subsequent chapters dealing with the dynamics of various neural processes shed considerably more light on the interactions that occur between modular systems.

WHAT DOES THE MODULAR HYPOTHESIS CONTRIBUTE TO TREATMENT OF PSYCHOLOGICAL CONDITIONS?

As we discuss in detail next in Chapter 5, memory is a complex modular system. The available data show that there are several relatively independent memory subsystems, each specialized for the processing of specific kinds of learning. These subsystems develop at different rates during childhood, and each is able to acquire the kind of knowledge peculiar to itself independently of whatever learning might take place in other systems.

It seems obvious that memory and learning play a role in personality development. But if we take another step and apply the modular hypothesis and evidence of the existence of multiple memory systems to personality, it seems that logically we must conclude that *different* memory systems contribute to the development and maintenance of different aspects of personality. If one wishes to provide effective therapy for a specific problem, one must understand the nature of the memory system that supports that problem and design one's intervention accordingly.

SUMMARY AND CONCLUSION

The brain is a hierarchically organized, modular distributed system. Complex cognitive, perceptual, and behavioral activity consequently also is modular in nature, reflecting the setup of the underlying neural substrate. This idea was well developed by A. R. Luria, who preferred to speak of *functional systems* rather than functions. He was concerned that the term "function" might convey the idea that the thing referred to was unitary. Equally problematic is the likelihood that the "thing referred to" might be considered a *thing* rather than a complex set of distributed processes. Disruption of any component of a functional system results in a specific type of pathological performance, and only when that is understood can we grasp the nature of both normal and psychopathological functioning.

In this chapter we have discussed the organizational complexity of two functional systems: vision and movement. With respect to vision, we focused primarily on the distribution of various cortical visual areas and their relations with one another. In covering movement, the main aim of our narrative was to describe the kinds of functional deficits observed following various injuries to the motor system, and also to describe in general terms the contribution of different neural structures to the complete motor act.

Although it may seem somewhat remote or perhaps even overly abstract, the concept of modularity—of both structure and function—is important for understanding human behavior in general and for clinical work in particular (Grigsby & Schneiders, 1991; Grigsby et al., 1991). Next, in Chapter 5, we address the organization of memory, a subject with profound implications for how one understands psychopathology and its treatment. A modular architecture also provides the basis for understanding certain aspects of such disorders as dissociation, passive–aggressive behavior, and borderline personality disorder. Moreover, various psychological functions, such as impulse control and reality testing, can be better understood by examining the neural basis of their various subcomponents.

5

MODULARITY OF MEMORY

INTRODUCTION

Consider the following scenarios. Each involves memory, yet each is somewhat different from the others in one or more important ways. These illustrations represent a wide variety of memory processes and different kinds of content, and (as might be expected), they reflect the anatomical and functional modularity of our capacity for experience-dependent change in the nervous system.

1. An 18-month-old child seems to have learned that if he cries loudly and hits himself with his fists, he will get his mother's attention.
2. A 9-year-old girl is taking music lessons and becoming proficient at playing the piano.
3. A 78-year-old veteran of combat in the Pacific in World War II continues to have recollections of the war that are so vivid he almost feels as if certain events are happening again.
4. A 4-year-old boy is learning how to read and write.
5. A 32-year-old man comes across as arrogant in most of his interactions with others.
6. A woman looks up a telephone number and remembers it long enough to dial it.
7. Conductor Arturo Toscanini had perfect recall for every note of each part performed by every musician in his orchestra for the scores of more than 100 operas.
8. A patient in psychotherapy says that although he is somewhat sketchy on the details, he remembers several incidents from his childhood when his father humiliated him in front of his friends.

Each of these cases can be distinguished from the others on the basis of several criteria. The content, the processes involved, and the neural networks that underlie those processes are not the exactly same in any two examples. What they have in common is that each is a manifestation of changes in functioning that occur as a result of experience. The phenomena subsumed under the category of memory vary considerably from one instance to another. This variety of memory systems is not yet fully understood; the categories that have been proposed by different researchers are not always clear, and frequently they seem somewhat arbitrary. Despite this lack of clarity, abundant evidence exists to support the presence of multiple memory systems that differ from one another in terms of the specific processes and the neural substrates they involve. Like vision and motor functioning, memory appears to be a complex set of modular processes instead of a unitary phenomenon.

BRIEF OVERVIEW OF THE MODULAR NATURE OF MEMORY SYSTEMS

The study of a patient referred to in the neuroscience literature as H. M. led to the recognition that relatively independent memory systems exist for the retention of events and information, on the one hand, and for the acquisition of skills, on the other. N. J. Cohen and L. Squire (1980; also Cohen, 1984) adopted the terms *declarative* and *procedural* learning from the artificial intelligence literature to refer to these two different mnestic processes. It is now known that memory is composed of a number of different systems. These vary as a function of whether there is content to be recalled, the nature of the content, and the specific sensory modalities involved. They also vary along the lines of temporal duration, with some memories lasting only milliseconds and others a lifetime.

Declarative memory involves some kind of content (images, information) that can enter awareness. In contrast, procedural learning is the acquisition of the ability to engage in specific processes, especially skills and habits. Unlike declarative memories, ordinarily no real "content" is involved in procedural learning. Instead, this system is involved in learning to do things so that with practice such actions or processes may be performed automatically and unconsciously. Procedural learning is especially important for understanding the aspect of personality often referred to as "character," as we discuss later in this book (Chapter 15).

There appear also to be systems specialized for memories of pain and for emotional memory. For example, recent data suggest that a vivid representation of the experience of pain may be subject to recall under somewhat extraordinary circumstances, although not in ordinary waking life. In fact, some published reports indicate that the experience of pain may be held surprisingly clearly in memory. There also are data suggesting that emotional memories—especially those involving fear—may be consolidated entirely independently of memory for the event(s) with which they were associated.

One distinction made frequently in memory research is that between *explicit* and *implicit* memory. Explicit memory involves the retention and recall of material that is consciously experienced, whereas implicit memories may be acquired without awareness of their acquisition. While some procedural learning is implicit, not all implicit memories are procedural and many involve some kind of content.

Another memory system that we will address briefly here (and in somewhat more depth in the Chapter 12 on consciousness) is the working memory system. Working memory—the temporary storage of information in awareness—is the term for the most widely held theory of short-term memory. Working memory involves consciousness of those cognitive and perceptual phenomena of which one has been aware for the past 10–20 seconds. Thus, the contents of working memory are essentially the contents of consciousness. This conscious, short-term memory system has a rather limited capacity, but (as we discuss in Chapter 12), it plays a very important role in personality functioning.

Most psychotherapy deals with memories in one way or another, so it is essential that clinicians understand both the architecture of memory and the relationships between the different memory systems. Since much of personality is learned, therapeutic approaches to personality change must take into consideration the nature of the relevant memories (e.g., procedural or declarative), and the relationships among the various memory systems, in order to devise an effective method of treating specific problems.

"H. M." AND THE DISSOCIABILITY OF MEMORY SYSTEMS

In 1957, Scoville and Milner published a paper describing the postsurgical status of a patient known ever since in the neuroscience literature by his initials, "H. M." In 1953, Scoville had performed a bilateral medial temporal lobectomy on H. M. in an attempt to eliminate his medically intractable seizures. Part of the temporal cortex, as well as the amygdala and hippocampus (structures now known to be important for different kinds of memory), were removed from both sides of H. M.'s brain. Although H. M.'s seizure disorder was not cured, the frequency of his seizures decreased significantly. H. M. has become well known as a subject of scientific study but not because of the effect of surgery on his epilepsy. Instead, H. M. is famous for other reasons, which brings us to a general principle of neuroscience: as a rule, unless you *are* a neuroscientist, it's not a good thing to be famous among neuroscientists or to have them think you fascinating.

Because substantial portions of both temporal lobes were removed, H.

M. demonstrated a persistent, severe anterograde amnesia after surgery (B. Milner, 1962); that is, he was unable to remember events or information subsequent to the time of his surgery. Although his intelligence remained in the high average range—he obtained Full Scale IQ of 118 on the Wechsler Adult Intelligence Scale (WAIS), placing him at the 88th percentile rank— H. M. had extremely limited recall for new events and information. He was unable to remember "words, digits, paragraphs, faces, names, maze routes, spatial layouts, geometric shapes, nonsense patterns, nonsense syllables, clicks, tunes, tones, public and personal events" (N. J. Cohen, 1984, p. 83). In addition, he did not know "his age, the date, the place where he lives, [and] the recent history of his mother and father." At the time of H. M.'s surgery, there was insufficient information about brain functioning for the surgeon to have predicted this unanticipated outcome. It is virtually inconceivable that anyone today would perform a bilateral temporal lobectomy to treat epilepsy, as it is now known that even a unilateral hippocampectomy can leave a patient with some additional memory deficit.

Despite his severe deficits, H. M. demonstrated normal or near-normal recall of certain kinds of new perceptual, motor, and cognitive skills. B. Milner (1965), for example, reported that H. M. was able to learn to copy geometric figures while only able to see the movement of his hand in a mirror—thus requiring him to learn to make the movements backward and upside down. H. M. improved with practice until he performed the task normally, and he retained this ability over time. He also showed other types of procedural learning, including the acquisition of other motor skills, a task called mirror reading (i.e., reading the mirror images of words), and a problem called the Tower of Hanoi. Interestingly, H. M. has no memory of having learned to perform those tasks at which he had become proficient. When presented with them, he does not recognize them but nevertheless goes on to perform normally.

H. M. has been studied by neuroscientists for the last 40 years. His amnesia is so severe that he cannot remember any of these people. A researcher can sit with H. M. for an hour administering tests, then leave the room for 2 minutes, and when she returns H. M. will introduce himself as though he has never met her before. In contrast, his recall of events and information prior to the surgery remains intact.

DISSOCIABILITY OF PROCEDURAL AND DECLARATIVE LEARNING

Cognitive neuroscientists determine whether two related functional systems (or components of functional systems) are independent of one another by looking for evidence of dissociations between them. For example, a considerable amount of data have accumulated to support the idea that amnestic patients may have severe declarative memory deficits in the context of pre-served procedural learning. More compelling evidence, however, is obtained when one is able to demonstrate the existence of *double dissociations*. In the case of declarative and procedural memory, this means that there also are some persons who demonstrate impaired procedural learning but intact declarative memory, a pattern opposite of that affecting H. M.

The double dissociation of these two memory systems has been demonstrated recently by Knowlton, Mangels, and Squire (1996). They tested 12 amnestic patients with bilateral hippocampal or thalamic midline damage, 20 nondemented patients with Parkinson's disease (PD), 15 control subjects who were matched with patient groups on age and educational level, and 10 patients with injuries to the frontal lobes. Using a test of declarative memory and a second test involving the acquisition of nonmotor habits, they found that the patients with PD were unable to learn nonmotor habits but performed "entirely normally" on the declarative memory measure. The amnestic patients showed the opposite pattern of performance, performing more poorly on the declarative memory measure than either the patients with PD or the control subjects, whereas the amnestic patients learned the procedural task as well as the control subjects did. Such findings, in concert with data derived from amnestic patients such as H. M., illustrate the existence of multiple dissociable, relatively independent memory systems.

DECLARATIVE MEMORY

Declarative memory, which is defective in the amnestic syndrome, is also dissociable into different subsystems. It generally is subdivided into two other subtypes of memory: *episodic* memory, or recall of subjective events in one's life, and *semantic* memory (or knowledge), the recall of objective facts and other nonpersonal information. Episodic memory involves representations of events that are temporally coded with reference to various autobiographical "landmarks." These may be single events (e.g., "the day Delbert was evicted from his mobile home"), or they may be time periods with a clear association to other events that date memories ("when I was in third grade," or "during the war"). For both kinds of memory, it is thought that the patterns of neural networks underlying a specific memory are prone to change somewhat over time (Squire, 1987) and that "each retrieval of information most likely changes its contents" (Markowitsch, 1995, p. 123). This propensity of networks, or memories, to change over time is extremely important. If memories were immutable, it is difficult to see how psychotherapy could ever be effective.

According to Squire (1992), declarative memory "is fast, accessible to conscious recollection, and is flexible, i.e., available to multiple response systems" (p. 237). The idea that declarative memory is "fast" refers to the fact that it is quickly encoded. Many events, some of which may seem trivial, nonetheless are remembered for a lifetime, even without much thought. Accessibility to conscious recollection means that such memories involve some content of which a person is able to be aware. By flexibility, Squire means that what is learned is generalizable, applicable in situations outside the context in which it was learned.

Tulving (1995) argued that the episodic and semantic memory systems differ both in content and with respect to the specific processes involved in recall. According to Tulving, the semantic system is at a lower level of the memory hierarchy than is the episodic system. While many authors have argued that both kinds of memory are impaired among persons with amnesia, others agree with Tulving that double dissociations may be found among amnestic individuals, causing some persons to show exclusively episodic impairment, whereas for others "a selective memory impairment in the knowledge domain is likely" (Markowitsch, 1995, p. 119).

An interesting phenomenon known as "source amnesia," in which an individual can recall information learned in the recent past but cannot remember the source of that information (D. L. Schachter, Harbluk, & McLachlan, 1984), supports the hypothesis of the dissociability of the episodic and semantic memory systems. Source amnesia occurs among many amnestic persons who have some preserved ability to retain new information. Source amnesia is not present in all amnestic persons, but among those who experience it, it is consistent. Squire has suggested (1987) that for these individuals, the inability to remember the source of learning reflects an impairment of episodic memory.

The precise neural substrate of declarative memory varies, depending on the task at hand. The specific areas of cortex involved may differ from one situation to another. For example, the occipital cortex is necessary for storage and recall of visual material, the temporal cortex for auditory memory, and the parietal lobe for memories having a somesthetic component. In addition to the involvement of different cortical areas in the recall of different types of material, certain invariant regions of the brain appear to be essential for declarative memory.

H. M.'s unfortunate experience suggests the importance of an intact hippocampus for processes essential to declarative memory, and while the matter may not be entirely settled, a sizable body of research has demonstrated that resection of the hippocampal formation alone produces a significant memory deficit (Victor & Agamanolis, 1990; Zola-Morgan & Squire, 1986; Zola-Morgan, Squire, & Amaral, 1989). Lesions of the hippocampus and the amygdala, and of the cortex surrounding both these structures (the *perihippocampal* and *perirhinal* cortex) produce a more severe amnestic disorder (Zola-Morgan & Squire, 1990). Zola-Morgan and Squire argue that lesions of the amygdala itself do not contribute to a declarative memory deficit (although a damaged amygdala may affect other kinds of learning) but that the injury to the surrounding cortex exacerbates the problem.

Gaffan (1992) contended that data also support the importance of the fornix (a fiber bundle associated with the hippocampus) and the mammillary bodies (the termini of the fornix) for declarative memory, especially for recall of events. Other structures outside this network may be significant as well. These include the mediodorsal nucleus of the thalamus, which sends projections to the prefrontal cortex (Fuster, 1989; Gaffan & Murray, 1990).

DISSOCIABILITY OF ANTEROGRADE AND RETROGRADE AMNESIA

Ordinarily, amnestic persons demonstrate *anterograde* memory deficits. That is, they are unable to remember events and information that have occurred subsequent to the onset of their amnesia, although recall of events that occurred prior to the onset of amnesia remains intact (i.e., they have little or no *retrograde* amnesia). The converse phenomenon—significant retrograde amnesia with limited anterograde amnesia—is rather uncommon but has been documented in a few cases (e.g., by Kapur et al., 1996, and Markowitsch et al., 1993). The importance of these findings is that they demonstrate that the *acquisition* of declarative memories depends on different neural systems than those involved in *retrieval* of the same kind of memories.

An example of the dissociation of episodic and semantic memory was reported by Kapur and associates (1996), who discussed the case of a 20-year-old woman ("G.R.") who had sustained a severe head trauma in a car accident in 1977. Following the accident, she experienced approximately 6 months of posttraumatic (anterograde) amnesia. When examined in 1992, G.R. obtained Verbal, Performance (nonverbal), and Full Scale IQ scores on the Wechsler Adult Intelligence Scale—Revised (WAIS-R) of 91, 106, and 97, respectively. Her performance on memory tests of new learning suggested "a mild degree of impairment" but not severe amnesia.

Episodic memory was evaluated by means of a structured interview. This was preceded by an interview with G.R.'s mother during which the researchers obtained information on vacations, hospitalizations, job history, residences, education, family births and deaths, and weddings (Kapur et al., 1996). G.R. showed severe retrograde amnesia. For example, she could not remember having attended school, although she knew the names of schools she had attended (intact *personal semantic memory* in association with impaired episodic memory), having learned them from her family subsequent to the injury. She had no recall of a trip to Paris 5 years before the injury, nor did she recall travel in England (her home country) after that trip (but prior to the injury). She also could not remember two jobs she had held before beginning her university studies. In contrast, this young woman could remember many events that occurred following her injury in fairly clear detail (e.g., her brother's wedding, including the location of the reception, the weather that day, and so on). Procedurally learned motor skills acquired prior to the injury were preserved. She still could play the recorder, which she had learned at the age of 7 years, but could not recall having learned to play it (Kapur et al., 1996).

Kapur and colleagues (1996) presented the case of another individual, "S. P.," who showed similar severe impairment of retrograde episodic memory. S. P. was injured in 1992 in a motor vehicle accident at the age of 45. She could not recall meeting her husband or her marriage to him in 1972, nor could she recall the deaths of her brother and father (in 1982 and 1971). Unable to recall learning to drive, taking a driving test, or other events associated with driving, S. P. nevertheless was able to recall the registration numbers of several cars she had owned in the 5 years prior to her injury. Both G.R. and S. P. were found to have severe damage of the left temporal lobe (both the cortex and the underlying white matter), with smaller lesions of the right temporal lobe and relative sparing of the hippocampus.

The preservation of the hippocampus and associated medial temporal lobe structures probably accounts for the relatively intact ability to acquire new memories that is demonstrated by the cases just described. The hippocampus is not required for *retrieval* of declarative memories, nor is it the site where declarative memories are stored (Squire, 1987; Ungerleider, 1995). In most amnestic patients—who cannot recall new events and/or information—the hippocampus is affected more severely than in the cases discussed by Kapur et al. (1996), for whom the majority of the damage was to the lateral temporal *cortex*. This provides support for the proposal that the reactivation of a declarative memory is dependent on the integrity of those cortical areas involved in representing that memory, as well as of those leading to such activation (Alvarez & Squire, 1994; A. R. Damasio & H. Damasio, 1994; P. M. Milner, 1989). The above cases, along with other data, also strongly suggest that declarative memories are not stored in any specific site but are encoded in a distributed manner, by ensembles of neurons in different areas of the cortex.

Episodic and semantic memory systems may be differentially affected by lesions of the right or left hemisphere (Markowitsch, 1995). When the left hemisphere is the most severely injured, mnestic deficits primarily involve semantic memory. In contrast, right hemisphere injuries are more likely to impair the recall of episodic memories. Markowitsch linked the studies of brain-injured patients with studies of brain metabolism among normal subjects (Shallice et al., 1994; Tulving et al., 1994a, 1994b, 1994c).

In most of these cases, neurologically intact volunteers were examined using positron emission tomography (PET). Tulving and his associates proposed that the left hemisphere is involved in encoding *episodic* memories for storage and that the right hemisphere is involved in recall of those memories; in contrast, they argued that the left hemisphere is involved in recall of *semantic* memories.

These hypotheses regarding the lateralization of storage and retrieval processes in semantic and episodic memory have not received definitive support. In fact, Ungerleider (1995) referred to studies ostensibly demonstrating that "the left prefrontal cortex is commonly activated during encoding of information, and the right prefrontal cortex is activated during retrieval, regardless of whether the material is verbal or visual" (p. 773). Finally, there are data suggesting that different areas of the brain are activated during different types of retrieval: the medial parietal lobe apparently is active during episodic recall but not during retrieval of semantic memories (Ungerleider, 1995). Obviously, much remains to be done before this issue is settled. Still, even the complex and uncertain nature of the findings of research on this issue supports the concept of memory as a set of modular distributed systems.

Although there remains a good deal of controversy over the details, what is presently known about declarative memory strongly supports the hypothesis that it is distinct from "nondeclarative" (Squire 1992; Squire & Zola-Morgan, 1988) memory systems. Such distinctions may be identified at the levels of anatomy, process, and content. Moreover, semantic and episodic memory appear to be distinguishable from one another on the same grounds, as are the retrograde and anterograde aspects of both kinds of declarative memory. Therefore, memory is also usefully conceptualized as a set of systems and subsystems with a modular, distributed, hierarchical structure.

PROCEDURAL LEARNING: THE LEARNING OF PROCESSES

Declarative memory, as we have seen, has to do with the retention of events and information. Procedural learning, in contrast, has to do primarily with the learning of *processes*. These processes may be motor skills (e.g., gymnastics), perceptual abilities (e.g., visual pattern recognition), cognitive skills (e.g., solving mental arithmetic problems), cognitive-perceptual skills (e.g., reading), and more complex kinds of tasks (e.g., playing music or learning social and relational processes). Moreover, it has been argued that procedural learning is important in the development and maintenance of character (Grigsby & Hartlaub, 1994).

It should be noted that disagreement exists about what constitutes procedural learning. Some authors have construed the term narrowly, using it to refer only to the acquisition of motor skills, a definition that we believe is overly restrictive. Others have broadened the concept and even changed the terminology. Squire (1992) recently suggested that memories be classified as either declarative or nondeclarative, a distinction that seems to us to sacrifice specificity in the latter category; under this scheme, the term "everything else" could as well be substituted for nondeclarative memory.

Some investigators prefer to consider the declarative/procedural categories to be similar to (or a subset of) the classification of memories as either *explicit* or *implicit*. According to this dichotomy (D. L. Schachter, 1987, 1992), "explicit memory refers to intentional or conscious recollection of prior experiences, as assessed in the laboratory by traditional tests of recall or recognition," whereas implicit memory "refers to changes in performance or behavior that are produced by prior experiences on tests that do not require any intentional or conscious recollection of those experiences" (D. L. Schachter, 1992, p. 244). It is our intention to use the term *procedural learning* to refer to the learning of *processes*. These may range from simple habits through complex behavioral repertoires.

WHAT IS PROCEDURAL "KNOWLEDGE"?

N. J. Cohen (1984) described procedural knowledge as involving a memory system that does not permit access to knowledge per se (in contrast to declarative memory), and which does not allow the individual to convey one's accumulating experience verbally. Via procedural learning, "experience serves to influence the organization of processes that guide performance without access to the knowledge that underlies the performance" (N. J. Cohen, 1984, p. 96). Such processes may be learned independently of any content, and although some may be described in words, others are almost entirely unverbalizable.

Mishkin and his associates (1984) defined procedural learning as the retention of "habits," a phenomenon that may be observed in all animals. They hypothesized that habit memory is dependent upon connections between the cortex and basal ganglia (cf. Saint-Cyr & Taylor, 1992). Mishkin et al. noted that the putamen and caudate nucleus of the basal ganglia receive afferent fibers from most regions of the cortex. These in turn project to the globus pallidus and associated structures. The same authors suggested that "this system of projections therefore provides a mechanism through which cortically processed inputs could become associated with motor outputs generated in the pallidum and so yield the stimulus–response bonds that constitute habits" (1984, p. 74). Other data suggest that the cerebellum also may play a part in this type of learning (Glickstein & Yeo, 1990; Yeo et al., 1984). Certain kinds of procedural learning involve different task-specific neural regions as well. Learning to read, for example, presumably involves rather different neural processes than those involved in learning to hit a baseball or to solve square roots mentally.

Unlike the declarative memory system, the procedural system involves a relatively slow, incremental learning process. When a single powerful event is experienced (e.g., an attempt on one's life, or the bombing of Pearl Harbor or Hiroshima), it may be remembered for a lifetime. In contrast, it is impossible to become proficient at basketball by playing it only once. Rather, the development of any motor skill to a high level of proficiency typically requires months or years of intensive practice. The precise reason for the slowness of procedural learning in relation to declarative learning is unknown, but Nadel (1992) argues that "a long-term memory system containing distributed representations of many items cannot afford to undergo rapid changes in 'synaptic weights'—such rapid changes would destabilize the memory representations previously formed. Thus, in such a system incremental learning is essential. However, the information contained in an episode must be rapidly acquired somewhere in the system, if it is to have any impact at all" (p. 186). Therefore, procedurally learned behavior may be altered, albeit slowly, and it is relatively "resistant to decay" (Saint-Cyr & Taylor, 1992).

With repetition, performance of procedurally learned processes becomes increasingly automatic. Langer and Imber (1979) found that as activities become more automatic with practice, one loses one's ability to monitor those activities. Abilities such as writing, juggling, throwing a screwball, driving a car, and playing the organ all are instances of acquired procedural learning. In each case, the procedurally learned process may be dissociated from any declarative knowledge (as was true of Kapur and colleagues' case "G.R.," 1996, who could still play the recorder but had no recollection of having done so previously); however, in the neurologically intact human, procedurally learned skills or processes also may involve varying degrees of declarative knowledge. Studying music theory, for example, will not lead to the ability to play the cello, nor will practicing the piano by ear lead to knowledge of music theory. In most cases, however, the two go together, and declarative knowledge may be useful to a musician who is increasing his or her level of skill. Although the two memory systems are somewhat independent of one another, they normally function in concert, complementing one another. Markowitsch observed, regarding the complex interactions among memory systems, that "many memories are so complex—for example when composed of emotionally laden scenes or sequences of acts—that the final integrated recall will evolve from several different, distributed modules (or interdigitated neuronal nets widely distributed)" (1995, p. 120).

Not only does repetition of a task gradually improve one's ability to perform the task, it also is associated with changes in the precise regions of the brain involved in the performance of that task. For example, Seitz et al. (1990) taught normal volunteers to perform a sequence of 16 finger movements that involved touching the thumb sequentially to different fingers of the same hand. While performing this task, subjects underwent PET scanning. The results showed that during learning of the activity, prefrontal cortex was activated—a finding consistent with what is thought to be the role of this area in the performance of novel tasks, or of tasks that require deliberate conscious effort. Once Seitz and colleagues' subjects had learned the sequence, however, the locus of cerebral activation shifted from the prefrontal cortex to the motor cortex and basal ganglia—as might be expected in the performance of automatic and procedurally learned motor activities (Shallice, 1988). Ungerleider (1995) noted that the cerebellum, as well as the prefrontal cortex, may be activated during the conscious and effortful learning of motor tasks. Interestingly, a different pattern of shifting activation may be observed when people learn nonmotor skills (Raichle et al., 1994).

The dissociability of declarative and procedural learning, and the automaticity of well-learned procedural memories, both facilitate the efficient performance of many tasks. When an activity can be performed relatively effortlessly, without thinking about the process involved or referring to previously acquired factual knowledge, the activity can be carried out more quickly and efficiently. The evolutionary advantage conferred on animals through the acquisition of a capacity for procedural learning should be obvious. (The issue of automatic control and deliberate conscious control will be discussed in more detail in a later chapter on conscious and nonconscious functioning.)

BRAIN DEVELOPMENT AND THE MATURATION OF DIFFERENT MEMORY SYSTEMS

The roles of different memory systems in personality development are affected by the fact that many regions of the brain develop at different rates. For example, the prefrontal cortex of primates is rather slow to mature. Myelinization of neurons in the prefrontal cortex may take place over the first few years of life in monkeys (Goldman, 1976). In humans the process takes many years longer (Benes, 1989; Yakovlev & Lecours, 1967), and it has been estimated that full myelinization of the prefrontal cortex, ordinarily complete by the middle of the third decade, may continue even longer in some persons. Because the prefrontal cortex is important for certain aspects of memory, its delayed maturation may play an important role in changes in memory functioning over time (e.g., Diamond, 1991).

The timing of development of procedural and declarative learning demonstrates the relative independence of the declarative and procedural learning systems (Saint-Cyr & Taylor, 1992), and suggests that during the first few years of life personality development is more influenced by procedural learning than by episodic or semantic memory. For example, Bachevalier and Mishkin (1984) demonstrated that cortical areas important for declarative memory are immature at birth in the rhesus monkey and argued that learning is at first largely a function of the *habit* or procedural system. Other researchers have reported that the procedural and declarative learning systems develop at different rates in humans as well, and that the procedural system matures first (DiGiulio et al., 1994; Tulving, 1985).

To summarize, procedural learning involves the memory of processes that typically operate nonconsciously as important organizers of behavior. Procedural knowledge is acquired relatively slowly and incrementally, involving different processes and a different neural substrate than does declarative memory. The capacity for procedural recall develops prior to the episodic and semantic memory systems, a fact with considerable significance for personality theory. Grigsby and Hartlaub (1994) proposed that "character" may rely heavily on procedural learning. In addition, it seems likely that many of the basic patterns of attachment—and the social practices that identify individuals as belonging to one group or culture—are manifestations of procedural learning.

IMPLICIT MEMORY AND THE PHENOMENON OF PRIMING

We have defined procedural learning as the acquisition of processes and have emphasized that procedural learning typically operates more or less nonconsciously. Procedural learning often (but not always) is a type of *implicit memory*, a type of learning that occurs without awareness (D. L. Schachter, 1987, 1992). Another example of implicit memory is *priming*, which—like procedural learning—has been found to be intact even among persons like H. M. who have anterograde amnesia (Graf, Squire, & Mandler, 1984; Warrington & Weiskrantz, 1973).

Priming offers a compelling demonstration of nonconscious perception and learning. The phenomenon of priming can be demonstrated in the laboratory by determining whether prior experience with some unattended stimulus affects subsequent performance. For example, an amnestic patient might be presented with a list of words, then 5 minutes later asked to recall the words. Ordinarily the patient will remember few or none of them, and may not remember having heard the list in the first place. Later, however, recall may be cued by providing the patient with three-letter stems for the words from the list, and then asking the patient to say whatever word comes to mind in association with the cue. For example, the patient may have been presented with the words *forest, window,* and *mosquito,* among others. Later, she might be presented with the word stems *for, win,* and *mos,* and asked to name a word beginning with those letters. Although there are many words that begin with these stems, amnestic patients, at a level significantly better than chance, are liable to complete the stems by using the words presented previously despite the fact that they have no conscious recollection of having been exposed to those words. Priming effects can be demonstrated routinely in both neurologically intact individuals and those who are amnestic, in response to stimuli of which the subject may be either conscious or unconscious at the time of presentation. Since priming is exhibited in amnestic patients, it must not involve the hippocampal system. We will return to priming later, in Chapter 12 on conscious and nonconscious processing.

EMOTIONAL MEMORIES

Although our knowledge of the system mediating emotional memory is somewhat limited, considerable data exist regarding a form of memory associated with events that are physically or emotionally painful. Conditioned fear is one such emotional memory. As LeDoux and his colleagues have demonstrated, the conditioning of fear responses to both auditory and visual stimuli is mediated by subcortical pathways projecting from the sensory nuclei of the thalamus to the amygdala, a structure located deep in each anterior temporal lobe (LeDoux, 1995; LeDoux, Sakaguchi, & Reis, 1984; LeDoux et al., 1986, 1988; LeDoux, Romanski, & Xagoraris, 1989). LeDoux et al. (1989) noted that "this circuit bypasses the . . . cortex and thus constitutes a subcortical mechanism of emotional learning" (p. 238). In contrast, the amygdala seems to play no significant role in most declarative memory processes.

LeDoux and his associates (1989) surgically removed the visual cortex of rats, then assigned them to one of two conditions: (1) conditioning involving a visual stimulus (a flashing light) in association with an electric shock, or (2) random presentation of the lights and shock. The lesioned rats then were compared with rats who had undergone sham surgery (in which a portion of the skull was removed but the brain was not lesioned) and who experienced one of the two learning protocols. Both lesioned and sham surgery animals acquired the classically conditioned response, demonstrating fear when the light began to flash. Rats assigned to the groups with random occurrence of lights and shocks showed no such learning. The results supported the hypothesis that visual cortex is unnecessary for this kind of conditioned learning.

In the same study, after the animals had acquired this conditioned response of fear associated with a flashing light, the experimenters attempted to extinguish it. Though they continued to present the lights at intervals, the lights no longer were paired with electric shocks. Extinction did not occur for the lesioned animals, whereas the sham surgery rats showed a decrement in the learned fear response. In other words, "in the absence of the visual cortex, fear responses to visual stimuli persisted in the face of unreinforced presentations of the [conditioned stimulus] long after the responses began to extinguish in sham operated animals" (LeDoux et al., 1989, p. 241). These results suggest that the cortex, while unnecessary for the initial learning, *is* necessary for disruption of the fear response. In essence, this means that fear conditioning may be acquired without consciousness (since the subcortical pathway involved here presumably operates outside awareness); however, without consciousness it may not be possible to reduce a conditioned fear response.

The extinction of the fear response that occurred among the nonlesioned animals is interesting in itself and merits further comment. Ivan P. Pavlov (1927) was the first of many to demonstrate that extinguished responses may later recur for no obvious reason. Moreover, even reexposure to the unconditioned stimulus (such as electric shock) by itself may cause an experimental animal once again to become fearful of the conditioned stimulus (W. J. Jacobs & Nadel, 1985; Rescorla & Heth, 1975). This observation suggests that the neural pathways activated by the initial conditioning experience remain intact, retaining their ability to evoke the conditioned response even though extinction may occur over time. The strength of the synaptic connections in these pathways thus may change as a result of experience (e.g., absence of foot shock), but the neural networks do not themselves dissolve or disappear in the course of extinction. Although perhaps inhibited, they are capable of reactivation in certain circumstances. This finding has important implications for change and for the limits of change, subjects which are addressed in Chapter 17.

The conditioning of fear in association with otherwise neutral stimuli has been studied in other contexts. For example, M. Davis (1992a) used what is called the "fear-potentiated startle paradigm." Rats first were conditioned to experience fear at the presentation of a conditioned stimulus (e.g., a flashing light) by pairing the stimulus with a shock applied to the foot. After conditioning was completed, the rats displayed a stronger startle response to acoustic stimuli when the light was flashing than when it was not, since the perception of the light induced a state of fear. For these animals, the time required from the presentation of a startling acoustic stimulus until the startle response is ordinarily 6–8 milliseconds (Ison, McAdam, & Hammond, 1973)—too little time for any cortical activity to be involved in the startle reflex. Therefore, Davis and his associates suggested that the reflex is mediated by several brainstem structures and motor neurons in the spinal cord (Cassella & Davis, 1986).

M. Davis (1992b) also found that electrical stimulation of the amygdala (which may induce fear) enhances the startle reflex, whereas lesions of the amygdala can completely block fear-potentiated startle. The effects of electrical stimulation of the amygdala on startle behavior illustrate the importance of the animal's state in determining its behavior. In this case, the state is in part a function of activity in the amygdala. Although we might infer that the stimulated animal experiences fear, the *awareness* of fear is unnecessary in producing the behavior. The entire neural basis for this reaction occurs at a subcortical level, outside of awareness. The stimulation of the amygdala in effect tunes the nervous system in such a way that the intensity of the startle response is magnified, and it is likely that this phenomenon would occur regardless of whether the animal was aware of feeling afraid.

McGaugh and his collaborators studied the role of the amygdala in emotional learning, examining the effects of *neuromodulators* on the consolidation of emotional memory in laboratory animals (McGaugh, 1990; McGaugh et al., 1993). Neuromodulators are substances that affect the functioning of neurons without necessarily directly acting as neurotransmitters themselves. Opioids, for example, demonstrate neuromodulatory effects in certain pathways, affecting the probability of synaptic transmission in certain pathways. The same holds true for norepinephrine, which produces CNS arousal as one of its effects. When released by the adrenal medulla, norepinephrine acts on the sympathetic nervous system to produce arousal. By way of the vagus nerve, sympathetic nerve fibers stimulate release of norepinephrine within the amygdala.

McGaugh and his colleagues (McGaugh, 1990; McGaugh et al., 1993) found that norepinephrine administered at or near the time of learning (electrical foot-shock conditioning) facilitates learning of the conditioned–unconditioned stimulus pair and enhances the durability of the conditioned response. This effect suggested that arousal (as is likely to occur in many traumatic situations) may lead to more powerful learning and raised the question of whether norepinephrine antagonists acting in the amygdala might have the opposite effect. McGaugh and his colleagues found that in fact the beta-adrenergic antagonist *propanolol* inhibited avoidance learning when administered within about an hour of the training session. This led these authors to suggest that the administration of propanolol to humans who have experienced acute trauma might prevent the development of posttraumatic stress disorder (PTSD).

Other research indicates that the development of the amygdala/emotional memory system is independent of development of the hippocampal (declarative) memory system and occurs prior to it. Rudy and Morledge (1994) found that rats are able to learn tasks that require the amygdala but not the hippocampus at a younger age than they can learn tasks requiring the hippocampus but not the amygdala. These authors suggested that a similar lag in development of the hippocampus relative to the amygdala may account for such phenomena in humans as infantile amnesia. According to their argument, conditioned fear responses might be learned prior to the time a young child is able to consolidate long-lasting episodic memories (which are presumed to require hippocampal involvement).

As noted earlier, the capacity for procedural learning also appears to develop prior to the capacity for declarative learning. This means that templates for habitual behaviors may be acquired, and the behaviors may become relatively automatic and routine, before the child has an episodic memory system capable of remembering the events that produced these behaviors. In situations involving both fear conditioning and procedural learning, very young children are likely to experience a kind of learning (habits, conditioned responses) that is dissociated from the context. In other words, it may be impossible to recall—at least under ordinary circumstances—the events that led to the acquisition of certain types of behavior.

OTHER KINDS OF CONDITIONING

Other kinds of conditioning also may occur independently of declarative memory (Weiskrantz & Warrington, 1979). One common paradigm for such conditioning involves pairing a neutral conditioned stimulus (e.g., a sound) with an unpleasant unconditioned stimulus (e.g., a brief puff of air directed at the eye). Over the course of a number of trials, individuals exposed to this experimental manipulation develop a conditioned blinking response at the presentation of the sound in order to avoid an unpleasant and intrusive puff of air. Weiskrantz and Warrington showed that this reflexive behavior, which is dependent on the involvement of the cerebellum (Yeo et al., 1984), could be acquired by amnestic human patients, again without cortical involvement.

MEMORIES OF PAIN

Memories of pain appear to rely on a somewhat different neural foundation than do the kinds of memory discussed so far, and a number of studies point to the role of the thalamus in mediating memories of pain. Some of these findings have come from the use of stereotactic thalamotomy with human patients. This is a neurosurgical procedure sometimes used for the treatment of persons with a serious, medically intractable involuntary movement disorder. The patient is fully conscious during this procedure, which is performed using a local anesthetic while the surgeon uses a stereotactically guided microelectrode to stimulate discrete areas of the thalamus with electrical current prior to making therapeutic lesions.

In a series of papers, Lenz and his associates (Lenz et al., 1993a, 1993b, 1994, 1995) reported finding that neurons in the ventrocaudal nucleus of the thalamus respond to painful stimulation and that when they are stimulated directly they also may produce sensations of pain. One such patient discussed by Lenz et al. (1995) was a 36-year-old man with a long history of panic disorder, undergoing thalamotomy for treatment of severe essential tremor. During panic attacks, this patient typically experienced unpleasant, severe, atypical chest pain. In the course of thalamotomy, electrical stimulation of an area just posterior to the ventrocaudal nucleus induced pain which the patient experienced as almost indistinguishable from what he felt during his panic attacks. This pain occurred within 1 second of application of the current and lasted for the duration of stimulation. On a scale intended to measure "unpleasantness," ranging from 0 ("no pain at all") through 10 ("most unpleasant sensation imaginable"), the patient rated each stimulation that produced this chest pain as a 10. The experience of pain in each case was associated with a very strong emotional response. Having ruled out the possibility that the patient was experiencing cardiogenic angina, Lenz and his colleagues concluded that thalamic stimulation had activated a circuit mediating a memory of spontaneous chest pain associated with a powerful emotional reaction.

Similarly, K. D. Davis and associates (1995) reported their work with a patient who, in response to thalamic stimulation, experienced severe pain associated with labor and delivery. In this case as well, a very strong affective coloring to the pain was present. While it is not unusual for an unpleasant emotional reaction to be associated with pain, the two do not necessarily coincide. Lenz et al. (1995) reported that among other patients "stimulation-associated pain with a strong affective dimension never occurred in patients who had no previous experience of spontaneous pain with a strong affective component" (p. 912).

An interesting aspect of this research is that the patients experienced their pain as though it were occurring in the present. As such, this was not a memory of the sort that might cause a person to say, "this reminds me of how I felt during labor and delivery," but rather, "I feel as though I am having a baby at this very moment." Also of interest is the fact that experiences such as these ordinarily appear to be inaccessible to consciousness. Nevertheless, during the surgical procedure, repeated stimulation of the same regions reliably produced the same sensations.

The representation of such a painful experience itself presumably is stored in a distributed network involving cortical sites (the somatosensory cortex, the secondary somatosensory cortex, the inferior parietal lobule, the anterior insular cortex, the cingulate gyrus, and possibly other areas) as well as subcortical ones, including the thalamus (Lenz et al., 1995). Thus far, it appears that only thalamic stimulation will produce these very dramatic experiences of pain; stimulation of the somatosensory cortex produces a variety of sensations, but pain is not among them.

THE WORKING MEMORY SYSTEM

The final memory system we discuss in this chapter is *working memory*. Working memory is composed of a set of processes or capacities that provide a medium for the contents of consciousness. It allows us to keep track of what is going on at any given moment, binding the present instant with the moment just past and with our intentions for the immediate future. The theory of working memory (Baddeley, 1986, 1992) has become the most widely accepted conceptual framework for understanding short-term memory.

As with the other memory systems discussed so far, working memory is thought to be a modular distributed system. According to this model, short-term memory involves a central processing system (what Baddeley termed the *central executive*) and several *slave systems,* or modality-specific sensory input *buffers* ("buffer," a term borrowed from computer science, in this case refers to a system specialized for short-term storage of information). Baddeley identified two such buffers: the *visuospatial sketchpad,* and the *phonological short-term store.* The former handles visual information and appears to comprise subcomponents that deal with (1) the appearance of visual stimuli and (2) their location in space (Baddeley, 1992; Mecklinger & Müller, 1996). The phonological buffer comprises two subcomponents: a passive aspect that retains the traces of verbal information one has just heard, and a more active *articulatory loop.* This articulatory loop refers essentially to one's ability to talk to oneself internally and may be thought of as *inner speech* (Vygostky, 1934/1986). Each of these subsystems itself is likely to have a modular structure.

To understand the distinction between the two phonological systems, let us consider performance on a free recall test of memory. Assume that you are asked to listen to and to repeat a list of 15 unrelated concrete nouns presented at the rate of one per second. As the examiner begins to read the list aloud, you are able to rehearse the first few words actively, repeating them silently to yourself ("ointment–ungulate–infundibulum–obstreperousness"). By about the fifth word, it becomes impossible to repeat the entire list with each addition of a new word, so you begin to try just to listen to the words. As the examiner finishes, you can almost hear the last few words in your mind.

According to Baddeley's theory of working memory, during the first part of the list you were using your articulatory loop to rehearse the words actively. By the end of the list, your passive short-term store was maintaining the sound of the last three or four words. These two subsystems are responsible, respectively, for the *primacy* and *recency* effects noted in memory research. That is, we tend to remember the first (primacy) and the last (recency) words from a long list but not those in the middle.

There are other sensory buffers for the working memory system, but these were not part of Baddeley's original model, and they have not been studied in detail. For example, olfaction, touch, position sense, and nonverbal auditory stimuli all presumably are served by relatively discrete subsystems. These working memory buffers are the systems responsible for representation of all perceptual input and imagery for each sensory modality—that is (in simplified form), the visual cortex, the auditory cortex, and so on. The individual sensory buffers ordinarily function in concert, and neuroscientists must devise clever means of separating them in order to test the integrity of specific subsystems.

SUMMARY AND CONCLUSION

A full appreciation of the phenomenon of multiple memory systems can shed interesting and clinically useful light on a number of aspects of personality functioning. Some of the implications of the modularity of memory for understanding personality are developed further in later chapters. For example, we explore the hypothesis that character—which is composed of those things that people do routinely, automatically, and nonconsciously, and which make us knowable and predictable—can be understood as a manifestation of procedural learning. If character emerges from procedural learning, some of the well-known difficulties associated with psychotherapeutic efforts to modify character might be conceptualized more clearly and perhaps come to be addressed from a more enlightened perspective. The limited success in treating character reported by most approaches to psychotherapy probably reflects ignorance of the memory system responsible for its development and maintenance. We believe that the model we propose can facilitate our understanding of the nature of character and hence lead to effective approaches to character change.

Understanding the existence, nature, and interaction of multiple memory systems offers some new ways of describing and comprehending certain paradoxical human behavior. For example, the theory of procedural learning provides a way of conceptualizing the processes involved in the acquisition of habits of all kinds, and of typical modes of interpersonal interaction in particular. Many of the fundamental "rules" of interpersonal participation and interaction are discerned implicitly early in life, and become organized and expressed behaviorally through the operation of procedural learning. Many of the other interpersonal processes and social practices one acquires during maturation also are likely to operate on such an automatic, nonconscious level. Although awareness may have been associated with the initial learning of such interpersonal processes, once they have become procedurally learned, conscious awareness is no longer needed. Elsewhere (Grigsby & Stevens, 2000) we discuss interpersonal relationships from the perspective of multiple memory systems, examining relationships in general, as well as issues related to transference and countertransference.

The limited capacity of working memory necessitates that the vast majority of information processing at any given time must occur non-consciously. Awareness of all the sensory and other types of data required for even the most mundane tasks would place excessive demands on the brain and on consciousness. Thus, procedural learning may represent one of the brain's strategies for meeting the emerging demands of adaptive behavior without overburdening working memory. As we saw in Chapter 4, the majority of the tasks required of the brain are farmed out to a large number of specialized, distributed subsystems for automatic processing. The importance of the functioning of these multiple memory systems is clarified when we consider the extremely limited, albeit critical, role of consciousness in relation to human behavior.

Finally, the existence of multiple memory systems may illuminate certain types of psychopathology. For example, PTSD is noteworthy in large part because of the importance of memory in the syndrome. Most theorists and practitioners have been especially impressed by the often sensational nature of vivid posttraumatic episodic memories, but classical conditioning has been identified as playing an important role as well, with conditioned hyperarousal (Kolb, 1984; Kolb & Mutalipassi, 1982) and emotional memories of the type discussed by LeDoux and his collaborators. PTSD clearly involves the concerted activity of multiple memory systems; thus an effective approach to therapy should involve a deeper understanding of the dynamics and interrelationships of these systems.

6

DYNAMICS

INTRODUCTION

The pressures of natural selection produced human beings characterized by the capacity to adapt to widely divergent, endlessly shifting environmental demands. These adaptations required the extremely intricate, ongoing synchronization of diverse processes. Earlier, we discussed the brain's modular architecture, a kind of organization that is associated with a very plastic, self-organizing capacity. In this chapter we begin by following the lead of the increasingly numerous scientists in many fields who are interested in *dynamics* as a way to describe the relationships between processes that generate complex phenomena and to understand the behavior of complex systems. For many years, classical dynamics dealt primarily with relatively simple physical and chemical systems. More recently, the dynamics of complex biological, economic, social, and psychological processes have become the focus of considerable research.

The French mathematician, Poincaré (1905/1952), argued that the objective of science is to understand the relationships among things, and not simply the individual things themselves. Hence we have the study of *dynamics*, which focuses on the processes that take place within and among the components of a system, placing process on an equal footing with the nature and structure of the components themselves. Dynamics is concerned with *change* and with the order that characterizes physical and chemical *processes*. Because our model emphasizes processes at different levels of abstraction, and because many of the ideas of dynamics also provide us with a way of describing some of the fundamental principles of neural and psychological activity, we discuss several basic ideas of dynamics in this chapter.

While it is obviously important to understand the structure of the brain, it is essential not to give short shrift to the *processes* by which those structures interact with one another, with other organ systems, and with the environment. From the vantage point of dynamics, biological structures become important especially insofar as the nature of their organization establishes potentialities and constraints on the activities of a system. The hippocampus, for example, seems to be necessary for consolidation of new memories. It is able to perform this role in part because of its unique pattern of afferent and efferent connections. So while the hippocampus as a structure is essential in the acquisition of memory, it functions through its involvement in an ongoing set of dynamic relationships and processes with many other regions of the brain. Dynamics offers us a way to understand these processes and the relationships between them.

In the present context, dynamics refers to processes and phenomena that are more fundamental than what usually is intended by the term *psychodynamics*. (The latter may be interpreted broadly as the role of unconscious motivation in behavior.) When applied to neuroscience, dynamics focuses on spatiotemporal patterns of neural activity at levels of analysis ranging from the subcomponents of cells (e.g., receptor sites, ion channels, or mitochondria) through the brain as a whole. We are especially interested in complex patterns of brain activity organized at the neurophysiological level (and including transactions with the environment), from which emerge human personality and psychology. In later chapters, we argue that *personality* is most accurately conceptualized as reflecting *nothing but* processes—a set of emergent properties associated with the brain's self-organizing activity. Mind and behavior are the emergent properties of self-organizing processes operating in the here and now, on the edge of chaos. They are not a set of structures.

Describing how the brain organizes itself in its ongoing process of adapting to environmental circumstances requires a dynamic perspective. Only by studying its dynamics is it possible to begin to understand how the nervous system might produce psychological activity. On the psychological level, most cognition and behavior involves the activation of various patterns of processes, so that here, too, processes represent elemental units of description.

An emphasis on process is not a new idea in psychology (James, 1890; Werner, 1937) or in neuropsychology (Goldstein, 1939, 1942; Goodglass & Kaplan, 1972; Kaplan, 1983; Luria, 1966, 1976, 1980), but with certain noteworthy exceptions it has not been applied systematically to the neuroscientific study of personality. A model based on the observation of processes offers a very useful approach to the way questions about personality are formulated and researched (Grigsby & Schneiders, 1991; Grigsby et al., 1991).

Below we introduce some basic concepts from dynamics, which, as we have noted, is concerned principally with describing the emergent order that characterizes various kinds of processes. Most natural processes tend to form regular patterns and may be characterized by the way in which they occur across time. Thus, some processes appear to be random, whereas others are periodic, quasi-periodic, or simply recurrent. We discuss below how the activity of a dynamic system can be described mathematically and how its functioning can be classified into patterns known as *attractors* and *repellors,* concepts useful in describing both neural and behavioral activity.

The language of neural dynamics is in large part a language of probabilities. Because dynamics is concerned principally with change and with the order that characterizes various kinds of processes, the language of dynamics can be understood as a way of discussing the probabilities associated with the occurrence or outcome of certain processes. At the level of personality and behavior, the study of dynamics can help to organize our observations about the conditions that facilitate change.

We intend to address what it means when certain kinds of systems are said to operate "on the edge of chaos," in "far-from-equilibrium conditions," or in states of "self-organized criticality." In essence, these expressions mean that the activity of any complex system reflects a delicate balance between repetitive, stereotyped activity and a tendency to engage in rather different, orderly, and yet sometimes apparently random and basically unpredictable activity ("deterministic chaos"). Such a balance permits maintenance of adaptive functioning in stable environments, as well as the capacity to adapt to changed or novel conditions. Adaptive functioning is enhanced—and perhaps even made possible—by operating on the edge of chaos. But we also discuss *fluctuations* and *bifurcations,* and the idea of a *phase portrait,* which provides a useful heuristic for conceptualizing the activity of nonlinear systems.

One important aspect of biological systems is the way in which they are conservative in their use of energy and unique in their relationship to entropy. Entropy, a fundamental characteristic of all matter, refers to the tendency of systems to become progressively more disorganized over time. Entropy in biological systems differs from entropy in nonorganic systems in that organisms use energy in such a way that they temporarily maintain order in the face of disorganization. When an organism dies, the rate of change in the system associated with entropy is markedly accelerated and the organism decays.

Organisms, efficient in their use of energy resources, minimize energy expenditure and take the path of least resistance in their functioning. Biological systems thus are able to operate with low levels of energy input from the outside. The propensity of organisms to minimize energy use is important in the context of the probabilistic functioning of neural networks, since those networks with the greatest probability of activation in any given situation are those most likely to become active. Changes in the state of the organism (e.g., such factors as emotional state or the general activity level) may affect these probabilities significantly. We close the chapter by noting some of the ways that an understanding of dynamics is relevant to an understanding of the processes associated with psychological emergence.

PERIODICITY, QUASI-PERIODICITY, RANDOMNESS, AND CHAOS

Things change over time. The nature of those changes and the intervals over which they occur are relatively enduring characteristics of the activity of a system. Certain configurations of the nervous system, such as death, or seizures induced by exposure to certain toxins, may occur only once no matter how long one observes that system. In contrast, some epileptic disorders involve the repeated occurrence of stereotyped seizures irrespective of whether someone ingests a poison. Other systems, like the swinging of a clock pendulum, certain patterns of brain wave activity, or phases of the sleep–wake cycle, recur more or less regularly and predictably. Such processes may be described using a number of basic concepts from the theory of dynamics.

Periodicity

In some clocks, the movement of a pendulum drives the gears that control movement of the clock's hands. Tension on the mainspring, maintained by winding the clock, provides the force that keeps the pendulum swinging. Ideally, the frequency (the number of swings in a given period of time) and amplitude (the distance through which the pendulum moves) of the clock-driven pendulum remain constant, so the clock will accurately keep time. Because of the force supplied by the mainspring, the pendulum returns to approximately the same point at the end of each sweep from side to side (i.e., the amplitude remains constant). If you trace the path of a clock-driven pendulum through time, assuming that you always wind the clock regularly, you could describe the movement of the pendulum as *periodic*. In other words, the pendulum oscillates at a regular rate, completing the same number of oscillations in a given period of time.

In the case of a free-swinging pendulum—to which no external force (such as that of the mainspring) is applied—the forces of gravity and friction (owing to air resistance and friction at the point of attachment of the pendulum to its swivel) eventually act conjointly to bring the pendulum to rest. If the path of a free-swinging pendulum is traced, the amplitude of each swing is found to be smaller than that of the previous swing—

eventually bringing the bob at the end of the pendulum to rest at the lowest point on its path.

Attractors

The general behavior of each of these types of system is predictable; each tends to follow a regular routine. When a system demonstrates a tendency to fall into such routine behavior, the pattern characterizing that behavior may be referred to as an *attractor*. It is as though the physical systems were attracted consistently to a specific pattern of activity: periodic oscillation for the clock-driven pendulum, and a state of rest for the free-swinging pendulum. Both these systems represent *stable* attractors, irrespective of starting conditions. Given sufficient time, each system will settle into its own specific attractor. Moreover, if either of these systems is perturbed in some way (e.g., by an extra force applied to the swinging pendulum), it will relatively quickly return to this stable attractor. In other words, the clock-driven pendulum will recover so that the force applied by the mainspring continually counteracts gravity and friction, whereas the free-swinging pendulum eventually will stop swinging altogether.

The activity of the clock-driven pendulum is characteristic of what is called a *periodic attractor* or *limit cycle attractor*. After such a regular system has run for a while, the probability is very high that its behavior will have evolved to a state that is regular and predictable. The activity of the free-swinging pendulum is characteristic of what is called a *point attractor*, which represents the behavior of a system at static equilibrium (a concept illustrated in Figure 6.1, discussed below). For both point and limit cycle attractors, every possible starting point for the system will, with time, evolve to the attractor (Abraham & Shaw, 1992). That is, *the attractor is invariant with respect to the initial conditions of the system.* No matter where it starts, the system will always end up in the same attractor.

Figure 6.1 provides an illustration of point and limit cycle attractors. In Figure 6.1A, the dominant attractor of the system is always static equilibrium at a single point. Unless energy is added continually to the system, the system will *always* end up at that point, regardless of the starting conditions. In Figure 6.1B, the attractor of our hypothetical system is always precisely the same path, with the same amplitude and frequency.

Chaotic Systems

A third type of attractor is known as a *chaotic* or *strange attractor*. Behavior characterized by a strange attractor may appear to be regular or may appear essentially random (depending in part on how it is viewed), but in either case its behavior remains essentially unpredictable. Since chaotic systems are extremely sensitive to changes in even seemingly trivial environ-

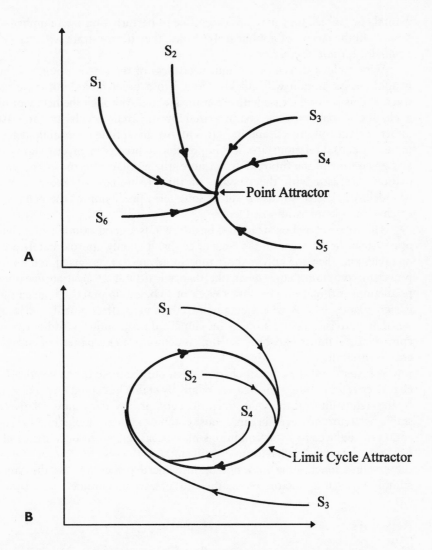

FIGURE 6.1. (A) Point attractor. The single point at the center of convergence of the surrounding six paths is the attractor. For a system with a point attractor, regardless of the starting conditions (S_1 through S_6), the system will always end up at the same point. This would be the case, for example, with a free-swinging pendulum. No matter what the amplitude or frequency is initially, gravity and friction will bring the pendulum bob to rest—the point attractor. (B) Limit cycle (periodic) attractor. The ellipse is the attractor in this case, while the other curves show paths with different starting conditions that all settle into the limit cycle attractor. For a system with a limit cycle attractor, regardless of the starting conditions (S_1 through S_4), the system will always end up in the same periodic pattern. This would be the case, for example, with a clock-driven pendulum. As long as the clock is wound, no matter from what position (or with what force) one starts the pendulum swinging, it will quickly settle into a pattern with constant amplitude and frequency.

mental conditions, they may be susceptible to perturbation by a number of factors. In the jargon of nonlinear dynamics, they demonstrate *sensitive dependence on initial conditions.*

With a clock-driven pendulum, regardless of the starting point of the pendulum, its motion will quickly settle into a predictable limit cycle attractor. This is not the case with a chaotic system. Although the behavior of a chaotic system may be characterized by apparent regularity (at least under certain conditions) and its status at any given time is certainly determined by causal relationships, it is impossible to predict its precise status at any given time in the future. Furthermore, the amount of error in any prediction increases with the passage of time (Abraham & Shaw, 1992; Mandelbrot, 1982), so that accurate long-term prediction of the behavior of chaotic systems is impossible.

The weather, as Lorenz (1963) has shown, is a good example of a chaotic system, or a system on the edge of chaos. It is only approximately predictable, and then for only a short time in advance. Even given extremely powerful computing equipment, the theoretical limit of accurate weather predictions is thought to be only a week or two, and in practice it generally is significantly less. A wide range of variables may affect global and local weather patterns. For example, the climate during summer ordinarily is consistently summer-like, but over time it demonstrates a pattern of considerable variability.

A system "on the edge of chaos," as in our example of the weather, is characterized by conditions that are relatively stable but could be perturbed by the right stimuli at the right time. Most complex systems show relatively stable behavior; however, because most complex systems are highly nonlinear, even slight changes in conditions may occasionally produce major effects on the system's behavior in certain states of the system. At other times the system's functioning may not be influenced perceptibly by the same stimuli, or even by factors of significantly greater magnitude.

Repellors

The converse of an attractor is a *repellor.* While an attractor can be conceptualized as a state of relatively stable functioning (and to anthropomorphize a bit, one might say that the system finds that state attractive), a repellor is a highly unstable configuration of the system. One might say that the system avoids the kinds of activity characteristic of a repellor. The rings of Saturn provide an interesting example of attractors and repellors working together. Saturn has several rings composed of orbiting particles ranging in size from microscopic dust through massive boulders. Separating the various rings are gaps in which few such objects are found. For the most part, these gaps remain relatively stable over time and may be considered repellors. Because of gravitational interactions among Saturn, its rings, and its moons, the particles that compose the rings do not find these attractive places in which to orbit the planet; instead, they are attracted to those regions in which ring material is found. Because of gravitational resonance effects, the spaces between rings represent highly unstable orbits, and thus few objects are found there. This means that there is no ring structure per se and no agent dictating the positions of the particles that compose the rings. When one looks at images of the rings from a distance, they appear to be solid. In contrast, viewed close-up the individual objects composing the rings clearly are separate from one another and in fact move around within the rings in relation to one another. The rings spontaneously organize themselves.

The concept of a repellor is illustrated schematically in Figure 6.2. Here we see a pair of two-dimensional attractors (a_1 and a_2) separated by a repellor (r_1). A ball placed at precisely the highest point of the repellor (a point known as a *separatrix*) could roll into the basin of either attractor. The direction of its movement may be unpredictable, but it reflects microscopic deterministic processes of various kinds. For example, the microscopic structure even of a ball bearing that has been smoothed to an extremely fine tolerance shows striking nonuniformities that could bias the direction of motion. There also may be slight variations in air currents in

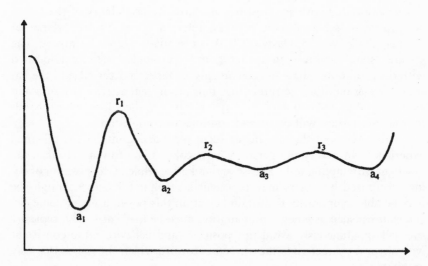

FIGURE 6.2. Schematic illustration of attractors and repellors. Attractors are labeled a_1 through a_4, and repellors r_1 through r_3. Attractor a_1 has a deep basin of attraction, and hence there is a high-energy barrier at the *separatrix* (repellor r_1) that stands between attractors a_1 and a_2. Repellor r_1 represents a very unstable state relative to repellor r_3. As a process moves back and forth between attractors a_3 and a_4, it will pass through r_3, which is likely to be manifested less transiently than is repellor r_1. Attractors a_3 and a_4 both have shallow basins of attraction and are likely to be less stable across time than is either attractor a_2 or a_1.

the room, produced perhaps by slight inhomogeneities in the distribution of heat (which itself reflects the average speed of movement of air molecules in a given region of space). In any event, with a great deal of effort, one might balance the ball at the separatrix, but its placement would be unstable, so that even slight undetectable perturbations of the system (perhaps even the rotation of the earth, assuming all others could be controlled) might cause the ball to roll into one or the other attractors. Once the ball has started to move in one or the other direction, it is said to have fallen into a particular *basin of attraction.*

As a general rule, attractors lie at relative energy minima. In the same way, neural processing tends to favor "relaxed" states involving lower-energy configurations (Abeles, 1991). Therefore, neural networks that involve high levels of energy (that have the lowest probability of occurrence) are inherently unstable and may be thought of as repellors. The time course of very high-energy networks ordinarily is short lived, since neural activity tends to be drawn into surrounding energy "valleys," which are more stable lower-energy basins of attraction in the *phase space* (discussed below).

Repellors and basins of attraction are useful concepts for describing certain physiological (and psychological) phenomena. For example, it appears likely that the nervous system sometimes may "learn" to have seizures. That is, the repeated occurrence of the synchronous neuronal discharge associated with seizures may increase the probability of the future occurrence of seizures. This process, referred to as *kindling* (Pinel & Rovner, 1978; Wada & Osawa, 1976), is essentially a kind of learning. The seizure "state" becomes an attractor, and neurological activity associated with the prodromal phase of such an episode represents the edge of the basin of attraction of the seizure. Once that prodromal activity (an aura and associated neural phenomena, perhaps) has begun, there is a high probability that the seizure will begin and continue to completion.

Other states of the system represent repellors. Consider the dilemma experienced by a very shy person who is called upon to put herself in the limelight. Attempting to be at ease and talkative while in the position of being scrutinized by others may represent a repellor for her. Although she may be able temporarily to sustain herself in this position under some circumstances (such as when a presentation must be made at work), typically she will spontaneously avoid this position, and behavior more consistent with shyness characterizes the attractors toward which she nonconsciously gravitates.

Nonlinear Systems and Unpredictability

In general, complex systems are inherently *nonlinear* in character. Both conceptual and mathematical ways of discriminating linear from nonlinear systems exist, but here we will focus primarily on the former. According to

Langton (1988), linear systems "are those for which the behavior of the whole is just the sum of the behavior of its parts, while for *nonlinear systems,* the behavior of the whole is *more* than the sum of its parts" (p. 41; emphasis in original). While the various subcomponents of a linear system may be analyzed independently and their contribution to the operation of the whole thus may be understood, this is not the case for nonlinear systems. Again, according to Langton (1988), "the key feature of nonlinear systems is that their primary behaviors of interest are properties of the *interactions between parts,* rather than being properties of the parts themselves, and these interaction-based properties necessarily disappear when the parts are studied independently" (p. 41; emphasis in original).

Although they may demonstrate regular, relatively predictable behavior across a range of conditions, nonlinear systems at times demonstrate discontinuities and abrupt shifts in functioning (bifurcations) that cannot possibly be predicted a priori. Despite the fact that such changes in activity are not predictable, they nonetheless are deterministic—they are the products of complex transactions within and between systems.

Chemical Equilibrium

The concept of equilibrium is essential for an understanding of nonlinear, self-organizing systems. Because equilibrium is primarily a physicochemical phenomenon, thermal equilibrium and chemical reactions may serve as a useful means of illustrating this issue. For example, in a simple acid–base reaction such as the addition of aqueous acetic acid (CH_3COOH) to water, a molecule of acetic acid loses one hydrogen ion (i.e., it gives up a proton without an accompanying electron). This proton is accepted by a molecule of water (H_2O) to form what is called a hydronium ion (H_3O^+). The molecule of acetic acid, having lost a proton (the hydrogen), is transformed into an acetate ion (CH_3COO^-).

The reaction products are not fixed and immutable. Instead, each of the products has a certain probability of being converted back into the original reactants. As the reaction progresses in time, the forward reaction rate slows down while the reverse reaction rate accelerates. Eventually, the two rates become equal and equilibrium is established. Thus, at equilibrium the reaction goes both ways. That is, once the acetic acid has had time to establish an equilibrium with the water, roughly as much of the two ions is converted into water and acetic acid as acid and water are converted into hydronium and acetate ions.

At that point, the mixture is in a state of dynamic equilibrium, characterized by continuing chemical activity in which roughly equal numbers of molecules are converted either from reactants into products or from products into reactants. Consequently, although from the outside it appears that little is going on in the solution, the ratio of reactants to products in the solution does not remain precisely constant but fluctuates. Because chemical reactions, over time, tend to evolve toward such a state, Prigogine and Stengers (1984) describe chemical equilibrium as an "attractor" state.

Quasi-Periodicity, Apparent Randomness, and Chaotic Systems

Although many physiological systems (which are likely to have fixed point, limit cycle, and chaotic attractors depending on the conditions; Kelso, Ding, & Schöner, 1992) frequently show apparent periodicity in their functioning, closer examination may reveal otherwise. Superficially, the heartbeat, respiration, the sleep–wake cycle, the REM/non-REM sleep cycle, and fluctuations in serum cortisol through the course of the day all can appear to represent periodic attractors. In fact, this is a simplifying assumption often used in describing physiological functioning—an assumption that is not quite accurate.

Consider the human heartbeat. Even at rest, a well-conditioned middle-distance runner whose average resting pulse is 50 beats per minute will show fluctuations in heartrate. For example, he may have an irregular heartbeat known as a respiratory sinus arrhythmia, in which case his pulse increases when he inhales and slows when he exhales. The acceleration in his heart rate is striking when he sprints the last 200 meters of a 1,500-meter run, after which it gradually slows over the hour or so following the race. There also may be many subtle fluctuations occurring across time that have no clear relationship to known or easily identifiable stimuli and which seem to occur randomly.

Such apparent randomness is frequently characteristic of chaotic systems. Consider the electroencephalogram (EEG), which measures changes in certain brain electrical potentials measured at the scalp, demonstrating a complex pattern of activity. Much of this activity is quasi-periodic, such as the wave forms known as delta, theta, alpha, and beta activity, but a great deal of what is observed in the EEG appears entirely random. Some neurophysiologists, however, maintain that this "random" activity actually is chaotic (Babloyantz & Destexhe, 1986; Freeman, 1987; Skarda & Freeman, 1987), meaning that it is deterministic rather than truly random. Some even have argued that chaotic activity may be essential to normal brain functioning (Skarda & Freeman, 1987).

SELF-ORGANIZED CRITICALITY: SANDPILES, EARTHQUAKES, AND BRAINS

Bak (1996) argued that complex systems spontaneously evolve toward *self-organizing critical states*. Much of the time they are at equilibrium, when perturbations of a system may have little effect on its overall functioning.

As a system evolves toward a critical state, however, its behavior becomes more complex and perturbations of the system may have more significant consequences. Much of Bak's work has involved studies of the behavior of sandpiles, a simplified model that has yielded insight into a wide range of processes.

How could a sandpile be a self-organizing system? Well, actually it needs a little more help from the outside than do biological systems, but the model goes something like this. Imagine that you are dropping grains of sand, one at a time, onto a flat surface. Slowly they accumulate, forming a pile that grows with an increasing slope. As grains fall onto the pile, they occasionally will cause small avalanches, but for the most part the pile continues to grow until it reaches what geologists call the *angle of repose,* "the steepest slope angle in which a particular sediment will lie without cascading down" (Press & Siever, 1978, p. 611). As it approaches this angle, the pile is in a critical state. As one continues to drop grains of sand on the pile, avalanches become more likely and, over time, avalanches of all sizes may be observed. As each grain of sand is dropped, it is impossible to predict whether (and to what extent) a slide will occur. An observer will note many occasions when no slide is produced, as well as a large number of small slides of varying degrees of magnitude. Eventually, one grain of sand will generate a major avalanche, causing the slope of the pile to fall below the angle of repose, and the system then resumes its evolution back toward the critical state. In such a case, a minor event, indistinguishable from countless other such events, results in far-reaching consequences and a redistribution of the entire sandpile.

As complex systems go, sandpiles are pretty simple. They are especially useful as models of self-organizing criticality, however, since there are a minimal number of variables that must be controlled. In nature, plate tectonics and the occurrence of earthquakes offer a more complicated but analogous process. The crust of the earth is formed by a number of *tectonic plates,* gigantic puzzle pieces that move around in relation to one another, driven by convection currents in the molten rock of the upper mantle. The forces driving tectonic plates cause enormous strain to build between them, but at the same time enormous amounts of friction prevent them from slipping along one another. If it were not for these frictional forces, slight movement would occur continually along a fault line and there might be no major earthquakes. What actually happens, however, is that the forces evolve toward critical states all along a complex set of fault lines. The threshold for slippage along a fault line is greater at some points than at others, and as Bak noted (1996, p. 172), "a rupture starts from the weakest site in the crust with the minimum barrier strength. When the site breaks, the stress in the neighborhood changes. Rupture propagates as long as the new barriers are weaker than the threshold for rupture. The earthquake stops when the minimum barrier becomes stronger than the threshold."

Depending on the state of the entire fault system, the tectonic situation where the rupture occurs, and the forces involved, the resulting quake may be detectable only by seismographic monitoring or it may be a massive earthquake. In either case, when things subsequently settle down, the fault line resumes its evolution toward a new critical state. There is no external guiding or organizing force behind this evolution—it is self-organizing (Bak, 1996). As Kelso noted, "spontaneous pattern formation is exactly what we mean by *self-organization:* the system organizes itself, but there is no 'self,' no agent inside the system doing the organizing" (1995, p. 8). A difference between inorganic and organic self-organizing systems is the fact that nonbiological systems do not demonstrate adaptive behavior (change as a result of experience), and do not incorporate information about the environment (learning).

Catastrophic events—large earthquakes, avalanches, manic episodes, and bifurcations of other sorts—may have their genesis in minor perturbations of local conditions. In a sandpile avalanche, for example, one grain of sand falling in a small area of the pile may generate a cascade that takes a large percentage of the total pile down with it. In an earthquake, the slippage along a fault occurs at the point with the lowest barrier to such movement, then propagates from there. In a generalized seizure, the epileptiform activity begins at some focal point and spreads to most of the brain.

Global order is created by the joint operation of the individual elements of a system, all interacting locally, and their behavior in turn is regulated by the order in the system. Only because the global system is in a critical state do small local perturbations (such as that of a single falling grain of sand) produce major bifurcations. As Bak suggests (1996, p. 112), "complexity, like that of human beings, which can be observed locally in the system is the local manifestation of a globally critical process. *Complexity is a consequence of criticality*" (emphasis in original).

CHARACTERISTICS OF THE SELF-ORGANIZED CRITICAL STATE IN ORGANISMS

Behavior of biological systems in a critical state has been described as being "on the edge of chaos" (Langton, 1991), or at the "boundary" between equilibrium and far-from-equilibrium states or between stability and chaos. This may be better understood if we more closely examine equilibrium and nonequilibrium conditions.

When close to equilibrium, systems demonstrate relatively stable, predictable behavior. A system may be perturbed by various stimuli so that frequent random fluctuations occur, but these are quickly damped. As a system moves farther from equilibrium, the importance of such fluctuations increases. In the vicinity of the critical state, the behavior of a system becomes more complex and even small local fluctuations in the system may produce global effects.

Organisms are organized in such a way that local fluctuations are readily communicated to other regions of the organism. The nervous system, by maintaining itself in a critical state, facilitates neural communication and adaptive action. As Bak puts it (1996, p. 177), "the brain must operate at the critical state where the information is just barely able to propagate. At the critical state the system has a very high sensitivity to small shocks." The problem, then, is one of communicating what must be conveyed without repeatedly sending the system out of control. According to Bak (1996, p. 177), "the input signal must be able to access everything that is stored in the brain, so the system cannot be subcritical, in which case there would be access to only a small, limited part of the information"; on the other hand, the brain cannot operate in a *supercritical* state, "because then any input would cause an explosive branching process within the brain, and connect the input with essentially everything that is stored in the brain."

The solution to this kind of problem can be found to some extent in the nature of the interconnected organization of different brain regions; in part, it lies in the balance of excitatory and inhibitory neurons within and between neural networks (e.g., Abeles, 1991). The ratio of inhibitory to excitatory neurons in the brain lies precisely in a small range that prevents the nervous system from running out of control in response to stimulation and from dampening its activity to the point that a response is prevented. (In Chapter 7 we discuss these neurodynamic issues in greater detail.)

FLUCTUATIONS AND BIFURCATIONS

The constant dynamic activity of the brain is marked by countless fluctuations. Although these may appear random, in all likelihood subtle changes in internal and external conditions continually produce such fluctuations. When a system is in a stable, noncritical state, these local, transient changes in activity are likely to have no significant effect on the global system. On the other hand, when that system is in a critical state (on the edge of chaos), even slight fluctuations may perturb the symmetry of random or routine activity, producing a striking change in the system's functioning. These changes are referred to as *bifurcations*.

An important characteristic of any dynamic system is the ease with which its functioning either is restored following a perturbation or leads into another attractor or into chaotic activity. Kelso et al. (1992) refer to the time required for such a system to return to a relatively stable state as the *local relaxation time*. As a general rule, stable attractors are characterized by relatively shorter local relaxation times and by smaller fluctuations from the attractor state in response to local forces. Those systems with the deepest basins of attraction (i.e., the most stable attractors) tend to have shorter local relaxation times.

According to Kelso et al. (1992, p. 411), "often a small change in some parameter results in a small change of the dynamics. However, at certain critical points, the dynamics may also change qualitatively, e.g., the stability of an attractor is lost." Under such circumstances, systems may undergo marked changes in activity, called *bifurcations* or *nonequilibrium phase transitions*.

An example of a simple bifurcation is the phase transition that occurs when water freezes at 0° Celsius or turns to steam at 100° Celsius under standard atmospheric conditions. This happens because the interactions between water molecules depend on the temperature of the water. As a solid (ice), water molecules are locked into a crystal matrix, with bonds formed between specific molecules. When water is in the liquid state, its molecules essentially slide around in relation to one another, held together as a liquid by relatively weak chemical bonds which, in aggregate, make large numbers of water molecules stick together. Each molecule in a fluid is attracted by surrounding molecules in all directions, but it is not bound to other specific molecules. When water becomes a gas, the energy of the water molecules overcomes the weaker attractive forces that characterize a liquid. The greater the temperature of a gas, the faster is the average velocity of the molecules in that gas. The average distance between individual molecules in a gas is large in comparison with their dimensions, and their attraction to other molecules is minimal. Molecules bond with each other during collisions, and even though the number of collisions increases with temperature, increased heat also makes bond formation extremely unlikely in a gas. These phase transitions—solid to liquid to gas, and so on—all represent bifurcations. Someone who had never seen ice would have no way of predicting that if the temperature dropped sufficiently, water suddenly would become hard and solid, or that the nature of its behavior would change so significantly.

Bifurcations occur not only in chemical or physical processes but in biological systems as well. According to Glass and Mackey (1988, pp. 25–26), "the local stability of a steady state or limit cycle is determined by perturbing with small stimuli. If a steady state or limit cycle is reestablished, then they are *stable*. If, on the other hand, a small perturbation induces a change in the dynamics so that the original dynamics are not reestablished, then the steady state or limit cycle is called *unstable*." As these authors point out, the nature of biological systems is such that they continuously experience small perturbations, in response to which it is important that organisms maintain local stability. Certain phenomena, however, represent such significant changes in the control parameters of a system that bifurcations occur, giving rise to chaotic, aperiodic dynamics (Glass & Mackey, 1988).

Bifurcations may be relevant to an understanding of certain personality processes, although this point will not be developed in detail in this chapter (more on this in Chapter 8). Consider, however, that a shift in behavior associated with a change in neurophysiology may represent a bifurcation, as when eight or nine beers entice an otherwise reserved person to sing *Volaré* in a karaoke bar. The pattern of certain developmental unfoldings of a psychological kind also may reflect a process of bifurcation. Jean Piaget, for example, described how cognitive development did not occur in an orderly linear fashion across time (see Thelen & Smith, 1994). Instead, acquired cognitive capacities appear to achieve a certain level of stability, and the world (at least along certain dimensions) may be seen through a certain set of lenses until the eventual onset of periods of dysregulation and relative unpredictability. A bifurcation occurs as new cognitive competencies or capacities develop (in conjunction with neural development), leading to a change in one's representation of the world, now seen in the light of the newly acquired capacity or construct.

ENERGY EXPENDITURE AND THE "LAW OF COSMIC LAZINESS"

We wish to make two important points here. First, when a system is in a critical state, bifurcations may occur that range in magnitude from trivial to catastrophic. In contrast, when the system is closer to equilibrium it is characterized more by relative stasis, and if change occurs it tends to occur slowly. As Bak argued (1996, p. 61), "things happen by revolutions, not gradually, precisely because dynamical systems are poised at the critical state. Self-organized criticality is nature's way of making enormous transformations over short [timescales]."

The second point is that natural processes are initiated when the minimum amount of energy required to produce them (in a given set of circumstances) is present. In an earthquake, a fault ruptures when the strain on the weakest part of the fault exceeds some critical level. In a chemical reaction producing more than one product, those reaction products that require a greater amount of energy for their formation are less likely to be produced than those requiring less energy, and the former will be produced only in small quantities. If you heat the reaction vessel, the percentage of these less stable products may increase, but as the vessel cools, the probability of their formation decreases; the equilibrium may shift back in the opposite direction, and more stable compounds predominate in the mixture. Physical, chemical, and biological processes tend to occur in such a way that they use the minimum amount of energy that is necessary and available—a phenomenon similar to what has been described as a "law of cosmic laziness." As Max Planck noted, "Nature does not permit processes whose final states she finds less attractive than their initial states" (1925, p. 16). This basic principle, which is associated with the second law of thermodynamics (which concerns entropy, discussed in the next section), will be crucial for understanding the dynamics of the brain, of memory, and of behavior.

Because neural processing tends to favor "relaxed" states involving lower energy (Abeles, 1991), as a general rule neural processes occur with the expenditure of as little energy as possible. Those neural networks that require little energy for their activation or maintenance have a high probability of occurrence and may be thought of as attractors. Conversely, neural networks that require high levels of energy for their activation or maintenance are inherently unstable and thus have a low probability of occurrence. These may be thought of as repellors.[1] Repellors often occur at *saddle points* separating attractor states. The activation of very high-energy, unstable neural networks ordinarily is short lived, as neural activity tends to be drawn into surrounding energy "valleys," which are lower-energy basins of attraction in the phase space.

At the level of personality processes, what is implied by this principle of conservative energy expenditure is that people are most inclined to do those things that require the least energy. It must be remembered, however, that the energy with which we are concerned is energy expended at the level of neurons and populations of neurons, and not necessarily at the level of the organism's overt behavior. A hyperactive child engages in a great deal of physical activity. Yet, at the level of neural networks, it probably requires less energy to behave in that way than would be required for inhibition of the hyperactivity. Certain neural networks are more readily activated (for the hyperactive child, those involved in increased activity) than are others (those that might inhibit irrelevant physical activity and permit more focused attention).

Consider again a shy person who finds herself in a stressful interpersonal situation with unfamiliar people. Although the number of possible behaviors in which she could engage is large, those that are most likely are behaviors mediated by neural networks that have the highest probability of activation (i.e., those requiring the least amount of energy). Such behaviors probably will involve withdrawal or interpersonal reserve. The neural networks mediating behavior consistent with shyness are those most readily activated, whereas neural networks that might support more outgoing, even histrionic behaviors would require considerable deliberate effort and energy expenditure for their activation. Hence the latter types of behavior have a low probability of occurrence.

It is important to keep in mind that we are discussing probabilities. Rarely is anything in either the brain or behavior a foregone conclusion—

---

[1]Under certain circumstances, the state of a system may change sufficiently that networks which are repellors under normal circumstances may become attractors.

instead, neural and psychological processes have different probabilities of occurring. Changes in either the internal or external environment may alter significantly the likelihood that a given stimulus will elicit a specific response. Although this may seem trivial, it is of fundamental importance. Specific mnestic, cognitive, perceptual, and behavioral processes all possess probabilities that are altered almost continually as a result of changes in an individual's state and in the environment (G. G. Globus, 1992).

SELF-ORGANIZING BIOLOGICAL SYSTEMS AND ENTROPY

In physics, the second law of thermodynamics (concerning entropy) has to do with the fact that over time a system becomes disordered. Energy is not perfectly conserved, but instead is lost as heat. Without a constant infusion of energy from outside a system, the process of disorganization increases irreversibly. On a cosmic scale, the universe is running down. It is thought that even protons decay over a very long period of time; if so, one of the basic constituents of matter will some day disappear. Everything wears out.

As Serway and Faughn (1989, p. 326) put it, "isolated systems tend toward disorder, and entropy is a measure of that disorder"; moreover, "a disorderly arrangement is much more probable than an orderly one if the laws of nature are allowed to act without interference." Apropos of our discussion of the law of cosmic laziness above, "the second law of thermodynamics is really a statement of what is most probable rather than of what must be" (p. 126).

Previously we discussed plate tectonics and one of its emergent properties—earthquakes—to illustrate self-organized criticality. Biological systems, however, represent a much more complex kind of system than do such inorganic systems as plate tectonics or the formation of sandpiles. Prigogine (1980) suggested that the former are systems which function far from equilibrium, whose departure from conditions of equilibrium leads both to instability and the development of new, complex behaviors. He referred to such biological systems as *dissipative structures*. The term *self-organizing systems* also is used commonly to describe them. Self-organizing systems consume energy from the environment and use it in such a way that they maintain a high degree of organization in the face of entropy. Living things are self-organizing—a human being might be able to live for 80 years or more, but in the absence of life a body begins to decompose immediately.

Biological systems operate in far-from-equilibrium conditions, but unlike ordinary chemical systems, they combine both activity and order (minimizing entropy). Organisms are open systems, dependent on the environment for their maintenance. They must, for example, take in food from their surroundings. They also show considerably more structural and functional complexity than do inorganic equilibrium systems. As Prigogine noted (1980, p. 83), for even very simple cells "the metabolic function includes several thousand coupled chemical reactions and, as a consequence, requires a delicate mechanism for their coordination and regulation. In other words, we need an extremely sophisticated *functional* organization." In addition, the amounts of reagents available within cells and their component organelles are quite small, and the temperature at which cells live is relatively low, chemically speaking. Both of these factors discourage chemical reactivity, and cells therefore must produce, as well as ingest, specific enzymes that will catalyze biochemical processes that otherwise would occur too slowly and too seldom to sustain life.

Dissipative structures function in conditions far from chemical equilibrium—according to Prigogine, the only conditions in which the order characteristic of organisms can exist. "Far from equilibrium, new types of structures may originate spontaneously. In far-from-equilibrium conditions we may have transformation from disorder, from thermal chaos, into order. New dynamic states of matter may originate, states that reflect the interaction of a given system with its surroundings" (Prigogine & Stengers, 1984, p. 12).

CONTROL PARAMETERS AND REGULATION OF COMPLEX SYSTEMS

There is no internal or external agent responsible for regulating the behavior of a complex self-organizing system. With respect to the brain, this means that there is no "ego," "self," "will," or other function or functional system that actually controls and directs brain and personality functioning. The "self-organization" that occurs is spontaneous, an emergent property of the transactions of the components of the system among themselves and with the environment. The functioning of the system is, however, sensitive to the influence of certain *boundary conditions* or *control parameters*. According to Prigogine and Stengers (1984, p. 106), these boundary conditions "describe the relation of the system to its environment." The terms "control parameters" and "boundary conditions" are used to refer to specific aspects of the organism and its environment, and the relationship between them, that affect the activity of the organism.

Thelen and Smith (1994) describe a control parameter as a specific variable of the organism–environment system "to which the collective behavior of the system is sensitive and that moves the system through different collective states" (p. 62). They note that the control parameter "does not control the system in any conventional sense; it is only the variable or parameter that assembles the system in one or another attractor regime. . . .

In biological systems, any number of organismic variables or relevant external boundary conditions can act as control parameters" (p. 62). A control parameter leads by establishing conditions conducive to or associated with the activation of certain attractors. The indirect nature of the control exerted by these variables was emphasized by Kelso (1995), who noted that a control parameter "does not prescribe or contain the code for the emerging pattern. It simply leads the system through the variety of possible patterns or states" (p. 7). In simple physical or chemical systems, such factors as temperature, gravity, or electromagnetic field strength may serve as important control parameters. For biological systems, the relevant variables are likely to be significantly more complex. Any number of organismic variables or relevant external boundary conditions can act as control parameters.

The specific control parameters involved in any neural or psychological activity differ as a function of the nature of the activity, the specific relevant regions of the brain involved (and the interactions among those regions), the nature of the environment, idiosyncrasies of individual brain organization, and many other factors. For example, the control parameters associated with the development of seizure activity are quite different from those associated with the production of fluent speech, with maintenance of a manic state, or with a change in character.

Consider the problem of jet lag. Our brain activity is regulated to some degree by a pacemaker that operates on roughly a 24-hour schedule, alternating between waking and sleeping. Although an endogenous rhythm exists, it is influenced by the timing of day and night. Should one travel by air from Peoria, Illinois, to Tashkent, Uzbekistan, the external clock would be shifted ahead by nearly half a day: the phase of the day–night cycle is shifted by almost 180°, and yet the physiological rhythm continues to operate on the old schedule. Exposure to daylight in the new setting will *entrain* the rhythm to a new schedule over the course of several days, but in the meantime it may be difficult to sleep at night or to stay alert during portions of the day. We might hypothesize that those control parameters involved in resetting the physiological rhythm in response to jet lag would include the phase differential between one's rhythms in Peoria, on the one hand, and the clock in Tashkent and exposure to light at appropriate times of the day in Central Asia, on the other. On the behavioral level, adjustment to the new regime might be affected by the time when one last slept, whether one sleeps during the day upon arrival, and whether there is deliberate exposure to light at those times most likely to entrain a new schedule.

To further illustrate the concept of control parameters, we'll examine attention-deficit/hyperactivity disorder (ADHD). Although the relevant control parameters have not been elucidated for the behavior characteristic of ADHD, there are some data to support the idea that the activity of neurons in the caudate nucleus is associated with an individual's activity level and with the ability to maintain attention without distractibility. Thus, it might be argued that activity related to the caudate nucleus serves as an organismic control parameter that may be modulated by administration of dopaminergic stimulants. Certain environmental conditions, however, also appear to be associated with behavior in persons with ADHD. These boundary conditions may be altered by changing the nature or intensity of sensory stimulation, hence affecting behavior.

Assuming the accuracy of our illustration, for both of these control parameters the effects on functioning are unlikely to be linear. For example, changes in activity in the basal ganglia (and caudate nucleus) might potentially be adaptive up to a certain point, at which time the individual's behavior becomes increasingly disorganized. Similarly, for some individuals increased sensory stimulation may facilitate the organization of behavior, whereas other types of stimulation may have deleterious effects. The effects of fluctuations in control parameters thus are somewhat unpredictable, except in probalistic terms.

THE PHASE SPACE: A USEFUL TOOL
FOR GRAPHICALLY REPRESENTING PROCESSES

Another important basic concept of the study of dynamics is the *phase space* or *state space,* a means of graphically depicting the functioning of a single system or group of interacting systems. A phase space is a representation of the instantaneous state of different dimensions of the system at multiple points in time. Over a long period of time these points will define the *trajectory* of the system. If the system's behavior is more or less regular or periodic, this will be apparent from inspection of the graph itself, which is referred to as a *phase portrait.* In a phase portrait, "the region in space in which almost all initial conditions converge to the attractor" (Kelso, 1995, p. 54) is known as a *basin of attraction.* Figure 6.3 illustrates such a phase portrait (derived from the EEG of a person in stage 4 sleep), consisting of a set of points showing the most probable activity of the system (or the most probable values of the relevant components of the system). The attractor in this case is chaotic. The rest of the space in the graph can be taken to represent unstable configurations of the system, since the system has an extremely low probability of having those values when allowed to run over an extended period of time. A phase space may contain several different basins of attraction simultaneously, a situation referred to as *multistability.*

Consider a simple two-dimensional phase space showing variability in an individual's body temperature over time. If temperature were measured over a sufficiently long period, it would show occasional spikes during fevers or periods of physical activity, and occasional lows that fall below the range we typically regard as "normal." These variations would represent

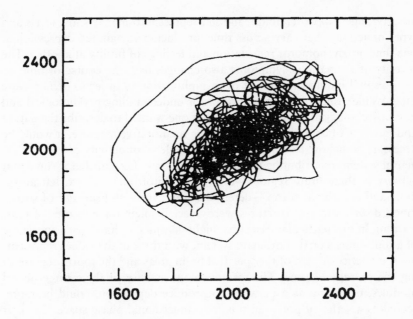

FIGURE 6.3. Two-dimensional phase portrait derived from the EEG of a person in stage 4 sleep. Note that the neurophysiological activity tends to occupy only a circumscribed region of the state space, while it never ventures into surrounding areas. The former region is an *attractor*, whereas the latter area might be a *repellor*. In a state other than stage 4 sleep, it is likely that one would observe neither this particular attractor nor the associated repellor. From Babloyantz (1990, p. 43). Copyright 1990 by Springer-Verlag. Reprinted by permission.

only transient perturbations of the system, which returns to its quasi-periodic attractor as these transients die out (e.g., as one recovers from influenza). By adding a third axis to such a graph, we could illustrate a slightly more complex three-dimensional phase space showing the change in two variables over time—temperature and diastolic blood pressure, for example.

Phase spaces can facilitate understanding of certain complex neural and psychological phenomena. The psychological state of depression, for example, is not a monolithic, one-size-fits-all state of mind. Depression typically varies from one individual to another, and within a given individual from day to day or even moment to moment, however subtly. Numerous factors may influence the specific character of one's depression at any given time. Some of these factors may be environmental (such as the number of hours of daylight, the nature of available psychosocial supports, or the experience of an insult to one's self-esteem). Other factors may involve various changes in parameters of the physiological system itself. Neural networks involved in regulating level of arousal, level of physical activity, anxiety, anger, appetite, libido, and self-representation may show levels and types of activity that vary across time, producing an agitated depression at one time or psychomotor retardation and feelings of futility at another. The severity of the various symptoms also changes over the course of time.

We will indulge in a bit of oversimplification in order to demonstrate the possible utility of a phase portrait for understanding psychological and neuropsychological activity. Assume that one wanted to describe the nature and intensity of depression by means of a quantitative measure. It would be necessary somehow to assign a value to the level of activity of each of the neural systems contributing to the depressed state. Let's further assume that activity in three brain regions—the right orbitofrontal cortex, left amygdala, and entorhinal cortex—determines the nature and severity of such a mood disorder (these structures were selected solely for purposes of illustration). In this particular case, one might consider a phase space consisting of a four-dimensional coordinate system, with three of the values representing the activity in each of the specified brain areas and the fourth representing the passage of time. The instantaneous activity of these three neural modules, operating as a network to produce depression, could be represented as a series of points in this four-dimensional phase space. Thus, at time 1, depression might be characterized as an ordered quadruplet such as $(1, 3, 6, -4)$, and at time 2, it might have changed to $(2, 3, 7, -5)$. The number of possible combinations of the variables would be infinite, but even if data were collected over a very long period of time, the phase portrait still would be constrained to a restricted region of the phase space—the attractor. Likewise, there are certain combinations of values that are so unstable they would never occur or would occur only rarely (these represent repellors). Thus, if we took such an extremely fine-grained view of depression, we would observe an infinite variety of nuances in depressed states, while on the psychological level we would find it difficult to make more than a handful of distinctions.

EXPERIENCE ALTERS THE PROBABILITY OF ACTIVATION OF SPECIFIC NEURAL NETWORKS

As we noted in Chapter 3, the probability of activation of a specific neural network is changed as a result of experience. Such neural plasticity makes the activation of some neural networks (and hence the occurrence of some behaviors, memories, perceptions, emotions, or ideas) more likely than the activation of others. At any given time, the overall physiological state (discussed in Chapter 9) of the individual—an emergent property of the predominant mood, activity level, level of arousal, amount of fatigue, and other factors—establishes the probability of activation of different neural networks. Thus, for example, when an individual is depressed, the likelihood is greater that he will experience thoughts and expectations consistent with that mood than is the likelihood he will experience a sense of lightness, euphoria, and optimism (this phenomenon is consistent with mood congruent memory). If his state changes and he now feels happy and relaxed, he is unlikely to experience thoughts about being worthless or a sense that all his efforts in life will amount to nothing.

We will illustrate this concept by revisiting our earlier discussion of chemical reactions, introducing into our model the concept of *energy of activation*. The energy of activation (E_{act}), a fundamental concept of chemistry, is the amount of energy (usually heat) that must be put into a mixture in order to produce a specific reaction product. When the compounds required for two different reactions are present in a reaction vessel at room temperature, the reaction with the lowest E_{act} is the one most likely to proceed to completion. Even if the mixture is allowed to stand (at equilibrium) for a very long time, there will be only a small percentage of the products requiring greater energy. This is shown schematically in Figure 6.4.

A similar situation exists when any of several neural networks are candidates for activation in a given situation (which is analogous to saying that any of several behaviors is possible in that situation). Neurons respond to incoming stimuli when the total amount of stimulation exceeds some threshold. Neural plasticity may alter those thresholds, either lowering or raising them. When there are several possible networks that might be activated, the one with the greatest probability of activation and maintenance is the one that currently has the lowest energy of activation. Hence, dysphoric associations emerge in the mind of the person who is depressed because such associations have the lowest energy of activation. The activation of this low E_{act} network is not an absolute or foregone conclusion, because the system operates in a probabilistic manner and any number of factors may alter the probability or otherwise affect the outcome. It is possible that several factors may converge in a given situation to produce a bifurcation. For example, in the psychotherapy of a depressed person, one might see the unexpected development of an expansive train of thought despite the fact that the individual is in a predominantly depressed mood. The emergence of such a line of thinking in turn might shift the patient's mood, or awareness of the mood, momentarily.

SELF-ORGANIZED CRITICALITY AND PERSONALITY

The concept of self-organized criticality can be applied to psychology and will be developed more fully in later chapters. Anticipating that discussion, we present the following example. Psychological functioning, mediated as it is by neurobiology, is characterized by the development of self-organized criticality. Depending on a number of factors, including the in-

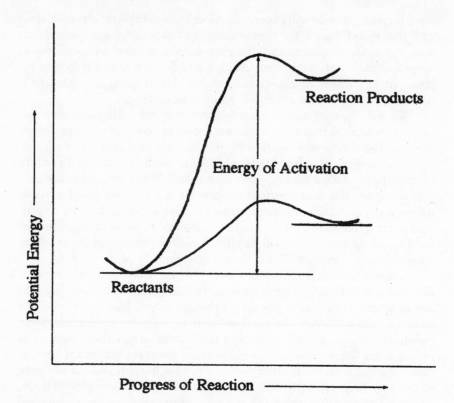

FIGURE 6.4. In a mixture of compounds that could yield two or more products, the proportion of the products is determined in large part by the energy of activation (E_{act}) of the competing reactions. That product which requires the least energy (usually in the form of heat) for it synthesis will predominate in the final mixture. In this schematic drawing, the lower of the two curves represents the reaction with the lowest E_{act}, which is the reaction that would yield the greatest quantity of product. This analogy is used to illustrate certain aspects of the dynamics of the nervous system. If two different neural networks might be activated in a given situation, that network most likely to be activated is that with the highest *probability* of activition (i.e., with the lowest barrier of activation, as is the case with E_{act} in chemical reactions).

dividual's state at any given time and the nature of the environment, that person's representations of the world and of other people may be more or less disposed to change. For example, a husband is likely to have developed such stable and reasonably accurate representations of his wife that he generally can anticipate her reactions to various events. The stability and accuracy of his representation of his wife may play an important role in guiding participation in transactions between the husband

and wife, leading to a shared feeling of consistency and intimate familiarity. Yet, at times these representations may be less than adaptive. The fact that the brain dwells in or near a state of self-organized criticality allows the husband to accommodate to new or atypical behavior and to recalibrate his representation of his wife when appropriate, as might be the case when the two of them face a novel and difficult situation and she is in need of some form of relatedness other than what is typical of him. Self-organized criticality allows him to see his wife in a new light and potentially respond to her accordingly.

Certain kinds of psychopathology may be characterized by a disequilibrium of self-organizing dynamics. An excessive rigidity and inability to respond to novelty may be at one extreme; thus, this same husband's representational processes may have limited flexibility so that he responds to his wife as though she is *always* doing a certain thing (e.g., he believes she is criticizing him even when she is not). His representation of her remains constant even in the face of considerable shifts in environmental conditions (in this case, changes in his wife's intentions). He cannot recognize new behavior as novel or different, nor can he see distinctions between different behaviors on her part. The consequence may be stereotyped behavior in relation to his wife.

For some persons whose representations of their spouse can be characterized as excessively volatile and unstable, minor shifts in their own state or behavior or that of the spouse can lead to highly divergent or idiosyncratic representations. For some individuals, varying individual representations may be quite inflexible and resistant to modification. Other persons may form representations too susceptible to change—essentially inconsistent and even chaotic. Representations of this sort would make it impossible to anticipate the behavior of the other. Such unstable representational processes could be psychopathological, thereby resulting in chaotic and unpredictable interpersonal behavior.

SUMMARY AND CONCLUSION

The way in which the brain's structures are organized and the processes in which these structures engage are of fundamental importance for understanding how the nervous system produces the entire range of psychological phenomena. The concerted activity of countless shifting, interconnected, self-organizing populations of neurons reflects complex dynamic processes that occur in a system "on the edge of chaos." Changes in organization of one sort might dampen brain activity, prohibiting the propagation of information necessary for adaptive behavior and locking animals into stereotyped activity. Changes of another sort might produce a system prone to surge wildly out of control. As it is, the brain has the capacity to stabilize functioning over significant periods of time while permitting bifurcations to occur that may lead to adaptive behavior in novel or demanding situations.

Next, Chapter 7 elaborates on the significance of neural and psychological dynamic processes. However, a few points of fundamental importance should be emphasized here.

First, specific behaviors have a probabilistic basis. That is, we tend to engage in a behavior because in a given situation (and assuming that we are in a specific physiological/psychological state) the likelihood of that behavior is greater (i.e., the energy of activation is lower) than is the probability of other behaviors. For example, if you are talking with your mother, the probability is great that you will automatically and nonconsciously behave in a way that differs significantly from the way you might behave with a spouse, an obnoxious neighbor, your boss, or a co-conspirator in a right-wing militia plot to overthrow the government. Change the internal environment (your *state,* in other words), however (e.g., by taking diazepam or getting drunk), and your behavior with your mother may change radically.

Second, people tend to operate in self-organized critical states. As is always the case, there probably are significant individual differences with respect to how these states are maintained. Some persons may have brains (and personalities) more consistently resistant to bifurcation in response to various kinds of perturbing stimuli, whereas others may have brains (and personalities) more easily destabilized (not always with adverse consequences). For the most part, we are relatively stable in our response to the slings and arrows of outrageous fortune. At times, however, events occur that lead to significant changes in functioning. Sometimes these are of major import (e.g., severe trauma); at other times they are subtle. Because people operate in critical states, even the subtle occurrences may produce major and lasting effects, whereas sometimes even horrifying experiences may produce few long-term changes in functioning.

Finally, regardless of how it is practiced, psychotherapy that produces change is likely to have taken advantage of self-organizing criticality. Even bad therapy is capable of producing significant functional changes of a deleterious nature. To a certain extent, successful therapy may facilitate evolution of a critical state, increasing the probability that even minor events inside or outside the therapy may lead to change. Sometimes, as in periods of emotional crisis, an individual is poised for rapid alterations in functioning because of the dynamics of the critical state. The neurodynamics underlying psychological functioning, if properly considered, can shed considerable light on processes of psychological development, stability, and change in new and hitherto unappreciated ways.

7

NEURODYNAMICS: NEURONS AND NEURAL NETWORKS

INTRODUCTION

In the previous chapter we addressed certain fundamental concepts concerning dynamics and self-organizing systems. In this chapter we apply some of those principles to the central nervous system (CNS), discussing how the brain operates as a self-organizing system. Specifically, we will emphasize the notion that the brain is anatomically structured and dynamically organized in ways that maximize its self-organizing potential. It is the brain's self-organizing capacity that allows for exquisite responsiveness to the diverse demands of biological and social adaptation. The presence of self-organization in the brain at different levels (physiological, dynamic, and psychological) reflects the fundamental importance and adaptive value of such activity. Self-organization ultimately engenders a dynamic balance between stereotyped activity and the capacity to respond to novel stimuli, a balance that is crucial for successful adaptation.

To understand the processes that characterize psychological development, stability, and change, we must understand the neural dynamics that constrain psychological functioning. Therefore in this chapter we consider the dynamic activity of interacting neurons and groups of neurons. Next, in Chapter 8, we move on to the psychological level of analysis, examining the implications of the brain's dynamic activity for the study of personality.

The nature of the connectivity of neurons in the brain is responsible for the emergence of complex organismic activity. Every area of the brain is directly or indirectly interconnected with every other area, yet the connections between neurons within any given area are relatively sparse. Neurons essentially weave together disparate areas of the brain through these synaptic connections, providing the structure necessary for maintaining the delicate balance between excitatory and inhibitory neurons essential for stable neurological functioning. The balance of excitation and inhibition in the cortex represents a basic, highly efficient process, an example of the brain's dynamic tendency to evolve toward a state of self-organized criticality.

The activity of individual neurons occurs within the context of larger assemblies of cells. The pattern of discharge of a single neuron is meaningful only because it is a part of a population of neurons. Complex psychological properties—movement, representations, intentions—are emergent properties of patterns of activity within neural networks. At any given time, the silent neurons may be as important in this regard as are those that are firing actively. Thus, although neurons represent a basic functional/structural unit in the brain, it is the activation of different *networks* of neurons—and not specific neurons themselves—that seems to be associated with psychological phenomena. The continual process of establishing and modifying these networks of neurons represents a fundamental expression of the self-organizing dynamic activity of the brain. The distributed, unguided functioning of neural networks, weaving together the brain's diverse anatomical structures into coordinated processes, yields the mind as an emergent process.

NEURAL CONNECTIVITY

Estimates of the number of neurons in the human brain vary, but there are probably about 50 billion of them. Depending on how one classifies them, there may be as few as two major kinds of neurons (Abeles, 1991) or as many as 10,000 (Kandel, 1991a). As a function of its type and location, each neuron receives input from and conducts signals to many others. It has been estimated that each cortical neuron receives stimulation from somewhere between 1,000 and 10,000 other neurons and projects in turn to a similar number. The density of connections between neurons in any given area of the brain is relatively sparse, however, as neurons typically connect with less than 1% of neighboring neurons (Freeman, 1995).

As discussed earlier, neurons communicate by transmitting signals unidirectionally from one neuron to another at a junction called the *synapse*. Each cortical neuron may have a direct synaptic connection with as many as 20,000 other neurons. Thus, the density of synapses is somewhere in the vicinity of 800 million to 1 billion per cubic millimeter of cortex (Abeles, 1991; Douglas & Martin, 1991). Given that about 10% of synapses are inhibitory and 90% excitatory (Abeles, 1991), an average cortical neuron may receive inhibitory input at about 2,000 synapses. It receives excitatory input at about 9,000 synapses from neurons in its own region, and at about 9,000 excitatory synapses from neurons in remote areas.

NEURONAL FIRING: THE ACTION POTENTIAL

Although some of the material in this section was discussed previously, we will summarize it again here for those readers unfamiliar with the working of neurons. In short, a neuron fires in an *all-or-none* manner: it either fires or it doesn't. Furthermore, apart from a few exceptions, the strength of each neuron's impulse is always the same. What varies in neural signaling is the *frequency,* or rate, of firing. If the incoming stimulation from all neurons or receptors that impinge on a neuron is sufficient to change the voltage of that neuron to a certain threshold level, it will fire (in technical jargon, it generates an *action potential*), propagating an impulse along its length with no loss of strength.

The input to a neuron usually consists of a combination of *excitatory* and *inhibitory* stimulation. Excitatory input *depolarizes* a neuron, increasing the probability that it will fire, whereas inhibitory input *hyperpolarizes* a neuron, decreasing this probability. The sum of all excitatory and inhibitory input over a very short period of time (a few milliseconds) determines whether a neuron will respond to the input. Thus, brief bursts of high frequency synchronous excitatory stimulation are likely to produce an action potential, whereas lower frequency stimulation, high levels of inhibitory input, or stimulation distributed over time are less likely to do so.

Whether a specific neuron fires at any given time is a probabilistic matter, and this probability is affected by a multitude of variables. For example, immediately following the propagation of an action potential, a neuron enters an *absolute refractory state,* during which time a second action potential cannot be generated. This, in turn, is followed by a brief *relative refractory period,* during which the amount of input required to produce an action potential is greater than when the neuron is at rest.

Neurons also receive input that is neither directly excitatory nor inhibitory, but rather is *modulatory.* Neuromodulation changes the state of a neuron in some way, altering the probability that a neuron will fire in response to incoming stimulation. Other variables (e.g., hydration, electrolyte balance, overall metabolic demand, mitochondrial efficiency, medications, ion channel state, or glial cell influences) constantly affect the readiness of neurons to generate action potentials. Thus the identical level and type of input at two different times—even in temporal proximity—may produce entirely different effects (the neuron fires or it doesn't). The activity of neurons thus reveals itself as highly nonlinear.

Synaptic strength refers to the probability that stimulation at an individual synapse will produce an action potential in the postsynaptic neuron. Synaptic strength generally is rather low, ranging from 0.000 to about 0.20. For neurons capable of influencing one another within a network, the mean synaptic strength is probably on the order of 0.003. In other words, just three times out of a thousand inputs, the synapse by itself will produce an action potential in the postsynaptic neuron. If we consider a presynaptic neuron projecting impulses to 5,000 other neurons, this means that each action potential in the presynaptic neuron will produce approximately 15 additional discharges in postsynaptic neurons (Abeles, 1991, p. 105). Abeles estimated that "in the cortex, a neuron receives input from about 100 neurons every millisecond" (1991, p. 188). On average, if 25 additional excitatory inputs are received within a millisecond (i.e., a total of 125 inputs in a thousandth of a second), the neuron will fire.

The resting voltage (or *membrane potential*) of neurons fluctuates most of the time, although it generally remains well below the threshold for firing. Hence, the probability that a neuron will be stimulated sufficiently to produce an action potential varies as the resting potential moves closer to or farther from the threshold. Nevertheless, most neurons are close enough to their thresholds that an inordinate amount of stimulation is not required to produce a discharge. According to Freeman (1975, 1992, 1995), by means of mutual excitatory connections, cortical neurons are maintained in a self-organized critical state just below their thresholds. He argues (1995, p. 56) that "their cooperative actions create an excitatory bias, which is mainly smooth, but which has a noisy ripple that takes now one, now another above threshold, but only briefly, and not in coordination with other neurons' firing. They give steady, unstructured noise," which appears to be random, but which actually may be deterministic in nature.

Most cortical neurons demonstrate a spontaneous firing rate of about five action potentials per second, but may be capable of more than 100 discharges per second given strong excitatory stimulation. This spontaneous and seemingly random activity is punctuated by increased rates of firing in response to appropriate stimuli. Thus, "there is always highly irregular *background activity* before and after a stimulus" (Abeles, 1991, p. 57). According to Skarda and Freeman (1987, p. 168), "the system is designed and built so as to ensure its own steady and controlled source of 'noise' (i.e., chaos). Most remarkably, 'signals' are not detected 'in' the chaos because the mechanism turns the chaos 'off' when it turns a signal 'on.'" It is as though the brain has a resting "hum" of background chaotic electrical activity, out of which emerges highly organized, synchronized neural activity yielding adaptive responses to shifting conditions.

EXCITATION, INHIBITION, FEEDBACK, AND OSCILLATION

The brain's architecture allows for the maintenance of the relatively delicate balance between excitatory and inhibitory neurons in the cortex. Excessive excitation can lead to an escalation of cortical activation, and in some disorders may be responsible for seizures, seizure-like episodes, and behavioral dyscontrol. Inhibitory neural activity serves to put the brakes on a potentially runaway nervous system. Yet too much inhibition may dampen overall brain activity and could lead to certain other pathological conditions.

Computer simulations of neural activity make it clear that stable neurological functioning demands a relatively close balance between excitation and inhibition. This balance is important for global functioning, but also for such specific functions as defining boundaries between objects or heightening contrast in visually perceived objects, a phenomenon known as *lateral inhibition* (Fahrenbach, 1985). Disturbances of this inhibitory–excitatory equilibrium are likely to manifest themselves in pathological functioning. For example, Abeles discussed computer models indicating that "any external interference with the delicate balance of excitation and inhibition can throw the cortex into saturated activity (epilepsy), depress its activity completely (spreading depression), or drive it into oscillations" (1991, p. 167).

Seizures thus represent one type of neurodynamic disorder. At the onset of a generalized *tonic–clonic seizure,* massive simultaneous firing of excitatory neurons occurs throughout the cortex. This synchronous discharge produces first the *tonic phase,* in which opposing muscle groups (e.g., extensors and flexors) both have greatly increased tone. After a short time, the seizure may enter a *clonic phase,* in which there is alternating contraction of opposing muscle groups with a resulting rhythmic jerky motion.

EXCITATION AND INHIBITION IN THE BASAL GANGLIA

The basal ganglia, a set of structures located deep in each hemisphere of the brain, illustrate a different and rather complex set of excitatory–inhibitory dynamic processes. Excitatory stimulation by cortical neurons forming synapses in the *caudate nucleus* and *putamen* of the basal ganglia cause neurons in these structures (known collectively as the *striatum*) to fire. The striatal neurons are inhibitory, and they form synapses with other inhibitory neurons in the lateral and medial *globus pallidus.* The net effect is that this second set of inhibitory neurons is inhibited from firing. Inhibition of inhibition produces a *disinhibition* of the neurons in the thalamus with which they synapse. Excitatory thalamic cells then produce increased activity in the cortical cells with which they form excitatory synapses. Meanwhile, some neurons from the lateral globus pallidus form synapses with the *subthalamic nucleus* (this is referred to as the *indirect* path), the net effect of which is to produce excitatory input to the medial globus pallidus. The balance between excitation and inhibition in these structures is maintained by self-organizing activity among these networks. Disturbance of this balance produces a variety of movement disorders, including in some cases involuntary movements (as in certain *dyskinesias*) and in others rigidity, reduced movement, and slow tremor (as in Parkinson's disease).

OSCILLATORY DYNAMICS

Mutually interconnected groups of excitatory and inhibitory neurons may produce patterns of oscillating activity. For example, a group of excitatory neurons may stimulate a group of inhibitory neurons and in turn be inhibited by them. Because the excitatory neurons then cannot stimulate the inhibitory neurons, the latter are released from the inhibition and can again generate an action potential, which will inhibit the excitatory cells once again. Oscillatory activity of this sort may be one of the brain's primary strategies for organizing, synchronizing, and integrating diverse processes. Many systems in the brain demonstrate oscillatory activity (see Buzsáki et al., 1979, 1992; Steriade, McCormick, & Sejnowski, 1993; Traub, Miles, & Wong, 1989). Different regions or populations of neurons are interconnected with one another so that the activity of each influences the activity of the others. This may result in large-scale patterns of periodic or quasi-periodic activation. Such mutually interacting oscillating systems are considered to be *coupled*.

The hippocampus, for example, demonstrates rhythmic, slow electrical potentials (Isaacson, 1982). Fibers from a midline region known as the *septum* are thought to be involved in driving this activity, although two hippocampal regions also seem to generate these rhythms. During deep sleep, the rhythms of these two hippocampal areas are in phase (positively correlated) with one another; but during waking and rapid eye movement (REM) sleep, which is associated with dreaming in humans, the rhythms are 180° out of phase (negatively correlated). Oscillatory neural discharge also has been found to be associated with various kinds of repetitive rhythmic movements such as chewing, walking, running, and swimming (Kelso, 1995).

Some oscillatory neural activity may yield unstable patterns of consistent behavioral activity. In one such pattern, a feedback loop may be established wherein an excitatory neuron stimulates inhibitory neurons, which in turn synapse with other excitatory neurons, dampening the latter's activity. According to Abeles (1991, p. 168), this process may represent "a [feedforward] activation of the inhibitory neurons that anticipates . . . increased excitatory activity and alleviates the problems that the extra delay of inhibitory feedback might cause." Another outcome of oscillation, observed in a simple positive feedback loop in which two populations of mutually interconnected excitatory neurons might repeatedly stimulate one another, would be the locking of the system in uncontrolled synchronous activity.

DYNAMICS OF RHYTHMIC MOVEMENT

Oscillatory behavior within populations of neurons and within the neuro-endocrine system is manifested in various kinds of periodic and quasi-periodic activity. Kelso (1981, 1984), for example, demonstrated that the performance of certain rhythmic movements is most stable when the movements are performed in certain ranges of speed. This is also illustrated by the gait of horses, which varies from a walk to a trot to a gallop. It is awkward and inefficient if a horse's legs make trotting movements at what normally is walking speed, whereas merely accelerating walking movements to a faster rate would be a poor substitute for a trot. Consider, for example, that race walkers expend more energy with a fast-paced walk than they would expend by jogging at the same speed.

Kelso reported some interesting research into dynamic mechanisms involved in coordinated movements of the hands. When both hands perform repetitive movements, these are most efficiently executed if the timing and direction of movement of the two hands is coordinated (in phase). It is quite difficult simultaneously to tap your left index finger at a rate of three taps per second while tapping the right index finger twice per second. Even skilled musicians who have practiced this kind of task may find it problematic, and for most people it is impossible (Tuller & Kelso, 1989). It is much simpler to tap both fingers together at the same rate (e.g., two or three taps per second) or to tap the right finger four times per second and the left two times per second. In the language of dynamics, coordinated in-phase tapping represents a stable attractor, whereas the two-per-second versus three-per-second regimen is a highly unstable state for all but those who have learned to perform the task after considerable practice.

FEEDBACK AND FEEDFORWARD DYNAMICS

The brain relies on complex feedback and feedforward systems for the regulation of various kinds of activity. Feedback, for example, might involve the assimilation of perceptual input into one's mental representation during the performance of an act, permitting modification of the act while it is in progress. An example of a simple feedback system is a thermostat, which constantly monitors the temperature. When the temperature falls below a certain set point, the furnace is switched on, and when the temperature has risen sufficiently, the furnace is switched off. Information on the state of the system (i.e., the temperature of the air in the room) is used to regulate the heating system.

The thermostat example is an oversimplification; in fact, feedback is not the simple linear process it might seem. Instead, feedback reflects the functioning of a complex self-organizing system. As Kelso noted (1995, p. 9), "there is no reference state with which feedback can be compared and no place where comparison operations are performed. Indeed, *non-equilibrium steady states* emerge from the nonlinear interactions among the system's components, but there are no feedback-regulated set points or reference values as in a thermostat" (emphasis in original).

Feedforward is the term used to describe the use of "input information to compute responses and corrections rather than waiting for feedback" (Szentágothai & Arbib, 1974). In some circumstances, feedforward might involve the use of a mental representation of the world to predict what is about to occur. In this process, a behavior may be initiated before an emerging situation is apprehended fully, as when movement perceived out of the corner of the eye leads to an initial defensive action, or when a tennis player makes her initial move toward the ball. Behavior based on feedforward activity then can be more finely tuned to the developing situation, as it is perceived more clearly, with the use of feedback.

Feedback and feedforward systems tend to act in tandem. Feedback generally provides more precise control of action than does feedforward, with the trade-off that feedback also requires more processing resources. Because of the need to integrate perceptual data continuously into ongoing neural activity, feedback therefore is slower than feedforward. According to Szentágothai and Arbib (1974, p. 348), "generally, gross feedforward is used to bring the system into the correct ball park and, then, simple feedback can correct for any errors." In baseball, when the batter makes contact with the ball, a good outfielder takes off in the direction of the baseball's trajectory almost as soon as the ball leaves the bat. Feedforward systems quickly take the fielder toward the anticipated destination of the ball. As the ball approaches the fielder, he begins to fine tune his movements in a complex feedback process that takes him closer to the ball but operates more slowly than the initial feedforward activity.

The processes of feedback and feedforward are simplified when the number of degrees of freedom of a system can be reduced. For example, walking involves synergistic patterns of movement that can be produced by electrically stimulating certain regions of the brainstem. It is not necessary to regulate each muscle contraction singly or consciously. Instead, an intention to move in a certain direction apparently initiates patterns (or synergies) of movement to produce the desired effect. If each muscle contraction or relaxation had to be controlled individually, the demand on the motor system's resources would be extreme.

The complexity of feedback and feedforward processes illustrates the necessity for exceptionally precise timing in the operation of interacting neural networks. The falcon in its dive toward moving prey is engaged in an elegant sequence of feedforward and feedback processes as it adjusts its trajectory toward its target. Events must be represented by all sensory modalities at exactly the same time in order to provide such a seamless perception of the world. The organism's own movement also must be precisely integrated with perception, and great athletic ability in part may reflect such exacting integration. Even very slight distortions of timing could introduce significant problems into the performance of all kinds of actions.

NEURAL NETWORKS

The activity of individual neurons occurs within the context of larger assemblies of cells. The pattern of discharge of a single neuron is meaningful only as part of a population of neurons—a neural network. In many ways, neural networks can be regarded as the fundamental units of most psychological processes. Complex psychological phenomena are themselves emergent properties of patterns of activity within these neural networks. Stated somewhat differently, a neural network is an interconnected assembly of neurons that yields a specific emergent psychological process when it is activated.

The neurons in most neural networks are involved in both parallel and sequential processing. Parallel processing means that different distributed neuronal groups process information simultaneously (Rumelhart & McClelland, 1986). For example, Luria (1980) suggested that vision represents simultaneous (parallel) processing of a large number of diverse stimuli (color, orientation, contrast, depth) to produce a unified visual image, whereas perception of language represents the serial integration of a large number of speech sounds in a process that rapidly decodes both semantic (word meaning) and syntactic (grammatical) aspects of language. Sequential processing means that neurons stimulate one another serially across time.

Most complex behavior involves massively parallel processing as well as sequential activation of neurons in a network. As performed by the brain, parallel processing is a very efficient means of integrating a variety of phenomena into ongoing activity (perceptual, motor, cognitive, emotional) while obviating the need for an executive system to keep track of the details. The result is a complete, multimodal experience of the world with which one can fully interact. For example, if you are involved in a serious automobile accident, you see the collision (visual processing) at the same time that you hear it (auditory processing) and feel it (vestibular and somesthetic processing). You may simultaneously have pain and an emotional response to the accident (e.g., anxiety, associated with activity of the amygdala), along with increased arousal (neuroendocrine influence on several cortical and subcortical areas), and all this neuropsychological activity takes place in conjunction with whatever behavior you may initiate in attempting to deal with the situation.

Synaptic strengths in neural networks are modified as a result of experience (Hebb, 1949). That is, experience changes the probability of activating a given neural network by increasing—or decreasing—the strength of the synaptic ties among the individual neurons composing the network. These probabilities change over time as a function of the individual's physiological state and learning history.

Most neural networks are not discrete sets of specific cells activated each time an individual engages in some behavior. Instead, large numbers of neurons are available to support a network and its associated behavior. Different ensembles of specific neurons may be activated in the performance of a single task, depending on a number of variables, such as the predominant state of the individual and important characteristics of the environment. Different networks mediating different aspects of a functional system nevertheless may have some overlap with respect to the specific neurons involved in each (and, conversely, there may be no such sharing of neurons). In any case, the specific neurons activated at any moment are a function of probabilities.

A few examples may help to convey the variability and flexibility characteristic of the functioning of neural networks. Consider the performance of a relatively simple, repetitive, highly overlearned activity, such as that of a pitcher throwing a curveball. Although the pitcher may have thrown a baseball several hundred thousand times in his career, with each pitch the specific situation is slightly different and therefore different neurons come to be involved in the pitch. The precise configuration of neurons activated for any given pitch is a function of such factors as the score, the count on the batter, the inning, the temperature, the presence of a breeze, the pitcher's experience of the umpire's perception of the strike zone, the importance of the game, the number of runners on base, the extent to which the pitcher can rely on the fielders, where the catcher places his glove as a target, the characteristics of the batter, the batter's history against the pitcher, the catcher's ability to throw out runners on base, the dimensions of the ballpark, the pitcher's recent performance, the pitcher's mood and level of fatigue, the pitcher's conscious decision to vary the speed of his pitch, and others.

Perception, even of the same object on two different occasions, also involves at least slight differences in the specific neurons activated, since it is highly unlikely that precisely the same set of cells ever would be stimulated twice, even given precisely similar stimuli. The lamp on my desk appears basically the same to me whenever I look at it, although it may be seen from a different angle, or the pattern of dust may vary from week to week.

Freeman has studied the response of populations of neurons to the presentation of various odors as stimuli. Discussing the activity of neurons in the olfactory bulb in responding to a specific smell (he called this "neuro-activity"), Freeman wrote that "sniffing an odorant activates a spatial pattern of firing like a constellation of twinkling stars, though it is never twice identical" (1995, p. 58). In the case of olfaction, such patterns of activation are distributed over the entire bulb, so that "by inference, every neuron participates in every discrimination, even if and perhaps especially if it does not fire, in that each spatial pattern requires both action and imposed silence" (p. 59).

Freeman noted that other factors affect the precise neural constellation activated by any single odor stimulus. For example, the turbulent flow of air within the nose means that even from one sniff to another, different ensembles of receptors are activated. Similarly, involuntary saccadic eye movements also ensure that the visual image falling on our retinas constantly stimulates different sets of visual receptors.

Freeman's research has demonstrated that despite the variability in the individual neurons that are activated, similar global patterns of activation are likely to recur for a given odor. Interestingly, the patterns he discovered were related to the *meaning* of the odor, not to the specific odor itself. He found, for example, that if a specific odor is associated with a reward (e.g., food), the pattern of activation for that smell is different than if it is not associated with that reward. Similarly, motor behavior appears to be directed to a great extent by the meaning of the behavior (e.g., walking to obtain food as opposed to walking to the gallows).

Other evidence that the activation of specific neurons is not necessarily required to mediate a behavior is demonstrated in the aging brain. Over the course of the lifespan, a significant neuronal loss occurs in many areas of the brain, including the thalamus, hippocampus, and prefrontal cortex (Adams & Victor, 1989; Fuster, 1989; Haug et al., 1983; Zatz, Jernigan, & Ahumada, 1982). This progressive depletion of cells is especially marked among the small neurons of laminae II and IV of frontal cortex. By the age of 90, as many as 50% of the cells in this area may be lost (Adams & Victor, 1989). Probably in association with this cell loss, there is a decrease in cerebral blood flow in the frontal regions of older persons (Gur et al., 1987), as well as an increased likelihood of eliciting primitive reflexes (L. Jacobs & Grossman, 1980). Although considerable evidence exists of some degree of cognitive impairment in people as they age (e.g., see Jacewicz & Hartley, 1987; LaRue, 1992; Salthouse, 1985; Schaie & Parham, 1977), the fact that many very elderly people continue to function well suggests that the loss of specific individual neurons need not degrade or disrupt the functioning of a neural network (although the loss of sufficient numbers of associated neurons may do so).

In short, within a neural network, a number of different neurons and potential subsets of neurons may mediate any given activity. Neural networks organize this shifting neuronal activity into organized and stable perceptions, representations, and behaviors.

THE DYNAMICS OF NEURAL NETWORKS

Work reported from Freeman's laboratory suggests that much of the brain's background activity is characterized by chaotic patterns of neuronal firing (Skarda & Freeman, 1987). In their research on olfaction, Freeman and his group implanted an 8 × 8 grid of microelectrodes on the surface of rats' olfactory bulbs (the structure in which odor information is first integrated), and the activity of neurons throughout the bulb was recorded. The animals were presented with both familiar and unfamiliar odors. In some cases odors were associated with a food reward, whereas in other no reward was forthcoming. What the investigators found was that upon presentation of a familiar olfactory stimulus, physiological activity shifted suddenly from being chaotic (and seemingly random) to being coherent and organized (a point or limit cycle attractor). Such a shift represents a bifurcation of the sort that "takes place when the system undergoes a major transition in its dynamics, equivalent to, for example, the transition from sleep to waking, or from normal to seizure activity" (Skarda & Freeman, 1987, p. 165).

Importantly, when the animal was presented with a novel odor, the neural activity did not converge to an attractor but remained chaotic (Freeman, 1995). In such novel situations, there was no existing attractor (i.e., no existing perception or memory) that the animal could recognize. Thus it seems that these point and limit cycle attractors themselves are associated with specific perceptions, memories, and thoughts. They represent steady states that involve minimal expenditure of energy. Settling into such a basin of attraction is analogous to recognizing a pattern.

Freeman and his collaborators argued that the presence of chaotic activity, punctuated by relatively stable attractors (themselves mediated by stable neural networks), has important implications for neurological and psychological functioning. For example, the maintenance of apparently random neural behavior may serve to prevent the brain from falling into the stereotyped patterns of synchronous discharge that characterize seizures. Moreover, such chaotic activity may keep the brain in critical states, "poised on the brink of instability where it can switch flexibly and quickly" (Kelso, 1995, p. 26).

Such self-organizing criticality may contribute significantly to the flexibility and adaptability of the nervous system. As Bak noted, "the small amount of random noise prevents the network from locking into wrong patterns, with too deep riverbeds, from which it cannot escape" (1996, p. 181). Again, to quote Skarda and Freeman (1987, p. 171):

> In the neural system, we postulate that the process of state change leading to the unstructured chaotic domain is essential for preventing convergence to previously learned patterns, and hence for the emergence of new patterned activity in the bulb and the corresponding ability of the animal to recognize new odors. In the olfactory system the chaotic background state provides the system with continued open-endedness and readiness to respond to completely novel as well as to familiar input, without the requirement for an exhaustive memory search.

A chaotic background "allows rapid and unbiased access to every limit cycle attractor on every inhalation, so that the entire repertoire of learned discriminanda is available to the animal at all times for instantaneous access" (Skarda & Freeman, 1987, p. 168).

In the nervous system, attractors (i.e., neural networks) are hierarchically organized. An individual's physiological state (mood, level of arousal, activity level, motivational status, type and intensity of emotion, and so on) may be thought of as a global attractor that interacts with the environment to yield many subsidiary attractors (specific perceptions, memories, thoughts, behaviors). The activation of any subsidiary attractors thus becomes a function both of the specific context and of the more global attractor (state). Freeman refers to these subattractors as "wings" to which one has access when one is in a particular state attractor.

An example may help to convey the hierarchical organization of these neural attractors. Take the case of an individual who is in a state of severe depression, characterized by a sense of futility, poor appetite, no libido, and psychomotor retardation. The hierarchical organization of associated attractors is suggested by the fact that the thoughts and behaviors with the greatest probability of occurrence are those associated with the basin of attraction of the depressed state—pessimistic expectations, a sense that everything is meaningless, and apathy, for example. Thoughts and behaviors incongruent with the depressed state—sexual interest, a desire for a good meal, an urge to get some exercise, and feelings of self-worth—have only a limited probability of occurrence unless something changes the state (e.g., antidepressant medication).

Behaviors emergent from a depressed state—precisely because they *are* emergent from the state—are likely to maintain the depression. Morbid grief, hypochondriacal concerns, reduced levels of activity, feelings of doom about the future, avoidance of others, and preoccupation with the possibility of failure are more likely to lead to behavior that sustains a depressive situation. Emerging experience also is perceived through the organizing lens of the depressed state, so that one is more likely to perceive emerging experience as entirely consistent with the state, further deepening the experience of depression. Thus, when one is depressed, the more barren and painful aspects of the world seem to be perceived more clearly and to be more real.

It is common, in fact, for many depressed persons to seek depressing stimulation, such as sad music, Ingmar Bergman films, or somber books. The perceptions, feelings, and thoughts associated with such stimulation are subattractors of the depressed state, and focusing on them may serve to exacerbate the intensity of the depressed attractor (to "deepen" its basin of attraction). In contrast, some individuals, when depressed, may turn to more upbeat stimuli, hoping this will "cheer them up." It sometimes is the case that these cheerful stimuli may induce a positive change in overall state. After all, the influence works both ways—not only does one's state determine behavior and perception, but the environment plays a significant role in determining the state.

Certain other phenomena serve to broaden the basin of attraction of a particular state (i.e., increase its likelihood of generalization). The emotional state associated with severe psychological trauma (e.g., posttraumatic stress disorder, PTSD), may be associated with a wide range of stimuli, many of which, superficially, demonstrate no apparent connection with the traumatic event. For example, in the 1980s a cover of *National Geographic* magazine showed a picture of the gorilla Koko holding a kitten in her arms. A Vietnam combat veteran saw the magazine at a newsstand and began to sob uncontrollably. The picture reminded him of an incident in which, while on watch at night, he fired at a shadowy figure in a kill zone who had failed to respond to his order to halt (given in both Vietnamese and English). Upon investigation, he found that he had inadvertently killed a familiar young Vietnamese woman and her infant. In other related instances, this veteran found that the sight of babies, mothers with babies, and similar stimuli provoked traumatic memories. It could be said that the traumatic state had a *broad basin of attraction,* or this phenomenon could be described in psychological terms as *stimulus generalization.* The first term emphasizes the neural dynamics; the second underscores the learning contingencies.

SUMMARY AND CONCLUSION

The brain shows a highly intricate and widespread connectivity among neurons. Although the single neuron is the basic signaling unit of the CNS, brain functioning is dependent on the concerted activity of large numbers of neurons composing neural networks. These networks organize input in ways that yield psychological experience and behavior as emergent properties. Information is conveyed by means of changes in the spatial and temporal patterns of activity across such populations of cells, so that cells which are silent at any given time may be contributing to the overall pattern of activity as much as are active cells.

The relative balance of excitatory and inhibitory neurons in the brain keeps the nervous system poised in a self-organized critical state. An excess of excitatory input can lead to runaway activation of the cortex and seizure-like activity, whereas an excess of inhibition may well dampen incoming stimuli and leave the cortex unresponsive. Mutually excitatory and inhibitory interactions lead to considerable oscillatory behavior by neural populations. Feedback and feedforward processes also are of fundamental importance to the regulation of various activities.

The background activity of the brain is chaotic—random in appearance, yet deterministic. Such chaotic activity allows the brain to respond quickly to incoming stimulation, which activates organized point and limit cycle attractors. The tendency of the brain to engage in chaotic activity permits rapid state changes, since the system is able to avoid entrapment in any particular attractor. Chaotic neural activity also serves to prevent seizures, which involve massively parallel synchronous neuronal discharge throughout the brain. Finally, a person's state, specific learning history, and a host of other variables (including the environment) affect the probability of activating any given neural network.

8

NORMAL AND PATHOLOGICAL DYNAMICS

INTRODUCTION

In Chapter 7 we dealt with the brain as a self-organizing system. Neurons and modules of different levels of complexity are linked together in distributed networks, the activity of which yields the entire range of emergent psychological processes. The brain's structure and physiology support the establishment and maintenance of states of self-organizing criticality, which are essential both for stability and a capacity for adaptation to shifting circumstances. The brain continually structures its activity in an improvised *pas de deux* with the environment, establishing and modifying countless neural networks, from the operation of which complex behaviors emerge in a self-organizing process.

Any complex behavior requires the synchronization of many widely distributed neural networks and their associated processes. In this chapter our aim is to focus on some of the ways the brain appears to integrate the array of processes required for survival and adaptation. The organizational demands on the brain, created by the drive to stay alive and well in the face of shifting internal and external circumstances, are staggering. Nevertheless, the brain accomplishes this in a way that, from the outside, makes many complex behaviors seem easy. Such a capacity for integration is an expression of the self-organizing tendencies of the brain.

In this chapter we turn our attention to certain dynamic processes that are essential for neural and psychological functioning. First, we discuss data suggesting that neurodynamics may be regulated by the qualities of sensory input. Too little stimulation (sensory deprivation), too much stimulation (sensory overload), or changes in the nature of stimulation may lead to bifurcations that drive the brain into altered states of functioning. We then consider the idea that a wide range of periodic and quasi-periodic biological processes are fundamental in shaping important aspects of psychological functioning. It appears that disruptions of the normal temporal dynamics of these biological systems can potentially have profound effects on cognitive, emotional, and perceptual functioning (Grigsby & Kaye, 1991, 1995).

Some disorders may have their origin in perturbations of *aperiodic* dynamic processes, and these disturbances of the brain's ordinary quasi-equilibrium may produce a variety of psychological changes. For example, some persons for whom neither the left nor the right hand/hemisphere has clearly established dominance over the other may experience disturbances of speech such as stuttering, and it seems likely that forced changes in handedness may induce alterations in psychological state.

Finally, we will discuss how even subtle variations in different physiological or psychological control parameters may produce significant effects on the overall system. These control parameters, which regulate the overall emotional and psychological state of the individual (and hence affect the probability of activation of different neural networks), may include such factors as activity level, level of arousal, predominant mood, emotional reactivity, capacity to tolerate intense stimulation, and capacity to respond appropriately to novel stimulation.

SENSITIVITY OF THE NERVOUS SYSTEM TO EXTERNAL STIMULATION

The cortex depends on incoming stimuli to regulate its routine functioning. Therefore, much of the brain's activity is organized by its transactions with the environment. Freeman's (1995) work suggests that perceptual input continually drives the brain out of chaotic activity into appropriate limit cycle and point attractors. The emergent properties of their activation are specific percepts, thoughts, states, and behaviors. The seemingly random behavior of the system prevents entrapment in any single attractor and permits a flexible response to all kinds of stimulation, including novelty. Because the chaotic behavior of the brain has the properties of a self-organized critical state, many of the perturbations thus affecting the system have the potential to lead to bifurcations and state changes. Thus, in certain situations sensory stimulation may have striking effects on neural and psychological functioning. There is probably a good deal of intra- and interindividual variability in this regard; the former reflects changes in state and in the specific character of the environment.

There are considerable data to support the hypothesis that significant change in the level or nature of sensory stimulation may produce a wide variety of psychological and neuropsychological phenomena. This has been observed in connection with sensory deprivation, for example, which for most individuals induces a mild alteration in conscious experience. Reports in the literature suggest, however, that a small subgroup of the population responds to sensory deprivation with anxiety, disorganized thinking, and peculiar behavior (Goldberger & Holt, 1958; Ruff, Levy, & Thaler, 1961). In sensory deprivation, the activity of the brain, in the absence of the external stimulation that regulates its functioning, undergoes a bifurcation. For some individuals the resulting state is very different from their "normal" state and is stable enough that it may persist for some time following the reintroduction of ordinary sensory stimulation.

Conditions of sensory overload might be expected to operate similarly, forcing the nervous system into a state of dynamic disequilibrium. There is a great deal of variability in individual response to increased stimulation: some persons seem to thrive on it, whereas others find it aversive. These individual differences probably reflect variations in cortical organization and in the capacity for habituation. Severe or chronic pain also may represent an anomalous sensory stimulus that perturbs the brain's dynamic equilibrium, and significant pain has been reported to interfere with performance on tasks of information processing and working memory (Grigsby, Rosenberg, & Busenbark, 1995). Among certain individuals, chronic pain could disrupt the ordinary dynamic patterns of brain activity, resulting in interference with the processing and integration of information.

PARAPHRENIA: LATE-ONSET PSYCHOSIS

The psychosis known as paraphrenia may illustrate the brain's dependence on incoming stimuli for maintaining its dynamic equilibrium. Paraphrenia occurs among elderly adults who usually have no prior history of psychosis but who begin to develop paranoid delusions and hallucinations for the first time after the age of 60. The disorder is poorly understood and may in fact represent a number of psychotic disturbances with varying etiologies. Pearlson and Petty (1994), after reviewing the literature on paraphrenia, concluded that there is no clear pattern of structural brain abnormality, as evaluated by computerized tomography (CT) and magnetic resonance imaging (MRI). Some persons with paraphrenia show evidence of cerebrovascular disease, but such a finding is not ubiquitous. While mild cognitive deficits may be present in some of these patients, frank dementia tends to be absent and, in the sample discussed by Pearlson and Petty (1994, p. 271), "if patients with obvious organic factors are excluded, the remaining patients do not have obvious dementia and most do not develop diagnosable dementing illnesses at follow-up."

An interesting characteristic of patients with paraphrenia is the high prevalence of sensory deficits, especially auditory and visual impairment (Pearlson et al., 1989; Cooper & Porter, 1976). According to Pearlson and Petty (1994), cataracts and conduction deafness are the most common sensory problems. Kathryn Kaye reports that in a series of paraphrenic patients nearly all had significant sensory deficits, especially hearing impairment (unpublished data, 1996). Interestingly, Eastwood, Corbin, and Reed (1981) found that paraphrenics with such sensory deficits respond well to treatment of the specific sensory problems. Kaye (unpublished data, 1996) has observed similar results.

Pearlson and Petty (1994) suggested that sensory impairment leads to social isolation, suspiciousness, and paranoia. Certain individuals may be predisposed to develop paraphrenic symptoms as a result of this isolation secondary to sensory loss. While there may be some validity to this analysis, Kaye (unpublished data, 1996) suggests that many cases of paraphrenia may represent a dynamic disturbance, the result of sensory deprivation (or distortion) in an aging brain that is somewhat compromised and easily perturbed. According to this model, normal sensory input is necessary to regulate brain functioning. For some persons, external stimulation plays a crucial role; in its absence, phenomena characteristic of extreme reactions to sensory deprivation may occur in susceptible individuals. While low-dose haloperidol often is beneficial, for many persons with late-onset psychosis, improved sensory functioning (e.g., by means of hearing aids and cataract surgery) may be the most efficacious treatment.

REFLEX EPILEPSY

The ability of specific sensory input to affect neural functioning is apparent in reflex epilepsy. It has long been known that seizures may be precipitated in certain individuals by any number of discrete perceptual or cognitive stimuli. Auditory triggers for seizures have included sudden noises, as well as specific sounds, melodies, or voices. One such case reported in the popular press in the early 1990s concerned a woman whose seizures were precipitated by the voice of a female announcer on a network TV program. Flashing lights are among the more common visual stimuli that will induce seizures (e.g., strobe lights; see Jeavons & Harding, 1975). According to Engel (1989), the causes of seizures among these photosensitive individuals include "(1) sunlight passing through trees or other regularly spaced objects as seen from a moving vehicle; (2) stroboscopic illumination; (3) flickering of the television set, which has its greatest effect when the patient is close to the screen and the image is out of focus (*television epilepsy*); and (4) video games" (p. 241; emphasis in original). Engel maintained that these stimuli will not cause seizures if they are perceived by only one eye. For stimuli of this sort, the flickering or intermittent perception of light with frequencies of 15–20 cycles per second seems most likely to induce a seizure (Engel, 1989), perhaps because it drives global brain activity into a synchronized pattern that is near the seizure basin of attraction.

Certain other visual patterns also may induce seizures in susceptible individuals (e.g., see Chatrian et al., 1970). Brinciotti et al. (1992) reported two families in which several members experienced seizures in association with certain visual stimuli. In one family, a 10-year-old girl had complex partial seizures "induced by viewing stripes or other spatially structured stimuli" (p. 88). Her mother, until the age of about 15 years, "had experiences of significant discomfort and nausea induced by looking at objects that presented vertical or horizontal stripes (shutters, patterned cloth)." In a second family, both a 9-year-old boy and his mother experienced partial complex seizures that were especially likely to occur in association with watching TV. These cases are interesting both because of the sensitivity of these individuals to visual patterns and because there appears to be a familial predisposition to develop seizure disorders associated with a specific kind of sensory stimulation.

Many other kinds of stimulation have been reported as precipitants of seizure activity. For example, a 2-year-old boy experienced seizures associated with his own singing or "his use of silly or witty language such as punning" (Herskowitz, Rosman, & Geschwind, 1984), and three cases were reported of persons who experienced seizures associated with the use of a *soroban*, a traditional Japanese abacus (Yamamoto et al., 1991). Some individuals have been reported who had seizures in response to playing such games as checkers, chess, or gin rummy (M. Siegel et al., 1992). One 25-year-old woman, who experienced generalized seizures associated with playing games of this sort, had a seizure during a game of checkers while undergoing video EEG monitoring. The same thing occurred during a period of monitoring 3 months later, following which Siegel et al. asked the patient to play checkers "for 10-min. intervals, alternating with 10 min. of rest. Although spike-wave discharges were recorded at all times of the day, a clear increase in discharge frequency was documented while [the patient was] playing checkers" (1992, p. 94).

In this case of "game-playing epilepsy," it appears likely that a particular type of cognitive activity may serve as the precipitant for a seizure (although it is conceivable that the visual pattern of the checkerboard served as a stimulus). The neural networks (i.e., the attractors) activated by specific stimuli are associated, perhaps as a result of learning, with the neural activity involved in seizure onset. They share basins of attraction. Game playing, or horizontal stripes, or other sensory stimuli may induce a state that greatly increases the probability of seizure initiation.

Howard, an epileptic patient with medically intractable seizures, reported that he experienced an "orgasmic" feeling at the onset of his complex partial seizures, which occurred several times a month and were always precipitated by looking at, thinking about, or buttoning his shirt. Simply discussing this with Howard could cause him to have a seizure. Because the onset of these seizures was so pleasurable, he had a long history of deliberately inducing them by staring at his own or others' buttons. He reported that sometimes in the evening, bored and lonely, he would deliberately induce a seizure. Over time these episodes increased in frequency, and Howard found that they could be elicited with increasing ease by this unusual stimulus.

As a child, Howard had discovered he could produce this orgasmic feeling, without any other features of a seizure, by watching the whirlpool in the drain as the water ran out of the bathtub. Because the sensation was so pleasurable, he frequently engaged in this behavior. When he reached adolescence, whirlpools no longer caused the feeling, but Howard began experiencing these auras, accompanied by other complex partial seizure phenomena, in association with shirt buttons. It seems likely that from early childhood he either had a predisposition to develop a seizure disorder or had minor partial seizures with no impairment of consciousness. By deliberately inducing (kindling) seizures, he essentially trained his nervous system, with repeated practice, to have seizures more easily. (Kindling is considered further in the next section.)

Finally, it is been reported that some seizures, under some circumstances, may be aborted or prevented by certain kinds of sensory stimuli, especially pain. Tempkins (1945) reported that, in the ancient world, the progression of seizures with motor manifestations beginning in a hand was sometimes stopped by placing a limb in cold water or by tightly binding the arm. Engel (1989) noted that strong or painful stimuli may interfere with the development of a seizure, especially when the stimulation applied projects to those areas of the brain associated with the genesis of the epileptiform activity.

SEIZURES AND KINDLING

The phenomenon of developing an epileptogenic focus in neural tissue as a result of repeated abnormal neural discharges, as just noted, is referred to as *kindling* (Wada, 1976) and is similar in many respects to long-term potentiation (Martin, 1991; McNamara, 1986). Experimental models of kindling demonstrate long-term physiological and structural changes in the CNS in association with the process (Wada, Sato, & Corcoran, 1974; Wada, 1976). It is not unusual for persons with a unilateral seizure focus in the medial temporal cortex to develop a *mirror focus* in the homologous area of the contralateral hemisphere, probably as a result of seizure impulses projected across the corpus callosum, the fiber tract that connects the two hemispheres of the brain (Engel, 1968). Howard inadvertently took advantage of kindling, increasing the frequency and ease with which he could have his pleasurable seizures, with the unintended result that his epileptic disorder became more refractory to medical treatment.

CIRCADIAN, ULTRADIAN, AND INFRADIAN PHYSIOLOGICAL RHYTHMS

Natural processes can be characterized by the ways in which they occur across time. Some processes are random or aperiodic, whereas others are periodic, quasi-periodic, or simply recurrent. These patterns of activity across time can be thought of as attractors. Periodic and quasi-periodic behavior takes place on a wide range of time scales, and is fundamental to such phenomena as movement, perception, learning, and circadian rhythms. Among humans, rhythmic oscillations in many aspects of physiological and psychological functioning have been observed.

Circadian rhythms, those that vary over a period of approximately 24 hours, include the sleep–wake cycle, fluctuation in plasma adrenocorticotropic hormone (ACTH) levels, variability in melatonin levels, and many others. The adaptive significance of circadian variability is suggested by the fact that it is nearly ubiquitous across evolution, with rhythmicity observed in species as diverse as unicellular organisms, bread mold, marine mollusks, fruit flies, mice, and humans. (Rather than reflecting a single mechanism conserved across evolution, it appears likely that circadian rhythmicity has evolved independently on several occasions.) *Ultradian rhythms*—which occur over periods shorter than 24 hours—include the 90-minute REM/nonREM sleep cycle. *Infradian rhythms*, such as the menstrual cycle, occur over periods longer than 24 hours. As noted previously, many neuronal systems oscillate with a very brief period (on the order of 25 milliseconds), and even certain isolated neurons have been found to demonstrate periodic functioning (Michel et al., 1993).

Research has implicated several factors in the regulation of periodicity, and there are many complex interrelationships between endogenous and environmental rhythms. In some instances, for example, the establishment of appropriate periodicity in some biological systems may require appropriate caregiving during infancy. The body also has a number of periodic rhythms that remain relatively constant over time (and that may run independently of one another), the regulation of which appears to be related to genes coding for proteins that have a pacemaker function. In addition, physiological rhythms seem to be influenced by regular variability in the secretion of melatonin, a substance that plays a significant role in circadian rhythmicity.

Many periodic processes are influenced by the timing of exposure to light and by changes in the daily pattern of light and darkness. For example, the findings of a number of studies support the idea that retinal neurons projecting through the optic nerve to the *suprachiasmatic nucleus* of the hypothalamus convey information about light and dark, thereby *entraining* animals to a sleep–wake cycle. The importance of light in setting this biological clock has been demonstrated by Czeisler et al. (1989), who reported that exposing subjects to three cycles of bright light over a 3-day period induced phase shifts of greater than 8 hours in a sample of 14 young adults. In contrast, without light exposure at appropriate times, such shifts occur significantly more slowly. As Czeisler et al. noted, "recent laboratory studies simulating the phase shifts required for adjustment to transmeridian travel or rotating shift work show that even after 9 days, the body temperature rhythm is still not fully realigned with the new sleep–wake schedule following a 6-hour phase-advance shift. Our results indicate that with properly timed exposure to bright light, ordinary indoor room light, and darkness, [physiological adaptation] to such a phase shift can be complete within 2 to 3 days" (1989, p. 1331).

A number of endogenous factors also may influence cyclic activity in the nervous and neuroendocrine systems. Their effects could be mediated either by direct influence on the oscillatory properties of neuronal groups or by inducing synaptic modifications, hyper- or hypopolarization, or alterations in membrane permeability and ion channel activity. The complexity of temporal physiological dynamics may be observed in the variable effects of internal and external stimuli on the organism as a function of the organism's immediate state. Even basic aspects of physiology may differ significantly at different times of the day. For example, Halberg et al. (1960) showed that a given amount of *Escherichia coli* endotoxin killed as many as 80% of mice treated at a certain time of day but that only 20% of those animals receiving an equivalent dose 180° out of phase (i.e., either 12 hours earlier or 12 hours later) subsequently died. Rusak and Zucker (1974) found that rats allowed to eat and drink only during the light phase of a schedule alternating 12 hours of light with 12 hours of darkness consumed less liquid than did animals who were allowed to eat and drink only in darkness. In a related finding, Margules and associates (1972) showed that norepinephrine used to stimulate a rat's hypothalamus may either increase or decrease food consumption, depending on whether it is applied during the light cycle or in darkness.

Circadian Variability in Human Cognition

Rhythmic variations in many aspects of normal functioning have been noted among humans. Ebbinghaus (1885/1964), for example, studied the rate of learning and forgetting of lists of CVC (consonant–vowel–

consonant) nonsense syllables and found that performance at 11:00 A.M. was 20% better than at 10:00 A.M. but deteriorated through the day by more than 30% until 6:00 P.M. Blake (1967), in a study of sailors between the ages of 17 and 33, administered several cognitive tasks at 8:00 A.M., 10:30 A.M., 1:00 P.M., 3:30 P.M., and 9:00 P.M. On several tests (complex reaction time, card sorting, speed of written calculations, and two tasks of attention) performance improved through the day (with the exception of the 1:00 P.M. testing, at which there was a postprandial decline in performance). The Digit Span test showed a pattern very similar to that found by Ebbinghaus, with an improvement of about 0.4 digits between 8:00 and 10:30 A.M., and with a decline of nearly 0.7 digits between then and 9:00 P.M. (most marked after 3:30 P.M.). In a study of working memory, Folkard (1975, 1982) found that maximum performance occurred between noon and 2:00 P.M., with a subsequent drop and second smaller peak at about 8:00 P.M. He concluded that performance on working memory tasks is at its best around midday, and he contrasted this with the 8:00 P.M. peak for nonmemory tasks reported by other authors (Folkard, 1982, p. 259).

Infradian Rhythms: Estrogen and Cognition

Research has demonstrated changes in cognitive and neuropsychological performance both as a function of the phase of a woman's menstrual cycle (Hampson, 1990) and as a consequence of hormone replacement therapy among surgically menopausal women (Sherwin, 1988). While the findings have been mixed and there apparently are no effects on such global measures as general intellectual functioning, higher levels of estrogen at the midluteal phase have been associated with improved performance on motor tasks (Hampson & Kimura, 1988) and articulatory rate (Hampson, 1990). In contrast, it has been reported that menstruating women perform better on tests of spatial ability than they do when estrogen levels are high (Hampson, 1990). Hampson and Kimura (1988, p. 458) concluded that, among the women they tested, "high levels of female hormones enhanced performance on tests at which females excel but were detrimental to performance on a task at which males excel." Sherwin (1988) reported that the performance on memory tests of women whose ovaries had been removed was inversely related to plasma sex steroid concentrations.

The Significance of Human Biological Rhythms

The existence of ultradian, circadian, and infradian rhythms in humans is significant for our model of personality functioning for a number of reasons.

First, it is important insofar as one's physiological state (Chapter 9) and certain aspects of state (e.g., arousal, activity level) may be variable and periodic or quasi-periodic. The overall state of an individual, although to some extent determined by the environment, also determines the probability of activation of various attractors (perceptions, memories, thoughts, and behaviors). If one's overall state varies periodically over time, it is to be expected that one's psychological activity will vary in a similar fashion. Although many of the effects of rhythmic variability may be subtle, the fact that the brain maintains itself in a self-organized critical state means that even subtle influences have the potential to produce significant effects.

Second, as proposed by Glass and Mackey (1988), rhythmic processes may become disrupted in a number of different ways, resulting in dynamic disorders. These disorders may involve loss of rhythmicity, appearance of rhythmicity where it should not occur, change in period length, or desynchronization of different rhythmic processes. Many sleep disorders, seasonal affective disorder, jet lag, and the irritability, fatigue, and malaise of rotating shift workers all represent such disturbances. There is some evidence that aging may be associated with temporal disorganization of rhythmic systems (Brock, 1991), a problem that may be especially apparent among older adults with sleep disturbances (Feinberg, 1974; Meguro et al., 1990).

Third, many kinds of psychological activity may be manifestations of a rhythmic process. Mice have been shown to have periodic fluctuations in such characteristics as "neurotic" behavior and emotionality, and while human behavior arguably is more complex than that of rodents (with certain possible exceptions), circadian rhythmicity may account for such things as variability in the severity of psychological symptoms or even the tendency of people to be somewhat more emotional in the evenings than in the morning (Poirel, 1982). Repetitive behavior or experiences, especially those that occur periodically or that tend to occur only at certain times of the day, should be considered as possibly reflecting temporal dynamics, in addition to (or as alternatives to) whatever learning theory or psychodynamic explanations might be adduced. For example, when a retarded man had a history of disruptive and violent behavior in different situations, with different people, and often without apparent precipitants—but always early in the morning—such a relationship was suggested.

DYNAMIC DISORDERS

Glass and Mackey (1979, 1988; Mackey & Glass, 1977; Mackey & Milton, 1987), and Crammer (1959) and Reimann (1963, 1974) before them, proposed the existence of *dynamic* or *periodic diseases,* which are disorders "characterized by abnormal temporal organization" (Glass & Mackey, 1988, p. 172). They argued that the following three types of changes in dynamics are possible and have been observed (pp. 172–173):

(1) variables that are constant or undergoing relatively small-amplitude "random" fluctuations can develop large-amplitude oscillations that may be more or less regular[, and thus] there may be the appearance of a regular oscillation in a physiological control system not normally characterized by rhythmic processes; (2) new periodicities can arise in an already periodic process; and (3) rhythmic processes can disappear and be replaced by relatively constant dynamics or by aperiodic dynamics.

Not all dynamic disorders need involve disturbances of periodicity; other dynamic factors that may affect functioning include decoupling of the activity of mutually interacting systems, and states of disequilibrium characterized by anomalous neural activity in one or more brain regions.

Glass and Mackey (1988) discussed several periodic disorders, some of which may involve disturbed periodic dynamics (e.g., atrial fibrillation), including conditions that are significant from neurological and psychological perspectives. These include premenstrual syndrome, certain quasi-periodic epilepsies, a subset of affective disorders (e.g., seasonal affective disorder), and jet lag. The abnormal dynamics of such diseases occur in the context of an apparently intact physiological system (Arbib, Érdi, & Szentágothai, 1998).

Disturbances of Periodic Functioning and Affective Disorders

There has been considerable speculation that certain affective disorders might reflect perturbations of periodic functioning. For example, Halberg (1968) suggested the "free-running" hypothesis of mood disorders, arguing that the rhythm of a pacemaker essential to the regulation of mood might escape from entrainment to a relatively fixed circadian cycle (probably the day–night cycle) and lead to cyclic affective disorders. Kripke et al. (1978) described a small group of rapidly cycling bipolar patients who showed such apparently free-running cycles, but the hypothesis has received only limited support. Kripke et al. (1978) also suggested the phase-advance hypothesis of depression, which ostensibly involves a stable (as opposed to free-running) shift in the phase relationships among various rhythmic systems.

Despite the methodological difficulties inherent in research on periodic phenomena, as well as the limited empirical support to date, several investigators have continued to pursue the importance of disrupted rhythms in affective disorders. Lewy and Sack (1987) reported successful treatment of depression by exposing patients to bright light over a period of days, presumably resetting certain physiological cycles. At least one condition—seasonal affective disorder—is reasonably well accepted as a periodic dynamic syndrome at this time and can be treated relatively effectively by properly timed exposure to light.

Further evidence supporting the possible relationship of depression to circadian dysregulation comes from studies of persons suffering jet lag and of rotating shift workers. Apparent phase shifting and desynchronization of different biological rhythms may produce malaise, insomnia, and gastrointestinal problems, among other symptoms (Monk & Gillin, 1984). Moreover, depression itself tends to have a circadian variability: patients frequently describe themselves as feeling more depressed in the morning, with some improvement in mood through the course of the day (Wehr & Goodwin, 1983).

It is interesting in this regard that electroconvulsive therapy (ECT) is effective with many persons who experience severe affective disorders. These observations are consistent with formulations that consider some affective disorders to be manifestations of disturbed neurophysiological phase relationships (Wehr & Goodwin, 1983). The precise mechanism of action of ECT is unknown, although given the literature suggesting a link between disturbed circadian rhythms and affective disorder, it seems a reasonable hypothesis that ECT might disrupt disturbed (possibly free-running) phase relationships, essentially wiping the slate clean and resetting them, allowing the normal phase relationships between periodic attractors to emerge. Over time, decoupling again may occur, necessitating repeated administrations of ECT.

Perseveration, Distractibility, and Confabulation

In addition to the three types of dynamic disorders discussed by Glass and Mackey (1988), we suggest that there are other kinds of dynamic disorders that may account for important aspects of pathological functioning. Unlike the disorders of temporal dynamics proposed by Glass and Mackey, these involve the mechanics of state changes. That is, they are associated with the ease or difficulty with which one activates, or shifts between, different attractors, and the degree to which such attractors are stable. Perseveration and distractibility, common sequelae of prefrontal cortex pathology, are disorders that might be considered in these terms.

Although there are different types of perseveration (Luria, 1965, 1980), in general *perseveration* can be thought of as getting stuck in a cognitive or behavioral rut—in an excessively and inappropriately stable attractor. E. Goldberg and Bilder (1987, p. 161) define perseveration as a behavioral situation "in which elements of previous tasks or behavior(s) fuse with an ongoing task or behavior, or when a behavior or operation cannot be terminated." When motor behavior is perseverative, a person may perform the same motor act continuously, long past the time when it would have been appropriate to stop and move on to something different.

Perseveration contaminates cognitive activity when elements of a previous task intrude on a new task that does not call for them. One patient, for example, immediately after performing several tasks that involved alternating tapping with his hands, was asked to shift between counting aloud and reciting the alphabet (i.e., "1 . . . a . . . 2 . . . b . . . 3 . . . c . . . "). He began tapping with his hands as he began the task, then became confused, and asked, "Should I be tapping? Do I have to take different hand positions?"

Perseveration reflects the brain's inability to escape from a specific basin of attraction. Frequently, input from another person is necessary to stop perseverative activity by an individual with a severe lesion of the prefrontal cortex. In dynamic terms, we might consider that a deficit in processes critical for prefrontal activation leaves the system with insufficient energy (i.e., insufficient neuronal input from outside the attractor's neural network) to activate a different network and hence escape from a basin of attraction. Another hypothesis is that change in background neural activity, perhaps a decrease in its chaotic quality, might leave an individual less able to shift out of an attractor in response to changing or novel conditions. The individual thus is unable to engage other attractors spontaneously or to initiate a less stereotyped form of activity. In contrast, the *distractibility* that sometimes is observed among persons with prefrontal lesions suggests an inability to settle into a single attractor without being captured by the basin of attraction of each new stimulus that comes along. The problem in this case is a difficulty establishing a stable limit cycle attractor.

In perseveration, the dynamic disturbance involves a change in one or more of the control parameters of the nervous system—possibly activation of the prefrontal cortex, which plays an important role in the regulation of purposeful behavior. Other neuropsychological control parameters could include (but are not limited to) the level of arousal, basal activity level, and speed of information processing. Depending on the level of analysis, other control parameters might be identified. Under normal circumstances, the prefrontal cortex may be activated when the brain is unable to activate a neural network appropriate for a specific situation, perhaps because the situation is unfamiliar. In the absence of prefrontal arousal, an inappropriate attractor (behavior, neural network) may be activated, or may remain perseveratively active.

Confabulation—the non-conscious and automatic filling in of gaps in memory by fabrication—may occur in conjunction with certain amnesic disorders. Neurologically impaired individuals who have both a severe memory problem and significant deficits in the executive cognitive functions (typically as a result of bilateral damage to the prefrontal cortex) may demonstrate this problem. Their recollection of past events, although fluent and often seemingly accurate, may be completely unreliable. Baddeley and Wilson (1986; also Baddeley, 1990) discussed one such patient who sustained a severe brain injury in a motor vehicle accident and who frequently gave "a very detailed but rather varied account of the accident, including verbatim and rambling descriptions of his conversation with the driver of the other vehicle" (Baddeley, 1990, p. 316). These descriptions had little likelihood of being accurate since the patient had been comatose for weeks following the accident. On one occasion, Baddeley (1990) noted, the patient described having written "a letter to an aunt in which he tells her of the death of his brother. In fact his brother was still alive and well. When this was pointed out, he explained the apparent inconsistency by claiming that after the death of his brother his mother had had another son and given the second son the same name" (p. 316).

Baddeley's patient wasn't deliberately making up details and information. Confabulation occurs without awareness or intention to deceive. It is somewhat like dreaming, in which ideas and images enter awareness spontaneously and are not evaluated critically. Even when they are recognized as bizarre, the dreamer usually rationalizes the bizarreness. The brain loses its selectivity in activating the neural networks (attractors) underlying specific memories and proceeds uncritically with whatever comes to mind. The outcome may be a floridly confabulatory syndrome. In dynamic terms, an almost unlimited number of neural networks mediating ideas and memories is accessible at any given time, but the brain activates and settles too readily into attractors that may be irrelevant. The brain's tendency to rationalize its actions, and to generate some sort of explanation of events, is likely to play a role in confabulation.

AMBIVALENCE AND INDECISION: A DYNAMIC BASIS?

Other psychological phenomena might be viewed from a dynamic perspective. Ambivalence, for example, could reflect vacillation between perceptions or thoughts mediated by neural networks that have shallow basins of attraction. In other words, when one is in a particular state, the probability of activating either of the attractors (e.g., a perception) or of shifting from one attractor to the other is high and roughly equal. It is easy to shift from one to the other. A change in state might alter the probabilities so that one alternative is more likely (or from a phenomenological perspective, more favorably considered) than the other, but a return to the initial state might be expected to restore the ambivalent or indecisive state of affairs.

The opposite situation (i.e., excessively deep basins of attraction) may contribute to other pathological conditions. For example, persons with certain personality disorders have a tendency to become deeply and unshakably entrenched in certain ideas or ways of perceiving other people. In paranoia, the dangers that lurk in the interpersonal world are constantly "discovered" and perceived. The paranoid person may have difficulty detecting novelty (such as the occurrence of a benign interpersonal situation) because of the depth and breadth of the basin of attraction associated with paranoid thinking. Rigid, unshakable perceptions may persist because their basins of attraction are very steep. Escape from them may require a change in state, which would be associated with a "resetting" of the probabilities of activation of the various neural networks that mediate such perceptions.

Metaphorically, the depth of a basin of attraction could be understood as analogous to the extent to which a specific neural network has been reinforced by learning. As a streambed is eroded and deepened by the constant or repeated flow of water, the attractor of a neural network might be deepened by repetition. Thus, with practice it becomes easy to activate the network (i.e., to move into a stable basin of attraction) necessary for the performance of a particular task. The breadth of a basin of attraction might be understood as the extent to which stimulus generalization has occurred in learning. A broad basin of attraction would be associated with a wide range of stimuli (as might be the case in mourning, in which there are myriad associations to the lost object of one's love), whereas a narrow basin of attraction would have few stimuli that might lead into it. Reflex epilepsy, for example, would have a very narrow basin of attraction.

The occurrence of such dynamic disorders could reflect some combination of biological predispositions and the consequences of experience and learning. In all likelihood, the relevant biological predispositions would reflect normally distributed variations in different aspects of neural organization. In the case of learning, variability may be intraindividual (e.g., reflecting differences in the intensity of a learning experience) or interindividual (reflecting differences among individuals with respect to the rapidity and robustness with which neural networks are modified by experience).

SENSITIVITY OF THE NERVOUS SYSTEM TO CHANGES IN ACTIVITY

Forced Shifts of Handedness and Stuttering

In the preceding section, we discussed periodicity and the manner in which certain disruptions of periodic dynamics may result in the emergence of pathological functioning. Disruption of periodicity may lead to pathology in part by upsetting the dynamic equilibrium of the brain, yielding different kinds of disturbed behavior. There are, of course, other ways in which the brain's equilibrium might become disorganized. In this section we examine how disruptions of cerebral dominance might yield pathology with a probable dynamic basis.

Several studies and a fair amount of anecdotal evidence suggest that at least some cases of stuttering may reflect incomplete lateral dominance (e.g., Curry & Gregory, 1969; Fox et al., 1996; R. K. Jones, 1966; Springer & Deutsch, 1981). That is, as children, some stutterers show no clear preference for the right or left hand. Orton (1925) was the first to propose that stuttering might be the result of conflictual interhemispheric dynamics, with neither side of the brain being fully dominant for speech. In Orton's time it was not uncommon for teachers and parents to force left-handed children to learn to write with their right hands, and among the stutterers he examined Orton discovered a number of such cases. The stuttering of these children was presumably of an iatrogenic sort, since when they were allowed to write with their left hands, the speech disorder resolved spontaneously.

More recently, Geschwind and Galaburda (1987) argued that stuttering and related problems are associated with a failure to develop right-handedness (i.e., to acquire left hemisphere dominance) and that the stuttering data "are compatible with the hypothesis that the influences that favor nonrighthandedness will in extreme cases lead to an increased frequency of learning disorders" (p. 86). The matter remains unresolved, and in any case it seems probable that there is more than one etiology for stuttering. Nevertheless, it is not difficult to find cases consistent with Orton's (1925) hypothesis. R. K. Jones (1966), for example, discussed a patient for whom a partial left frontal lobectomy cured severe stuttering, and three other patients in whom unilateral cortical hemorrhage (probably involving the frontal lobe) also eliminated stuttering.

A Dynamic Stuttering Disorder in an Adult

Marilyn was a 38-year-old student and medical technologist. She described herself as "ambidextrous" but said she was primarily left-handed. As a child she had used her left hand for drawing and other skilled tasks, but when she entered school her teacher encouraged Marilyn's parents to allow the child to use only her right hand for these same activities. At about that time, Marilyn began stuttering. Her parents expressed their concern to the teacher but were told she would "outgrow it"; in fact, within 12 months the stuttering stopped. Marilyn had no other history of neurological disorder or learning disability.

We serendipitously discovered that Marilyn was proficient at what is known as mirror writing (Orton, 1937; Streifler & Hofman, 1976; Trueman, 1965). That is, she could write either forward or backward, in mirror image, using either hand, and she could do it as quickly and legibly as she could write normally with her right hand. In fact, she could use her hands either individually or simultaneously, in the same direction or in opposite directions. Following our discovery of Marilyn's talent, we recruited her as a research subject, and over the course of a week she spent several hours writing with both hands. Within a few days she experienced a recurrence of stuttering, which had not affected her since childhood, and stated that she wished to discontinue the experimentation. Not only had she begun stuttering, but she was having frequent difficulty finding the precise word she wished to use, an unusual problem for this ordinarily very fluent woman. The testing was discontinued, and within 2 or 3 days the stuttering stopped.

We hypothesize that Margaret, who was naturally left-handed, originally may have had mixed dominance. As a result of intensive practice in school, she established the right hand as dominant, but this was associated with an easily perturbed dynamic equilibrium. Increased use of the left hand may have presented the brain with an unaccustomed pattern of neuronal activity, upsetting the balance between the cerebral hemispheres. This resulted in stuttering, which resolved spontaneously when the experiment was discontinued and a relatively stable state restored.

The study of persons who have undergone changes in handedness could yield some interesting data. One might, for example, study both right- and left-handed persons who have sustained injuries to or undergone surgery on their dominant or nondominant hand and subsequently are forced to use the opposite hand for skilled tasks. Whether changes in functioning would be observed among those who are strongly lateralized is an open question, but it is a reasonable hypothesis that those with mixed dominance might show a variety of interesting phenomena. Among persons with incomplete dominance, it may be that force of habit establishes a quasi-stable state that easily may be perturbed (with a subsequent bifurcation) as a result of altered patterns of activity in the cortex (i.e., by being forced to use the ordinarily auxiliary hand for skilled tasks). In such cases, one might observe a disorder that is dynamic in nature but to which one might be predisposed as a consequence of whatever developmental anomaly produced incomplete dominance.

SUMMARY AND CONCLUSION

A number of physiological processes are periodic, with a relatively regular period. These systems appear to be controlled by a kind of biological clock—entrained by environmental stimuli—that maintains periodicity. Such processes may be clinically important because the variability of the individual's state over time (which is affected in part by these rhythms) determines the probability that he or she will engage in specific behaviors. Moreover, disturbances in such processes may produce a number of clinical syndromes.

In this chapter we examined how either abnormal temporal organization or other disruption of the dynamic relationships between different regions of the brain may produce dynamic disorders. For example, oscillating systems may stop oscillating, may change their period, or may be out of phase with other systems with which they usually are coupled. In other cases, periodicity may appear where it previously was absent. In addition to these disturbances of timing, variations in the ease with which the system shifts into, out of, or between attractors may produce a number of pathological phenomena. Perseverative behavior may be an example of such a disorder.

Finally, we discussed data suggesting that the ordinary functioning of the nervous system may be perturbed by a wide range of externally and internally generated stimuli. Sensory deprivation (including that resulting from sensory impairment in older adults) and sensory overload may have significant deleterious effects on certain individuals, whereas they affect the overall state only minimally in other persons. Reflex epilepsy is a disorder in which a specific type of stimulation may lead to major perturbations in psychological and neurological functioning. Forced shifts in handedness among persons with incomplete dominance may produce stuttering and possibly other disorders.

9

THE PHYSIOLOGICAL STATE
AND THE BIOLOGY
OF EMOTION
AND MOTIVATION

INTRODUCTION

This chapter begins with a discussion of what we refer to as the *instantaneous physiological state* (*state*, or *physiological state*, for short), to which previous references have been made. We call it *instantaneous* because although it may appear stable, it continually fluctuates, and although the fluctuations may be subtle, one's state is never quite the same from one instant to the next. State is exquisitely sensitive to both the internal and external environments. The way we use the term it refers to the emergent property of a complex set of physiological factors affecting arousal, attention, activity level, affect, and motivational status. Some of these are more stable than others; many reflect circadian or other quasi-periodic variability; most of the neural processing affecting state occurs outside of awareness and beyond individual voluntary control.

The term *state* has been used in innumerable theoretical and colloquial contexts, of course, and it therefore is not surprising that the term means different things to different people. In this chapter we look at the concept of state from the perspective of dynamics: state is an emergent property of the self-organizing activity of the brain, acting as an organizer of experience, and influenced by experience itself in a variety of ways. State thus is understood to be a complex, multidimensional control parameter influencing behavior by affecting the probabilities associated with activation of specific neural networks, and influenced in turn on the biological level by the individual's psychological and behavioral activity.

In Chapter 8 we discussed a number of periodic, quasi-periodic, and aperiodic dynamic neurophysiologic processes, all of which are likely to interact with state in an ongoing way. In this chapter, after first analyzing some of the implications of considering state from the point of view of dynamics, we address several of the endogenous factors contributing to state. Specifically, we examine research on the neural basis of emotion and motivation—significant contributors to one's state—which suggests that significant aspects of emotional and motivational processing are likely to occur nonconsciously.

We then discuss some aspects of the functioning of the amygdala, the orbitofrontal cortex, and the hypothalamus. These structures are part of the neurophysiological architecture that support the emergence of states. Each is a sort of neurophysiological crossroads at which inputs from many different areas of the brain converge, interact with, and presumably influence one another. These same areas of the brain are involved in very complex, modular, self-organizing networks, the emergent properties of which are rather complex psychological phenomena. In later chapters we discuss several other psychological phenomena—including temperament, character, relationships, and conscious and nonconscious processing—all of which also interact with state in important ways.

STATE AS A DYNAMIC (PROCESS) CONSTRUCT

Considering state from the dynamic point of view has a number of implications. First, one's state is a *process* that has its origin in the nonlinear interactions and relationships of a large number of component processes and variables. Therefore, to one degree or another, one's state constantly fluctuates in concert with continually changing input from internal and external sources. A person's state therefore is not a *thing*, and neither is it static in nature, although it typically may be experienced and considered as stable. On the contrary, state is an emergent, constantly evolving process that plays its own particular role in the brain's self-organizing activities. Again, it is because of this moment-to-moment fluctuation in state that we refer to it as *instantaneous* physiological state.

States are important for a variety of reasons, but here we are concerned in particular with the fact that they influence the probability of activation of any given neural network. On the psychological level, this means that states are important in determining the likelihood that one will have certain thoughts, feelings, perceptions, memories, and inclinations toward behavior at any given moment. From the perspective of dynamics, state descriptions are thus, in part, assertions about probabilities. An individual's state—and the current environmental situation—establish the probability that a person will engage in a specific behavior, perceive the world in a particular way, or recall certain types of memories at any given moment. Moreover, in a nonlinear, recursive manner, a state acts as an organizer for the very same constituent processes that give rise to it. Thus, for example, while a number of influences may contribute to one's state, that state in turn provides a set of organizational and behavioral tendencies that influence one's experience of the multiple influences from which the state has arisen. If I am angry at the world and expect others to treat me abusively, my anger may lead me to behave in ways that provoke others to act shabbily toward me—a sort of feedforward process involving state, behavior, and the environment.

In common colloquial and clinical usage, the word "state" frequently is used to describe behavior deviating from some hypothetical "normal" baseline; state thus may be equated tacitly with pathology or deviation. Our concept of state should not be presumed to imply pathology. Indeed, from the dynamic point of view we can always describe any individual at any given moment in terms of his or her state. At some moments a state description may suggest psychopathology, but at other moments it may have no such implications. For example, a person can at one time be described as being in a "state of depression" or a "state of panic," whereas at other times an individual's state may have no particularly strong emotional valence.

Another implication of looking at state in terms of processes and their dynamics is that states, like other emergent properties of self-organizing systems, are characterized by fluctuations and bifurcations. We previously discussed the self-organizing behavior of a sandpile: recall that, as grains of sand are dropped onto the pile, there eventually comes a moment when a single grain leads to a major bifurcation of the system. Similarly, although the contributions of any given variable may have only minor effects on a person's overall state at any moment, there are likely to be times when a minor shift in the value of this same variable may lead to a major bifurcation (Figure 9.1). This appears to be the nature of nonlinear systems like the brain.

We previously noted how changes in processes across time can be represented graphically by means of a "phase portrait." This holds true for state as well and is a useful way of thinking about the contribution of different variables to state. For example, consider a phase portrait of a state as follows. Assume for the moment that the following 10 factors determine state: arousal level, point in the sleep–wake cycle, level of activity, mood, sympathetic nervous system activity, current emotional status, body temperature, blood glucose level, current status at that moment in a significant personal relationship, and short-term behavioral goals. (Most of these fac-

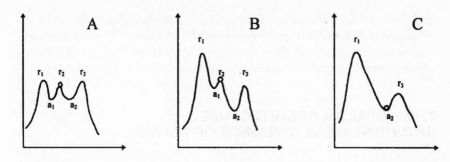

FIGURE 9.1. Schematic diagram demonstrating the realtionship between state and the probability of activation of different neural networks. Parts A, B, and C are used to illustrate the change in attractors and repellors over time. In Part A, the ball is balanced at an unstable point (r_2), which is a repellor. The likelihood of the ball moving into either attractor a_1 or a_2 is about equal. As the same control parameter changes, altering the overall state, a situation develops like that in Part B. Here r_1 has become a repellor with an even greater energy barrier (i.e., it is even less likely to occur). The basin of attractor a_1 now is more shallow than that of attractor a_2. While their probability of occurrence remains approximately equal, r_2 now is a repellor with a smaller energy barrier to attractor a_1, and when the ball rolls into a_1 it takes less energy for it to roll through r_2 into a_2. As the control parameter changes further (Part C), both attractor a_1 and repellor r_2 disappear. Now the probability landscape has changed so that attractor a_2 has the highest probability of occurring, while the probability of a_1 is essentially zero.

tors actually are complex functional systems reflecting the activity of numerous subsystems, each of which is composed of different complex neural networks.)

For simplicity, assume we can assign an integer value between –10 and 10 to each of these variables, representing the activity of specific neural systems. Then, at every instant we could describe a person's state by listing the set of numbers characterizing the activity in each subsystem; at one moment a person's current state might best be described as 7, –3, 2, 4, –3, 3, 4, –7, 0, 2. Fifteen minutes later it might have shifted to 7, –5, 1, 4, –4, 3, 4, –6, –1, 2. (These numbers, of course, are meant only for illustrative purposes.)

If at each instant we drew a graph in 10-dimensional space of an individual's ratings on these dimensions and followed them over a very long period of time, the resulting graph would form a phase portrait of the person's state over time. Out of the infinite number of possible configurations, our subject's phase portrait would be found primarily in only a few general regions of phase space, representing the fact that he or she tends to experience several broadly defined but recurring states most of the time. Some possible combinations would never be observed in a given individual (e.g., extreme mania), others would be highly unlikely, and others would be likely only under unusual conditions. Those states which cannot occur or which are highly unstable (extremely unlikely) and therefore short lived can be described as repellors; those states which are more likely to occur and which demonstrate relative stability can be described as attractors.

THE MODULAR ARCHITECTURE
AND NONLINEAR DYNAMICS OF STATES

We have noted that a person's state at any moment is a function of the complex interplay of a wide range of endogenous and environmental variables. Both the physical and social environment (e.g., ambient temperature and humidity, terrain, elevation, availability of food, familiarity of the culture, presence of family or friends, presence of guerrillas in ski masks with automatic weapons) play a significant role in determining state. Here we discuss several endogenous factors that influence state.

Previously we considered a number of periodic and quasi-periodic neurological and neuroendocrine processes that characterize human functioning: sleep–wake cycles, fluctuations in activity level during the day, the menstrual cycle, variability in serum cortisol, and so on. It seems obvious that these all are likely to influence one's state. If someone has not slept well for the past several nights, she may be more prone to doze off after lunch than if she is well rested. If she is susceptible to premenstrual syndrome (PMS), she may find that when she has PMS she is more likely to be withdrawn, or emotionally reactive, or simply to feel considerable physical discomfort that influences her feelings about herself and the world.

Periodic phenomena—infradian, circadian, and ultradian—also are likely to be important determinants of state (see Chapter 8). Two or more such periodic variables may occur in various phase relationships with one another. For example, a woman with cyclic mood variability and PMS may experience these in phase, in which case she may be at her most depressed at the same time that she is experiencing difficulty due to PMS. At other times, however, these cycles may be out of phase, in which case her overall state will be different than when they are in phase. The contributions of periodic physiological phenomena to state may be subtle or more overt, and probably account in part for such things as the variability of depressed mood throughout the day or the intensification of feelings of depersonalization and derealization at certain times. Such phasic variables combine with other more tonic influences to yield a continually variable overall state. And, to reiterate, as state varies, so does the probability of activating various neural networks and their associated behaviors, perceptions, and memories.

Various aspects of temperament also make a contribution to state (e.g., see A. H. Buss & Plomin, 1984; Gabbay, 1992; Tellegen et al., 1988). For example, basal level of activity appears to be temperamentally based and may differ considerably from one individual to another. Indeed, some infants have been observed to move nearly 300 times as much as other infants (Irwin, 1942). While such a level of activity may not be maintained, it nonetheless is likely to be an important determinant of a child's state. The same holds true for factors such as level of arousal, emotional reactivity, emotional intensity, chronic sympathetic (autonomic) arousal, sympathetic reactivity, and a number of other variables, all of which appear to be related to temperament and intraindividual constitutional variability.

Mood clearly makes significant contributions to state. Mood can be thought of as the manifestation of relatively persistent neurophysiological activity, determining the background emotional tone of a person's experience. Moods may be acute and short lived, or chronic and lifelong. They may vary periodically or quasi-periodically, probably in association with certain rhythmic physiological processes. Finally, moods establish a significant part of the context in which emotions occur in response to events in daily life. An individual who is chronically but mildly depressed may experience periods of happiness, but these are likely to be somewhat muted in their intensity.

Moods themselves are complex phenomena that demonstrate a modular structure. Among other factors, temperament is likely to be a powerful determinant of an individual's predominant mood states, so that some individuals seem to be predisposed to regular positive or negative mood states of varying degrees of intensity. Moods also are likely to be influenced significantly by environmental factors and experiences in relationships. Thus, parent loss or abandonment during infancy can result in a predisposition to depression. From the perspective of dynamics, repeated episodes of depression as an infant may serve to establish a neural network with a high probability of activation in a wide range of circumstances, through a process of "learning" much like the *kindling* that occurs in many seizure disorders (Post, 1992; see also Chapter 8). The depressive state thereby may acquire a basin of attraction that is deep (i.e., is difficult to get out of) and wide (i.e., may be induced by a wide range of stimuli).

Transient emotional reactions and shifts in motivational status also affect state. Happiness, elation, anger, sadness, fear, hunger, envy—all have both obvious and subtle effects on a person's state of mind. Certain emotions, as they arise, are especially likely (at least initially) to elicit species-specific patterns of automatic behavior. Fear, for example, activates the fight–flight–freeze system, so that a person who suddenly experiences fear is strongly inclined to become aggressive, to withdraw, or to "freeze up" and do nothing. Although such tendencies are modified by experience, they are likely to be especially compelling in determining state. As a rule, strong emotion in the presence of increased arousal disposes one to engage almost reflexively in relatively automatic behavior. The likelihood of conscious deliberation is minimized unless a person develops the habit of delaying a response to strong emotion, so it can be said that there is a high probability of acting without thinking under such circumstances.

Many other physiological variables also notably contribute to overall state. If you are mildly hungry, it may be possible to ignore the feeling for a while. Soon, however, you will probably find something to eat, and then hunger no longer will be a significant contributor to your state. So long as hunger goes unsatisfied, you will likely find your thoughts and actions organized around looking for food. Certain other physiological phenomena, such as sexual urges, may have a waxing and waning influence on state over time, having less urgency for the individual's survival than the more fundamental appetitive drives of hunger and thirst.

CONTEXT-DEPENDENT MEMORY

Context-dependent memory provides an interesting example of the role of state as an organizer of experience. It long has been held that certain aspects of the context in which learning occurs may affect subsequent recall (Baddeley, 1982; Overton, 1984; Teasdale & Fogarty, 1979; Teasdale & Russell, 1983). The adjectival terms *state-dependent, mood-dependent,* and *mood-congruent* have been applied to various aspects of this phenomenon. For example, an animal trained to respond in a certain way after injection of a particular drug may respond differently without the drug. In mood-dependent memory, knowledge acquired while an individual is in a particular mood is best recalled at a later date if that person is in that same mood; it is less well remembered if he or she is experiencing a different affective state (Bower, Monteiro, & Gilligan, 1978; M. H. Johnson & Magaro, 1987; Weingartner, Miller, & Murphy, 1977). The concept of mood-congruent memory suggests that the important variable in recall is whether the affective valence of information is congruent with one's emotional status. Thus, events and information learned or experienced while a person is depressed are best recalled when he or she is depressed again (Blaney, 1986). In this respect, state influences recall.

Although the concepts of mood-dependent and mood-congruent memory make intuitive sense and are consistent with much experiential data, research on the effects of context on learning and recall has yielded mixed results. In part this may be due to problems with methodology, including the means by which specific moods are induced in experimental subjects (the clear findings of the study of Weingartner et al., 1977, were obtained with manic psychiatric patients; most studies have used college students pressed into service as experimental subjects). In his analysis of the literature, Eich (1995) suggested that a major variable affecting mood-dependent outcomes is whether the events to be recalled are internally generated (e.g., thoughts or images) or externally generated (word lists read aloud by an experimenter's research assistant). When internally generated, a second variable involved in mood-dependent outcomes is the extent to which recall is facilitated by the environment. Note that these experiments controlled only a small number of the variables that contribute to state; uncontrolled variation in other important variables is liable to wash out some of the effects. In any case, it appears that an individual is more likely, in a specific mood state, to recall thoughts and images associated with that state. In the same way, when in a particular state, a person is more likely to behave in certain ways associated with that state than in various other ways not so associated.

HOW STATE INFLUENCES BEHAVIOR AND COGNITION: AN ILLUSTRATION

Hunger motivates people to find food. Hunger is a conscious feeling associated with an organism's need for the raw material needed to support metabolism. At a cellular level, hunger arises because cells' demand for nutrients outstrips supply of those nutrients in the blood. In response to certain molecular stimuli, periventricular and hypothalamic neurons apparently initiate processes which, among other things, stimulate the sensation of hunger, eventually leading the individual to develop a plan for obtaining food.

Although a hungry person has no awareness of what is going on in the neural substrate, as he or she goes longer and longer without food, attentional processes and perceptual gating may become altered so that sensory stimuli related to food become more salient. After 2 or 3 days of fasting, people become acutely aware of food-like odors. When you're hungry, a pizza may look and smell delicious. On the other hand, if you've just stuffed yourself, what's left of that same pizza may look and smell a lot like garbage. As a person goes longer without eating, the preoccupation with food may take on a sense of great urgency as distributed neural centers mediating affect are recruited. Yet, with all this neural activity taking place, even if a person fully understood the physiological processes involved in hunger, all he or she would be directly aware of would be the feeling of hunger and associated emotion. Such feelings are an emergent property of neural activity in response to the cells' need for food. Thus, the psychological experience of hunger reflects a series of neural processes that model one major aspect of an organism's physiological state. We neither experience directly nor need to know the physiological basis for our hunger.

The manner in which a state organized around extreme hunger may influence psychological functioning is graphically illustrated by the behavior of starving people. An example of this comes from the experience of the unfortunate men who accompanied U.S. Army officer A. W. Greely, who set out on the steamer *Proteus* to explore the Canadian Arctic in the summer of 1881. By August of that year, Greely and his two dozen crew members reached a point on Ellesmere Island about 600 miles from the North Pole. They left the *Proteus* locked in the ice, planning to spend the winter in a hut near the northern end of the island at a place called Fort Conger. The first winter passed relatively uneventfully.

Greely and his party had anticipated spending two or more winters in the Arctic, and had brought what they thought would be a sufficient supply of provisions. Nevertheless, a resupply ship was sent to meet them the following summer. Unfortunately this ship was blocked by ice from reaching Greely in August 1882, and he and his men were unable to obtain fresh food and supplies. This set the stage for a worsening situation in the summer of 1883, when events conspired once again to prevent them from obtaining adequate supplies for the coming winter. The already-short summer (6–8 weeks) ended early that year, and given that the sea already had frozen over, it was clear that more provisions would not be coming. The party therefore attempted to head south, and by October 1883 had arrived at Cape Sabine, where they settled in for another dark Arctic winter.

Now perilously short of food, the hungry crew became increasingly desperate. At one point, some men ate dog biscuits that previously had been thrown away by the party's physician, Octave Pavy, because, as Pavy noted in his journal, they "had been reduced to a filthy green slime." The group's condition was described by crew member Lt. James B. Lockwood, who wrote in his journal that "we are now constantly hungry and the constant thought and talk run on food, dishes of all kinds, and what we have eaten, and what we hope to eat when we reach civilization. I have a constant longing for food" (Berton, 1988, p. 465).

Lockwood wrote long memoranda to himself about what he had eaten, and what he intended to eat when he returned home. On November 23 he reported that he had eaten a raw fox's foot, and followed his mention of that meal with the phrase "pie of orange and coconut." On the 25th of November he made a list of foods he would keep in his room for late night snacks when he returned to Washington. There were 35 items, "ranging from smoked goose and eel to Virginia seedling wine and Maryland biscuit" (Berton, 1988, p. 468). In the end, only a few men survived, and they had at times resorted to extraordinary measures. Dr. Pavy, for example, had eaten parts of the corpses of 6 of the 19 deceased crew members, a behavior that one can only assume would have been somewhat less likely had his state been different than it was.

Changes in state need not be so extreme to produce significant alterations in the probability of specific behaviors, percepts, or memories. Even subtle changes in one or two control parameters potentially could result in rather different outcomes (although an urge to indulge oneself in cannibalism probably requires a pretty extreme state).

INTRODUCTION TO THE BIOLOGY OF EMOTION AND MOTIVATION

Emotions obviously serve an array of different and important functions, yet there is much about emotional processing that is poorly understood. The complexity of emotion and its various roles in human psychology were noted by Rolls (1995), who discussed the following "functions" of emotion: (1) eliciting autonomic and endocrine responses that prepare the body for action; (2) facilitating flexible responses to reinforcing stimuli; (3) motivating the individual to take action; (4) communicating; (5) social bonding; (6) determining how one evaluates events or memories; (7) facilitating the storage of memories; (8) producing persistent motivation and direction of behavior; and (9) triggering the recall of episodic memories. There may be others as well that Rolls didn't address.

Earlier in this chapter we defined *state* as the emergent property of a hierarchically organized system, itself constituted of a number of modular subsystems. Thus, a multitude of endogenous and exogenous factors contribute to a person's state at any given time. In this section and those that follow we take a closer look at some aspects of the anatomy, physiology, and neuropsychology of emotion and motivation. Consistent with our central thesis, we review findings suggesting that the systems associated with emotion and motivation have a modular architecture, widely distributed and hierarchically organized. We won't undertake an in-depth exploration of emotion and motivation. Any effort to address these topics comprehensively would take us too far afield from the main focus of this work. Our goals are more circumscribed. First, we wish to show how, to a significant extent, motivation and emotion are dissociable subsystems of a hierarchically organized, modular, distributed, self-organizing system. Next, we will review data demonstrating that the neural systems involved in motivation and emotion include both cortical and subcortical pathways, a design that contributes to the dissociability of emotion and motivation from awareness.

Emotions arise nonconsciously in response to internal and external stimulation. They may remain on the periphery of awareness, but when associated with increased arousal they tend to dominate conscious processing. Hence, people often feel before they *know what* they feel. The result, LeDoux argues (1996) is that much emotional experience has a nonconscious quality.

Finally, we consider research findings regarding several regions of the brain that appear to be important for processes associated with emotion and motivation. Although emotionality and motivation are widely distributed, hierarchically organized systems, certain specific cerebral structures appear to have particular significance for the complex dynamic processes involved in emotional and motivational processing. For example, some areas of the brain have been shown to be associated with different emotional and motivational states. Certain of these, when stimulated, appear to be rewarding, whereas others appear to produce unpleasant feelings. The relationship between these regions remains somewhat unclear, but they clearly belong to complex distributed networks that are essential to the experience of emotion.

LATERALIZATION OF DEPRESSIVE AFFECT

Given the complexity of the demands and tasks assigned to emotional functioning by the trial-and-error process of evolution, it is not surprising that the neurophysiological and neurodynamic underpinnings of emotionality are correspondingly complex. Research findings regarding the lateralization of depressive affect demonstrate some of this complexity.

It appears that the right and left hemispheres of the brain may be specialized for mediating pleasant and unpleasant affects, respectively. Schaffer, Davidson, and Saron (1983) found that the EEG of persons who were mildly depressed, compared with nondepressed persons, showed significantly lower levels of left frontal activation. The same observation was reported in another study among persons who were clinically depressed (Henriques & Davidson, 1991)— a pattern observed both when these people were depressed and in remission. In yet another study, examining a nonclinical sample of 100 subjects, Davidson found that persons with consistently "extreme" left frontal activation experienced more positive affect than did those with consistently "extreme" right frontal activation. These findings were consistent with those of Robinson et al. (1984), as well as other investigators, who have reported that persons with left frontal strokes are more likely to experience depression than are persons with right-hemisphere strokes.

Using positron emission tomography (PET), Drevets et al. (1992) took a different approach to the analysis of local activity in depression (see also Drevets & Raichle, 1995). These authors studied persons who had both unipolar depression and a family history of the disorder. They found increased cerebral blood flow in the left prefrontal cortex and in the left amygdala at the time subjects reported being depressed, but only in the left amygdala by the time the depression had remitted. In still other work, subjects were asked to induce feelings of sadness by thinking of sad thoughts or memories. Here again, blood flow was increased in the left prefrontal cortex (Pardo, Pardo, & Raichle, 1993). These results are consistent with the report of R. M. Cohen et al. (1992) concerning persons with seasonal affective disorder, but they are at odds with findings reported for bipolar depressed patients (e.g., see Buchsbaum et al., 1986).

Davidson explained this reported asymmetry in frontal activation by arguing that the right frontal cortex and left frontal cortex reflect "specialized systems for approach and withdrawal behavior, with the left frontal region specialized for the former and the right frontal region specialized for the latter" (1992, p. 40). Drevets and Raichle (1995) offer a somewhat more complex explanation for their own findings. In any case, whatever is going on with respect to the lateralization of emotion is certainly as yet unresolved. Why, among depressed persons, did Drevets and his associates find increased left frontal metabolism, whereas Davidson and his colleagues found decreased EEG activity in the same region? We don't know. Nevertheless, while the specific findings are difficult to interpret, the data provide support for the more general hypothesis that depression and positive affect may be mediated by different regions of the brain.

SEIZURES AND EMOTION

It has long been observed that seizure activity can perturb emotional functioning in various ways. Why this is so remains an open question, but findings concerning the relationship between seizures and emotionality are interesting. For our purposes, one important implication of this relationship is that it underscores the degree to which emotional functioning emerges from complex dynamic processes involving many distributed neural networks.

Epilepsy may produce a broad range of both transient and more enduring emotional phenomena. Some seizures, for example, involve laughing (gelastic epilepsy) and, less commonly, crying (Daly, 1975; Daly & Mulder, 1957; Engel, 1989; Gascon & Lombroso, 1971). Anger, fear, depression, embarrassment, sadness, and guilt have been reported as ictal phenomena, but so have pleasant feelings, including elation and euphoria, sexual sensations, and orgasm (Daly, 1975). There may be feelings of uncanny familiarity (e.g., déjà vu), as well as feelings that familiar things are strange and unfamiliar (jamais vu). Other somewhat more common disturbances of the sense of reality include depersonalization and derealization.

The interictal period (i.e., the period between seizures) of certain epileptics also may be marked by unusual emotional phenomena. Psychosis can occur, especially in conjunction with complex partial seizures (e.g., temporal lobe epilepsy). Decreased libido is common (Dansky, Andermann, & Andermann, 1970; Gastaut & Colomb, 1954; Lindsay, Ounsted, & Richards, 1979). Hyperreligiosity, sometimes accompanied by abrupt religious conversion (Dewhurst & Beard, 1970), and "deepened emotions" are among the personality traits most frequently attributed to persons with temporal lobe epilepsy (Blumer, 1975). The occurrence of these often discrete emotional states, as both ictal and interictal phenomena, is in some senses a spontaneous version of the elicitation of emotions by means of electrical stimulation, discussed later.

LEDOUX'S NEUROPSYCHOLOGICAL THEORY OF EMOTION

The precise manner in which emotion is mediated by the brain remains to be elucidated. There are, however, several theoretical formulations that account for many of the research findings (LeDoux, 1995, 1996; Rolls, 1995). We focus in particular on work done by J. E. LeDoux, who has studied fear, fear conditioning, and the amygdala, and whose thinking we will try to summarize in the following paragraphs.

A fear-arousing stimulus is perceived by the brain through both subcortical and cortical pathways. The subcortical pathways are very rapid, requiring 10s of milliseconds to respond, and they may prime emotional reactions to stimuli of which we are incapable of becoming aware (Zajonc, 1968, 1980, 1982, 1984; for a thorough review see Bornstein & Pittman, 1992). Fear conditioning, via the amygdala, occurs through these subcortical networks. In a threatening situation, the amygdala induces increased cortical arousal, in part through the nonspecific cholinergic effects of a forebrain structure called the basal nucleus, but also through brainstem arousal systems. These processes occur *preconsciously,* prior to clear awareness of the stimulus.

The amygdala also receives inputs from cortical areas involved in later stages of perceptual processing (LeDoux, 1996) and projects back to both earlier and later cortical processing areas. Because cortical processing involves more synapses in sequence than does the subcortical route, conduction through the cortical pathways, which have access to awareness, is slower than through the subcortical paths. The cortex, however, has access to a more accurate and fine-grained representation of the emotion-inducing stimulus than does the subcortical route. According to LeDoux (1996, p. 165), the subcortical input, which comes directly from the thalamus, "is unfiltered and biased toward evoking responses. The cortex's job is to prevent the inappropriate response rather than to produce the appropriate one." The two processes operate very much like feedforward and feedback systems.

These cortical and subcortical systems are dissociable. The amygdala has considerable access to the hippocampal declarative memory system, and hence the events associated with emotional conditioning may be consolidated as declarative memories. The declarative memories, however, are significantly more amenable to alteration over time, whereas emotional memories—at least at the subcortical level—appear to be "indelible" (LeDoux et al., 1989). The cortex may be able to inhibit emotional memories, but they are prone to reemerge intact in response to a variety of circumstances (e.g., see Jacobs & Nadel, 1985). The dissociability of memory systems, which was discussed in Chapter 5, has significant implications for the clinical situation (which we address later in Chapters 12, 15, 16, and

17). For now, it is sufficient to note that these findings support the existence of nonconscious emotional processing networks that may be inaccessible to introspection and that operate in parallel with conscious networks.

Cortically processed representations of the environment reach awareness in conjunction with feedback from the body. These include sensations associated with sympathetic arousal (increased pulse and respiration, sweating, and other phenomena), as well as others resulting from neuroendocrine response (e.g., the release of epinephrine). Different emotions are associated with various patterns of autonomic and endocrine response (Ekman, Levenson, & Friesen, 1983; LeDoux, 1996), and Levenson (1992) suggests that there are at least five different patterns of autonomic nervous system reaction associated with different emotions (see also Zajonc & McIntosh, 1992). These autonomic and endocrine processes, which are relatively slow to dissipate, are in large part responsible for the sustained feeling of an emotion.

According to Halgren and Marinkovic (1995), the awareness of an emotional response to an event also involves orienting (arousal), along with integration of the stimulus with associations in long-term episodic and semantic memory, and with "the current cognitive and emotional context" (p. 1138). People organize perceptions of the current situation through some process that includes categorizing the situation in terms of its emotional valence and in accordance with previous experience. The result is "an affective coloring and cognitive interpretation of even the most mundane events. The event, as encoded during event integration, is itself integrated with the context for action, resulting in voluntary (conscious) acts" (p. 1138).

LeDoux's neuropsychological theory differs significantly from "cognitive appraisal" theories of emotion (Arnold, 1960; R. S. Lazarus, 1984; Schachter & Singer, 1962), which maintain that emotion is a felt reaction to a cognitive assessment of a given situation. Cognitive appraisal theories hold that this assessment occurs at an early stage in the process of emotional reaction, and they rest in part on the assumption that we have introspective access to the causes of our emotions (LeDoux, 1996).

LeDoux summarizes the fundamental difference between the cognitive appraisal theories and his own thinking as follows:

> If emotions are triggered by stimuli that are processed unconsciously, you will not be able to later reflect back on those experiences and explain why they occurred with any degree of accuracy. Contrary to the primary supposition of cognitive appraisal theories, the core of an emotion is not an introspectively accessible conscious representation. Feelings do involve conscious content, but we don't necessarily have conscious access to the processes that produce the content. And even when we do have introspective access, the conscious content is not likely to be what triggered the emotional responses in the first place. The emotional responses and the conscious content are both products of specialized emotion systems that operate unconsciously. (1996, p. 299)

This is not to say that cognition is unimportant in emotionality. Despite the fact that cognition is minimally involved in the early stages of emotional reaction, cognitive processes can affect emotion, directly or indirectly. One may, for example, have a vaguely guilty feeling for reasons that are outside of awareness, and interpret it as a reaction to certain actions earlier in the day, perhaps with a consequent change in the affective color of one's experience. Psychotherapy is able to have an effect on emotional disorders in part because of the capacity of cognition to influence emotional state.

The dissociability and nonconscious nature of much emotional processing have significant clinical ramifications, explicated in greater detail in subsequent chapters, particularly Chapters 12, 15, and 16. In any case, it appears that people often don't know what they feel, even when they already may have started to feel something. Furthermore, emotional responses tend to take place primarily nonconsciously. This is not to say that affects and awareness are *necessarily* dissociated. Indeed, emotional functioning and awareness work in parallel. Rather, awareness in any case is likely to follow the onset of emotional processing, and much of this processing may remain nonconscious. In Chapter 12 we review findings suggesting that people often initiate actions nonconsciously and subsequently provide post hoc rationalizations for their actions.

Now we turn from this neuropsychological discussion of emotion to a consideration of different regions of the brain implicated in mediating emotional and motivational status. Most of the work that produced these findings involved either the placement of lesions in specific brain sites or the electrical stimulation of those sites. In particular, we are concerned with the medial forebrain bundle, septum, hypothalamus, orbitofrontal cortex, and amygdala.

INTRACRANIAL ELECTRICAL STIMULATION OF THE BRAIN

In the early 1950s, certain technical advances made it possible to implant wire electrodes that remained in place more or less permanently (i.e., unless they fell out) in the brains of experimental animals. This capacity allowed experimenters to deliver stimulation to relatively discrete areas of the brain and opened up the possibility of teaching animals to stimulate themselves by means of instrumental behaviors such as bar pressing. Many of these early studies dealt with the avoidance of unpleasant stimulation and attempts to obtain pleasurable stimulation.

Delgado, Roberts, and Miller (1954) were among the first to investigate these phenomena. They found that animals stimulated via an electrode in certain regions of the brain demonstrated fearful behavior when later returned to the same area of the cage in which they received the stimulation.

J. Olds and M. E. Milner tried to follow up on this earlier work, but a misguided electrode led to an unanticipated effect. Instead of avoiding the area of the cage in which it was stimulated, the animal seemed to loiter and even come back, apparently seeking more stimulation.

Intrigued by this behavior, J. Olds and Milner (1954) next trained animals to press a pedal that could deliver pleasurable stimulation to the brain. When no stimulation was given in response to a press on the pedal, rats were observed to press it fewer than five times an hour (J. Olds, 1958). On the other hand, "if the pedal-pressing produced a reward, the rate, even for the first hour, rose to 200 or more responses an hour; thus, 'reward' was clearly discernible. If the pedal-pressing produced punishment, the rate dropped radically; there were only two or three responses during the total experimental procedure" (J. Olds, 1958, p. 316). According to Olds, after only one inadvertently self-administered stimulus to a highly rewarding area, rats enthusiastically tried to figure out what had happened and how to reproduce it. Some rats learned to press the pedal at rates as high as 7,000 repetitions per hour (or nearly twice per second).

These results seemed to contradict Clark L. Hull's *drive reduction* theory of motivation (1943), which held that it is the reduction in intensity of a need state (or drive) that animals find reinforcing. The self-stimulation results suggested instead that the animals were pressing a bar because it felt good, and J. Olds and Milner (1954) theorized that the effect had to do with the activation of centers important for satisfying hunger, thirst, or sexual urges. J. Olds (1958), reviewing this work, noted that animals would endure painful foot shocks and sometimes forego eating in order to stimulate their brains; in fact, "when animals were run for periods of an hour a day, they usually maintained the same rate of self-stimulation throughout the hour and for as many days or months as they were tested" (p. 319). If allowed to continue stimulating themselves ad libitum they "continued to respond as long as physiological endurance permitted" (p. 319).

There were, of course, questions about whether the stimulation actually was pleasurable, or whether, for example, it simply might induce compulsive, repetitive behavior. A series of experiments suggested the former (although some regions, when stimulated, elicit seemingly compulsive and stereotyped behavior), and experiments on humans[1] established that some kinds of intense pleasure, including sexual feelings and even orgasm, could be elicited by stimulation of the appropriate brain regions (Delgado, Hamlin, & Chapman, 1952; Heath, 1964, 1972; Sem-Jacobsen, 1968; Valenstein, 1973).

---

[1]These were the halcyon days of human brain research, before messy informed consent requirements and meddlesome institutional review boards could get in the way of research on such once popular ideas as prefrontal lobotomy (e.g., see Freeman & Watts, 1946; Moniz, 1936).

THE MEDIAL FOREBRAIN BUNDLE
AND SELF-STIMULATION

Following this initial work, a number of researchers subsequently demonstrated that stimulation of various brain structures appeared to be highly rewarding (Carter & Phillips, 1975; M. E. Olds & J. Olds, 1963; Simon, LeMoal, & Cardo, 1975), whereas stimulation of certain others was aversive, sometimes extremely so. As might be anticipated, things turned out to be not quite as simple as originally hoped. For example, it was found that animals not only will work to attain stimulation but also will press a bar to terminate it when it is constantly turned on (Bower & Miller, 1958; W. W. Roberts, 1958). Moreover, some kinds of stimulation are more rewarding when an animal is in certain motivational states (e.g., hunger due to food deprivation) than in others (Conover & Shizgal, 1994; R. A. Frank & Stutz, 1984; Hoebel & Teitelbaum, 1962; Hoebel & Thompson, 1969). The most rewarding regions for self-stimulation appear to be in the *septum*, the *nucleus accumbens*, and the *medial forebrain bundle* (MFB), a tract that contains output fibers from hypothalamus to both the midbrain posteriorly and the septal area anteriorly. In large part, the areas that are rewarding when stimulated are associated with the neurotransmitter dopamine (Wise, 1980, 1996; Yeomans, 1982).

Brain sites most likely to produce punishing effects are fewer in number and are concentrated especially in the midbrain near the cerebral aqueduct (the *periaqueductal gray matter;* Delgado et al., 1954). The aversive quality of stimulation in these sites sometimes is attenuated by opiates (Kiser & German, 1978), and Reynolds (1969) found that analgesia can be produced by stimulation of the gray matter of the midbrain. While this analgesia has been reproduced in humans, it can be accompanied by vertigo and with intensely unpleasant sensations of suffocation and nausea (Isaacson, 1982; Richardson & Akil, 1977), suggesting that it is unlikely to catch on as a treatment for chronic pain unless a managed care organization is able to develop an inexpensive procedure for stimulating the periaqueductal gray matter.

Stimulation of human brains, including the implantation of self-stimulation hardware in humans, has produced some interesting phenomenological reports. In particular, the "rewarding" sensation frequently is said to be very pleasant but also very difficult to describe. Some subjects have said that they persisted in stimulating themselves in part to try to produce the sensation for long enough to be able to understand what it was really like, without much success (Valenstein, 1973). Presumably their pleasurable self-stimulation was done largely for the advancement of science.

The specific functions of these "rewarding" brain structures are obscured by the complexity of the research results. While septal stimulation generally is rewarding, animals with lesions of the septum demonstrate increased levels of rage and emotionality for 15–20 days following surgery, with subsequent decreased levels of aggression and a tendency "to interact well with other members of their species" (Isaacson, 1982, p. 144). They tend to avoid fights, and when a fight breaks out they usually are defeated by animals with an intact septum. Thus, as might be expected, animals that were socially dominant presurgically are likely to lose status after lesions are made in the septal area (Gage, Olton, & Bolanowski, 1978).

These findings demonstrate the importance of pleasurable and punishing sensations in motivating specific behaviors, and illustrate the complex modular distributed character of the networks underlying reward and punishment. All animals (including humans, of course) are strongly motivated to seek pleasure and to avoid what feels painful. From an evolutionary perspective this seems very reasonable. If certain adaptive behaviors (such as eating and having sex) feel very good, animals are more likely to engage in them, and hence to survive and pass on their genes. One only has to consider the anhedonic state of depression, for example, in which both libido and appetite may be diminished, to see the importance of this relationship for natural selection. Moreover, it is important to note that the pleasurable effects of many drugs commonly used for recreational purposes seem to be active in dopaminergic pathways, especially in the MFB and nucleus accumbens.

REGULATION OF APPETITE:
A MODULAR DISTRIBUTED SYSTEM

The hypothalamus is a small but complex structure involved in autonomic regulation of the viscera. It is bilaterally symmetric, divided into left and right sides by the third ventricle, and it can be further subdivided into periventricular (i.e., near the ventricle), medial, and lateral zones. The MFB passes between the medial and lateral areas, as well as through the lateral area (Isaacson, 1982). The hypothalamus secretes several hormones and also affects the secretion of hormones by the anterior pituitary. It has the capacity to produce changes in neural activity throughout the nervous system. Stimulation of the hypothalamus, especially the lateral portions, has been shown to produce pleasurable sensations, changes in motivational state, and various kinds of behavior. Lesions of different regions of the hypothalamus have been shown to produce a wide range of phenomena, including strong emotional reactions (Eclancher & Karli, 1971; Isaacson, 1982), neglect of stimuli on the side opposite the lesion (J. F. Marshall, Turner, & Teitelbaum, 1971), and disturbances of eating and drinking (Chi

& Flynn, 1971; Heatherington & Ranson, 1942; Teitelbaum, 1955; Teitelbaum & Epstein, 1962).

In the 1950s and 1960s, much research was done on the possible role of the hypothalamus in the regulation of eating behavior. Teitelbaum and Epstein (1962) demonstrated that lesions of the lateral hypothalamus (LH) caused rats to stop eating and drinking. Unless extraordinary measures were used to keep them alive, they died. If kept alive, they gradually recovered some spontaneous eating and drinking behavior but remained impaired in response to certain physiological challenges. Recovered animals never fully regained their presurgical weight and had a number of other physiological abnormalities. Curiously, this postsurgical outcome could be altered by depriving animals of food prior to lesioning (Powley & Keesey, 1970), in which case the postoperative feeding disturbance (aphagia) and drinking disturbance (adipsia) could be diminished or even nearly eliminated.

Heatherington and Ranson (1942) showed that while lesions of the LH produce aphagia and adipsia, lesions in the ventromedial nucleus of the hypothalamus produced hyperphagia (overeating) and extreme obesity (see also Snapir et al., 1976), and a similar syndrome was proposed in humans (Reeves & Plum, 1969). Stellar (1954) suggested that eating and drinking behavior reflected a sort of equilibrium in the activity between these two areas, which were presumed to be "feeding" and "satiety" centers, respectively. In simplified form, it was proposed that the LH was a sort of "on" switch that turned appetite on, whereas the ventromedial nucleus turned appetite off when the animal was satisfied. The theory sounded good—but as it turned out, it was wrong.

Part of the problem is that lesions created by researchers in the 1950s and 1960s were crudely made using the uninsulated tip of an electrode; tissue was destroyed in a fairly large area around the electrode tip. Thus, lesions of the LH also might destroy fibers of the MFB that run through the LH. These electrolytic lesions thus affected more widespread areas than was thought to be the case at the time, a fact which might account for the wide range of deficits, in addition to aphagia, observed among lesioned animals (Isaacson, 1982). The more recently acquired ability to make precise chemically induced lesions has led researchers to reexamine the LH syndrome (for a review see Winn, 1995). Winn and his associates (Dunnett, Lane, & Winn, 1985; Winn, Tarbuck, & Dunnett, 1984) found that using ibotenic acid instead of electrolytic lesions produced adipsia and aphagia in comparison with a control group, but the extent of the disorder was much less severe than that of an electrolytically lesioned comparison group. Moreover, nonfeeding disorders associated with electrolytic lesions of the LH (e.g., spatial neglect) were not observed in animals lesioned with ibotenic acid.

Arguing from his own data and the findings of previous work by

Lawes (1988), Winn (1995) proposed that rather than being a function of simple feeding and satiety "centers," eating and drinking behavior are controlled by "a series of interconnected structures that form a core within the brain, extending along the walls of the cerebral ventricles. Most importantly, nearly all structures included in this system are associated with some aspect of eating and drinking" (p. 186). There thus seems to be a complex distributed system that regulates the body's internal environment, signaling the need for eating or drinking. These structures include the LH, which, according to Winn, receives input from this system. The primary output of the LH is to the frontal cortex, which is involved in the organization of behavior. Thus the LH may be an "interface" between subsystems monitoring the organism's nutritional needs and behavior executed in order to meet those needs (Winn, 1995).

The brain processes information about hunger, as well as about the appearance, taste, odor, and texture of food. All these variables interact, and they apparently are processed at several hierarchical levels. For example, the basic components of taste (e.g., salty) first are processed in the nucleus of the solitary tract (Beckstead, Morse, & Norgren, 1980; Scott & Giza, 1992) and primary gustatory cortex (in the frontal operculum and insula); then in the orbitofrontal secondary taste cortex these basic tastes are integrated to yield complex sensations and are modulated by hunger for specific tastes. Thus, if an animal has had its fill of glucose, it may refuse more sweet food but may remain interested in other foods (Mora et al., 1979).

The rewarding value of a specific food at any point during hunger and feeding is reflected in changes in the activity of specific populations of neurons. As you fill up on dinner, neurons that initially fired rapidly in response to the smell and taste of the food decrease their rate of firing. When your desire for the foods served at dinner has waned, so has the activity of these neurons, although if you have not yet started your dessert, neurons responsive to sweet tastes may have a high rate of activity (in other words, the smell and taste of dessert remains rewarding despite the fact that otherwise you feel like you've had enough to eat). As is true for taste, the smell of food is processed hierarchically, first in the olfactory bulb, then in the primary olfactory (pyriform) cortex, and then in two or three areas of the orbitofrontal cortex, where it is integrated with taste, texture, and reward (see Rolls, 1999, for a review of neural control of eating and reward).

STIMULATION OF THE HYPOTHALAMUS AND ELICITED BEHAVIOR

Stimulation of the LH has been shown to cause experimental animals to engage in different kinds of stereotyped behavior, referred to as *elicited* behaviors. Sometimes all that is observed is an increase in activity, but certain behaviors which appear to satisfy no particular motives may be elicited by stimulation at levels too low to be rewarding. These include nest building, eating, licking or drinking, gnawing on wood, aggressive behavior, and sexual behavior (Isaacson, 1982).

One especially interesting aspect of these elicited behaviors is that stimulation at certain sites in the hypothalamus produces different behaviors depending on what objects are present. If she has rat pups available, a female rat may groom them. If a drinking tube is present, the rat may lick it—but if the tube is removed, the rat won't necessarily drink from a dish. If stimulation routinely elicits a particular activity (such as gnawing on wood) and the objects associated with that activity are removed, another stereotypical behavior may emerge as a function of other objects in the environment, but what it will be cannot be predicted. According to Isaacson (1982), if the laboratory animal has the opportunity to engage in a new elicited behavior for a while and then the old object is returned, the animal is likely not to give up the new behavior in favor of the old one. Mendelson (1972) reported a similar dependency on the environment for certain parameters of rewarding brain stimulation. Thus, not only is the motivational system widely distributed among a number of modular centers, but its manifestations in behavior frequently are very dependent on specific environmental conditions.

HYPOTHALAMIC STIMULATION AND AGGRESSION IN CATS

Flynn (1967, 1976; see also Chi & Flynn, 1971) found that cats receiving hypothalamic stimulation frequently engage in one of two different aggressive behaviors. In one ("affective attack"), the animal shows anger, hissing and arching its back. In the other ("quiet, biting attack," often observed in academic institutions), the animal behaves as though it were quietly stalking a mouse. Flynn also found that differences in the site of stimulation might produce differences in the precise behavior demonstrated.

THE ORBITOFRONTAL CORTEX

The orbitofrontal (or basal frontal) cortex is that area of the brain at the base of the frontal lobes, above the eyes. This area appears to integrate the regulation of behavior with emotion, motivational systems, and the autonomic nervous system. According to Fuster (1997), electrical stimulation of the orbitofrontal cortex produces alterations in "blood pressure, heart rate, cardiac dynamics, and skin temperature" (p. 145). Such stimulation also may cause decreased eating in some experimental animals (J. Siegel &

Wang, 1974), while lesions of orbital cortex, in both humans and laboratory animals, frequently lead to excessive food intake (Fuster, 1997).

The orbitofrontal cortex is characterized by dopaminergic fiber tracts that apparently are associated with brain centers important for pleasure, rewarding stimulation, and emotionality (Rolls & Cooper, 1974; Thierry et al., 1978; Wise, 1996). The orbital area also is perhaps the only *cortical* area that, when stimulated electrically, produces rewarding sensations for monkeys, presumably because this site is "normally somehow involved in the physiology of drive and motivation" (Fuster, 1997, p. 53).

A distinctive kind of euphoria is commonly associated with lesions of the orbitofrontal cortex. According to Fuster (1997), it is "neither constant in time, nor is it always characterized by a pure feeling of elation. Rather it usually occurs in sporadic or recurrent fashion and resembles the affect of the hypomanic state, with its nervous and irritable, sometimes paranoid, quality. It is usually accompanied by a peculiar kind of compulsive, shallow, and childish humor" (p. 171). Persons with lesions in this area tend to be disinhibited, irresponsible, and socially inappropriate.

Schore (1994) argued that the orbitofrontal cortex plays a crucial role in emotional development, the regulation of affect, and the capacity for social interaction. According to him, this region "represents the cortical system that is fundamentally involved in mediating the central autonomic manifestations of emotional behavior and in regulating motivational states" (p. 321). He noted that orbitofrontal activity is associated with "the pleasurable qualities of social interaction" (p. 132) and that this may be a function of the specific neurotransmitters found throughout much of this area (Kelley & Stinus, 1984; Panksepp, Siviy, & Normansell, 1985). Schore's work, which is too detailed to discuss in any but the most superficial terms here, represents an interesting and thorough analysis of the development of the basal frontal region as a result of experience in infancy; he also considers the consequences of that development for later personality functioning.

THE AMYGDALA

Thus far we have considered the amygdala primarily as an important structure in emotional memory (in Chapter 5 on modularity of memory), but it seems to be involved in regulating a range of emotional phenomena. After lesions of the dorsomedial amygdala, according to Isaacson (1982), "dogs ceased to be friendly and became fearful, sad, and sometimes aggressive. After a second lesion of the lateral area, the dogs became happy, played, showed affection, and enjoyed eating again" (p. 114). According to Fonberg (1973), this reflects the functioning of two antagonistic regions of the amygdala. In general, lesions of the amygdala produce a reduction in aggressive behavior, and it appears that among social animals with a dominance hierarchy, those that have undergone amygdalectomy are lower in status than intact animals (Bunnell, 1966; Dicks, Myers, & Kling, 1979; Fuller, Rosvole, & Pribram, 1957). Stimulation of the amygdala has been found to produce different effects as a function of electrode placement (Isaacson, 1982). Some animals become tame (Egger & Flynn, 1962), some show fearful responses, and others become rather aggressive (Ursin & Kaada, 1960). Fear is a common response, and it is thought that aggression and rage associated with lesions or stimulation of the amygdala may represent defensive reactions.

Careful analysis has shown that lesions of the central nucleus of the amygdala interfere with conditioning of experimental animals to fear-inducing stimuli (M. Davis, 1992a; Kapp, Pascoe, & Bixler, 1984; Kapp et al., 1990; LeDoux, 1995). In reviewing this research, LeDoux (1996) notes that "lesions of the central nucleus interfere with essentially every measure of conditioned fear, including freezing behavior, autonomic responses, suppression of pain, stress hormone release, and reflex potentiation" (p. 158).

Cortical and Subcortical Connections of the Amygdala

Understanding the results of older research on the amygdala is made difficult because of the recent realization that it is a very complex structure with a variety of subcomponents, inputs, and outputs. The amygdala receives sensory input directly from the thalamus and from the thalamus via the cortex. The former route is rapid, allowing for quick emotional responses to stimuli, but without the ability to make fine discriminations among those stimuli. The cortical route operates more slowly but permits such distinctions to be made. This led LeDoux (1996, p. 165) to argue that "the information received from the thalamus is unfiltered and biased toward evoking responses. The cortex's job is to prevent the inappropriate response rather than to produce the appropriate one." These parallel pathways thus minimize the time required for an alerting reaction to fearful stimuli (the subcortical pathway) while permitting the individual to choose among possible responses (the cortical pathway).

The amygdala also receives more complex information concerning the environment that has already been integrated by the hippocampus. This multimodal information provides the amygdala with data regarding the context in which events are taking place. Demonstrating the dissociability of these systems of amygdalar input, several studies (Kim & Fanselow, 1992; LeDoux, 1996; Phillips & LeDoux, 1992) have shown that lesions of the hippocampus do not interfere with learned fear reactions to a conditioned stimulus such as a noise but do prevent animals from associating the fear with the context in which they are conditioned (e.g., the conditioning apparatus itself). The implications of this finding for clinical work are extremely important.

Outputs of the Amygdala

Not only does the amygdala receive input of varying degrees of complexity in parallel from different sources, it also has several parallel outputs that produce separate autonomic and orienting responses. Projections to the central (periaqueductal) gray matter, LH, paraventricular hypothalamus, and pons produce the freezing response, changes in blood pressure, release of stress hormones, and startle responses (LeDoux, 1996). Clearly the amygdala is crucial in emotion and emotional learning (Kling & Brothers, 1992), and LeDoux has made it a centerpiece of his theory of emotion (1995, 1996). For a recent discussion of the complex hierarchical organization of the amygdala and of its functions, the interested reader should refer to Pitkänen, Savander, and LeDoux (1997).

THE NONLINEAR NATURE OF STATE

One's instantaneous physiological state is a major determinant of the probability that one will engage in a specific behavior. One's activity, however, in turn influences one's state, although in ways that may be somewhat less direct. For example, a state which has depression as a primary component may make depressive behavior, thinking, and perception more likely. As a consequence, the state may be maintained by these emergent properties. In other ways, the state may be changed by the processes in which an individual engages. Consider the example of EEG biofeedback, through which a person can alter the functioning of the brain and certain aspects of his or her state. It is important to bear in mind that, while the probability of activation of any neural network is, in large part, a function of state–environment interaction, the process is highly nonlinear, and the person's state may experience bifurcations with subsequent activation of other attractors as a result of the right kind of perceptual input, cognitive processing, or behavior.

SUMMARY AND CONCLUSION

An individual's state at any given moment is a function of the complex interplay of a wide range of endogenous and environmental variables. Both the physical and social environment play a significant role, as do such factors as mood, rhythmic phenomena (infradian, circadian, and ultradian), various aspects of temperament, current motivational state, and emotion. Certain patterns of activity in these systems recur with enough regularity that they can be considered stable attractors, whereas other patterns of activation are so unstable as to never occur or to occur only infrequently and transiently. One's state is an emergent property of the activity of these systems, and it influences the probability of specific behaviors, percepts, and memories.

Emotional reactions are nonconsciously activated, and although they may possess a nearly simultaneous conscious component as well, one may experience an emotion without having any knowledge of the stimulus that elicited it. The intensity and clarity of emotion is increased by the presence of arousal as well as by feedback from the body regarding autonomic and neuroendocrine activity. Although different primary structures and pathways probably mediate each basic emotion, it seems likely that rather than a person feeling a "pure" emotion, his or her experience is colored by varying degrees of activity in a distributed array of structures that mediate motivation and emotion. Complex emotions such as jealousy or grief are especially likely to involve these multifaceted patterns of neural activity, including a significant cognitive contribution.

Lesions in or stimulation of a number of structures can produce a range of emotional phenomena. Anger, fear, pleasure, and several complex disturbances of the sense of reality (depersonalization, derealization, *déjà vu, jamais vu*) are observed commonly in association with complex partial seizures, especially those having a focus in the medial temporal lobe. Stimulation of the amygdala, hypothalamus, septum, basal ganglia, orbitofrontal cortex, midbrain, and medial forebrain bundle may induce feelings of fear, rage, and smothering, as well as pleasurable feelings so intense that animals and humans will stimulate their own brains at high rates if given the opportunity to do so. Some sites produce feelings so aversive that further stimulation of them is avoided at all costs.

10

THE DYNAMICS
OF TEMPERAMENT

INTRODUCTION

Psychological theories of temperament view it as a biologically based set of personality traits, present from infancy, that forms a sort of template for the development of personality. Although there are a number of different formulations, and different researchers have proposed different characteristics as fundamental to temperament, it ordinarily is thought to include such traits as extraversion or introversion, "neuroticism," activity level, level of arousal, emotional reactivity, predominant mood, speed and capacity of information processing, ability to regulate one's own behavior, and the capacity to deal with novel situations. In this chapter we explore temperament from the point of view of dynamics and consider its role in the development and maintenance of personality. While research on personality traits as dimensions of temperament has been productive, we believe that it may be useful to shift the emphasis somewhat from traits to the subcomponent neural processes that determine those traits, examining temperament in terms of its probable effect on various neural networks when they are activated and hence on their associated emergent behaviors.

Temperament has a strong biological component, reflecting heritability and early developmental influences (including intrauterine and perinatal factors). At the extremes of temperament (e.g., marked shyness or gregariousness), it is likely that constitutional factors so dominate the picture that, barring exceptional experience, certain predispositions will have a strong and decisive influence on behavior and character that endures throughout the life of the individual. However, experience may modify certain aspects of the expression of temperament, and experience certainly accounts for much of the variability among persons with essentially similar temperamental styles. For example, research has demonstrated the importance of "goodness of fit" between the temperament of the child and the environment provided by the parents. Successful personality development involves the establishment of an adaptive interaction, with parents who are able to accept and deal with the child's temperament helping the child find a more or less harmonious place in the world. In many cases, this process fails because the parents have the expectation that they can change the child's temperament, because they cannot deal with the child's disposition, or because they don't understand the consequences of a poor fit between the child and the environment.

Cultural and socioeconomic factors also influence the likelihood that an individual will be able to develop an adaptive relationship with the world, by providing specific niches within which an individual's capacities can be satisfactorily expressed. A bright but hyperactive and distractible child, for example, may have considerable difficulty succeeding in certain educational environments but may have the capacity for success if an appropriate academic, occupational, and social niche is available.

Finally, assessing the respective roles of temperament and learning in producing specific personality configurations may permit realistic projections regarding what kinds of change might be possible through psychotherapy (i.e., through learning), as opposed to the kinds of change that might ensue from pharmacological interventions (through neuromodulation). For example, it may be that certain aspects of character are relatively immutable because what is required is an alteration of a more or less "fixed" aspect of the biological substrate, something that we have no effective means of doing (e.g., as in autism), whereas other characteristic behaviors can be altered by various means.

TEMPERAMENT AND DYNAMICS

From the vantage point of dynamics, temperament, like state, is an emergent property of a self-organizing system. As such, it can be described in the language of neurodynamics and probabilities. Temperament acts as a fundamental organizer for emergent psychological experience by affecting the probabilities associated with the activation of various neural networks. We are in fundamental agreement with Zuckerman's (1995) conclusion that "we do not inherit personality traits or even behavior mechanisms as such. What is inherited are chemical templates that produce and regulate proteins involved in building the structure of nervous systems and the neurotransmitters, enzymes, and hormones that regulate them. We are not born as extroverts, neurotics, impulsive sensation seekers, or antisocial personalities, but we are born with differences in reactivities of brain structures and levels of regulators" (pp. 331–332). Temperament thus is an abstraction, a representation of the activity of diverse neural networks, a way of describing basic personality orientations. From the vantage point of dynamics, temperament is content-free. What appear as temperamental traits (introversion, excitability, or whatever) are emergent processes expressing this underlying neural activity.

Emergent temperament is far from static. Temperament as a process is always undergoing modifications and shifts (albeit often subtle) as ongoing adaptation occurs. Like all emergent processes in the brain, temperament emerges from the activities of a brain with a modular distributed architecture. This means that many different streams of processing contribute to the expression of temperament at each moment. The constant dynamically shifting constitution of temperament on this micro level is the reason that people with a certain temperament may show a great degree of variability in the expression of a given aspect of temperament across time or across contexts.

Temperament is relatively stable because the neuropsychological factors that constitute temperament themselves represent relatively stable attractors. Thus, the probability is greatest that an individual's temperament would occupy a more or less predictable region of the temperament phase space—a shy child is likely to be shy most of the time. Nevertheless, the subcomponents of temperament are in fact only *relatively* stable; that is, they are subject to fluctuation over time, sometimes periodically or quasi-periodically, and sometimes aperiodically (depending on the specific process). The consistency of temperament is only apparent and reflects the probabilistic functioning of the nervous system.

From the perspective of dynamics, everyone's behavior is influenced to some degree by temperamental influences (i.e., by those biological factors that constitute temperament). Temperament may be more "noticeable" among those in one of the tails of the distribution, but temperament (or, more precisely, its subcomponent processes) influences even those who lie closer to the mean, whose expressions of temperament do not have a visible or defining "signature" such as hyperactivity.

GENOTYPE AND PHENOTYPE

In recent years there has been a dawning realization that the so-called nature–nurture debate, over which much ink and invective have been expended, is a pseudocontroversy. As it turns out, both genetics and the environment are important in the development of most complex human traits. People are not simply robots shaped entirely by genetic inheritance, but neither are they infinitely plastic. Human personality reflects an amalgam of heritable traits and propensities in association with much that is learned. Unless we understand the relationship between what is inherited and what is acquired, we can have no realistic theory of whether and how people are capable of change.

GENES AND BEHAVIOR

Plomin, Owen, and McGuffin (1994) have noted that there is evidence of significant genetic influence in nearly every psychological disorder that has been studied, and the same holds true for variability in normal traits (see also Bouchard, 1994; Bouchard et al., 1990). For example, genes have been implicated in the genesis of schizophrenia for many years, although the exact nature of this effect remains unclear. The risk of schizophrenia for children of schizophrenics is 13%, while the base rate of the disorder in the population is approximately 1% (Gottesman, 1991). In one of the early studies of familial patterns of schizophrenia, Heston (1966) found that among a group of 47 children who were adopted at birth, taken out of the homes of their schizophrenic mothers, 9.4% themselves became schizophrenic. In contrast, there was no schizophrenia among 50 adopted control subjects. Twin studies also provide support for the hypothesis, with monozygotic twins demonstrating significantly greater concordance for schizophrenia (about 45%) than dizygotic or "fraternal" twins, who have a concordance rate of about 15% (Gottesman, 1991).

Like schizophrenia, autism is a disorder with a high degree of heritability, and according to Plomin and associates (1994), other conditions influenced by genetics include specific language disorder, panic attacks, eating disorders, antisocial personality, and Tourette's syndrome. Fragile X syndrome (Hagerman, 1996), which is associated with a mutation on the X chromosome (a CGG [cytosine–guanine–guanine] trinucleotide expansion at a locus identified as q27.3), has a phenotype characterized by mental retardation in males, specific cognitive problems in females, and a fairly consistent pattern of emotional and behavioral traits (Hagerman, 1996; Kemper et al., 1986; Sobesky, Hull, & Hagerman, 1994; Sobesky et al., 1995).

Genes contribute to certain cognitive disorders, and account for a significant amount of variance in normal cognition, although controversy remains regarding the precise roles played by the environment and DNA. In general, the heritability of intelligence is estimated at approximately 50%—that is, about half of phenotypic variance is genetic in origin (Bouchard & McGue, 1981; Chipuer, Rovine, & Plomin, 1990; Devlin, Daniels, & Roeder, 1997). Even among octogenarian identical twins, for whom one might expect years of experience to have produced rather different patterns of functioning, one recent study estimated that more than 60%

of the contribution to general cognitive ability is genetic (McClearn et al., 1997; see also Pedersen et al., 1992). Conversely, however, up to nearly 40% of this ability is a result of environmental influence.

Just as normal intelligence has a clear heritable component, so do normal personality characteristics. Plomin, Owen, and McGuffin (1994) list extroversion, vocational interests, scholastic achievement, self-esteem, and H. J. Eysenck's trait of *neuroticism* as showing heritabilities ranging from 38 to 51%.

Recent data suggest that sexual orientation may be determined, to some extent, by genetic factors. Bailey and associates (1993) reported 48% concordance between monozygotic female twins when one twin was homosexual, with 16% concordance for dizygotic twins. Bailey and Pillard (1991) found concordance of 52% for homosexuality for monozygotic male twins and 22% for dizygotic male twins. Hamer et al. (1993) reported data suggesting that at least one subtype of male homosexuality is associated with a sex-linked form of genetic transmission (i.e., in conjunction with a site on the X chromosome, which men receive only from their mothers). The paths to attraction for same-sex partners may be varied, however, with environmental influences playing a role even among persons with a genetic predisposition.

The physiological processes determining sexual orientation are obscure, but certain findings are of interest. Gladue and his colleagues (Gladue, 1994; Gladue, Green, & Hellman, 1984), for example, reported anomalous responses to estrogen injections among homosexual men and women. Gay men tended to show elevated luteinizing hormone (LH) following the injection—not as great as that of women, but greater than that of heterosexual men, who generally don't respond to estrogen with increases in LH. In addition, for all men, testosterone level dropped following estrogen injections, but for heterosexual men it returned to normal levels more rapidly than for homosexual men. Among lesbians, the response to estrogen also was anomalous—the level of LH was significantly greater than that of heterosexual women.

Some neuroanatomical findings suggest that there may be structural differences distinguishing the brains of heterosexuals and homosexuals. These results are open to question on a number of grounds and require replication, but nonetheless are interesting. For example, differences in the corpus callosum, which connects the hemispheres of the brain, have been demonstrated for men and women (Allen & Gorski, 1991; Breedlove, 1992). Such findings suggested to researchers that similar differences might be present among members of the same sex as a function of sexual orientation. Although scant research has been conducted to date, Gladue (1994, p. 152) suggested that "the emerging neuroanatomical picture is that, in some brain areas, homosexual men are more likely to have female-typical neuroanatomy than are heterosexual men." Areas investigated in which differences have been found include certain hypothalamic nuclei and the anterior commissure, a part of the corpus callosum that connects homologous regions of right and left temporal lobes (Allen & Gorski, 1992; LeVay, 1991; Swaab & Hofman, 1990).

TEMPERAMENT

Fundamental species-specific similarities in human neural organization account for much of the interindividual consistency in our observations of both normal and pathological behavior, yet people differ widely from one another along certain dimensions of temperament and cognition. These dimensions include such phenomena as basic levels of arousal and activity, capacity to direct and regulate attentional processes flexibly, response to novel stimulation, autonomic reactivity, and others. Thomas and Chess (1980) described temperament as "a general term referring to the *how* of behavior" and note that people "may differ significantly with regard to the quickness with which they move, the ease with which they approach a new situation, the intensity and character of their mood expression, and the effort required by others to distract them when they are absorbed in an activity" (p. 70). Thomas and Chess (1980, p. 72) argued that different temperamental styles are all normal variants, with variability along the different dimensions that probably has something approaching a normal distribution in the general population. Temperament appears to be heritable to some extent, but while genetics probably plays a major role in determination of temperamental style, other biological and environmental influences on the developing organism cannot be ignored.

Several authors have proposed theoretical models or typologies of temperament that suggest ways in which temperament may influence subsequent personality development. Buss and Plomin (1975), for example, suggested a classification of people along four lines: activity level, emotionality, sociability, and impulsivity. Plomin and Rowe (1977) subsequently revised this system to a set of six personality traits, including activity, emotionality, sociability, soothability, attention span and persistence, and reaction to food. Thomas and Chess (1977, 1980) argued that there are nine stable dimensions of temperament, including activity level, rhythmicity (or regularity) of biological functions, approach or withdrawal to novelty, adaptability to new or changed situations, sensory threshold of responsiveness to stimulation, intensity of reaction, quality of mood, distractibility, and attention span and persistence. Regardless of which set of factors best corresponds to the personality traits that are heritable, these dimensions probably are not entirely independent of one another. To a certain extent their expression reflects the operation of complex functional systems having a modular architecture, and they tend to be somewhat intercorrelated.

The dimensions of temperament suggested by various researchers are primarily *psychological* constructs and are useful on that level of analysis. Just as one size doesn't really fit all, not all children can be pigeonholed in one of these groups; instead, there is variability among individuals, and these clusters represent idealized types. They are the emergent properties, however, of the activity of various distributed regions of the brain. To some degree, the subcomponents of temperament play a significant role in the regulation of the individual's overall state. Activity level and quality of mood are direct determinants of state, while most of the others affect the dynamics of state (i.e., stability, fluctuation, or bifurcation). These include rhythmicity of biological functions, response to novelty, adaptability to new or changed situations, sensory threshold, intensity of reaction, distractibility, and attention span and persistence.

INHIBITED AND UNINHIBITED CHILDREN

Kagan and associates (Kagan, 1989; Kagan, Reznick, & Snidman, 1988; Kagan & Snidman, 1991) have conducted research on various aspects of temperament, especially shyness, and have found marked stability along certain dimensions. Kagan, Snidman, and Arcus (1992) suggested that there are two kinds of shy children: (1) those influenced by experience alone (e.g., by parental rejection), who are inclined to avoid unfamiliar people, places, and things; (2) others born with a constitution predisposing them "to acquire an avoidant style to many unfamiliar events—people as well as nonsocial stimulus events. These latter children differ from the former in both autonomic functioning, affect, and physical features and belong to the temperamental category we call *inhibited*. In contrast, children who are born with a physiology that biases them to approach these same unfamiliar events are called *uninhibited*" (1992, p. 171).

According to Kagan and Snidman (1991), about 10% of Caucasian children are consistently shy and emotionally reserved in unfamiliar situations or with unfamiliar persons, during their second year. About 25% of the Caucasian children they examined were sociable, emotionally spontaneous, and generally free of fear in unfamiliar settings. When these two groups were compared on a number of physiological variables, the inhibited children demonstrated greater autonomic (sympathetic) reactivity, with increased pulse, dilated pupils, muscle tension, and postural change in diastolic blood pressure. Kagan and Snidman argued that these differences reflect variation "in thresholds of excitability in the amygdala and its projections to targets [e.g., hypothalamus] that participate in reactions to unfamiliar events" (1991, p. 40).

They reported, for example (Kagan & Snidman, 1991), that infants showing high levels of motor activity and crying were more fearful in response to novel stimulation than were infants who were less active and fretful. These findings were consistent across time, each group demonstrating similar behavior when tested at 9 months and at 14 months. In previous work, Kagan et al. (1988) reported findings from a longitudinal study of two cohorts of children selected because they represented extremes of either inhibited or uninhibited behavior. One group was examined four times between the ages of 21 months and 7½ years, whereas the second group was examined four times between the ages of 31 months and 7½ years. Temperamental styles remained very consistent over time.

CHILDREN WITH A DIAGNOSIS OF CONDUCT DISORDER

Lytton (1990), in a review of factors contributing to the behavior of boys with a diagnosis of conduct disorder, argued that "a biological predisposition to CD [conduct disorder] . . . operates in conjunction with environmental factors" (p. 693) to produce this disorder. The autonomic nervous system of these boys presumably is inadequately responsive in situations that other children might experience as threatening (Mednick, 1977; Raine & Venables, 1981; Schmidt, Solant, & Bridger, 1985). The behavior characteristic of boys with this diagnosis generally is stable over time (Loeber, 1982; Quay, Routh, & Shapiro, 1987). The same holds true for children diagnosed as hyperactive, who tend to demonstrate poor academic, social, psychological, and legal outcomes (August, Stewart, & Holmes, 1983; Gittelman et al., 1985; Lambert et al., 1987; G. Weiss et al., 1985). Loeber, Stouthamer-Loeber, and Green (1987) found an association between a child's behavior in preschool and subsequent delinquency in adolescence.

Zuckerman's review (1995) of some of the neurochemical findings associated with specific temperament traits is a useful introduction to the issue of temperament and its biological basis. Our current state of knowledge regarding these matters is rudimentary. The relationships are complex, and there is much to be learned. The findings nevertheless strongly suggest the importance of biochemical factors in determining basic personality orientation.

TEMPERAMENT AND ENVIRONMENT

Temperament is a manifestation of the phenotype, heavily influenced by genetics, stable yet malleable within limits that are imposed by biology, and showing some variability across time. It is a sort of template of organizing tendencies which shape a personality that is further refined by learning. As an emergent property, temperament is composed of a set of self-organizing, biological, dynamic processes. Although it appears to be stable across time, temperament is not immutable. For example, a hyperactive, impulsive, and distractible child is unlikely to become quiet and compliant, although he may do so briefly in specific contexts. Similarly, the very shy child is a poor candidate for the development of a gregarious personality.

Some temperamental characteristics are probably more readily altered than others. A boy diagnosed with attention-deficit/hyperactivity disorder (ADHD) is liable to maintain a relatively stable personality style into adulthood. His character will be shaped to some extent by experience, and he in turn will have a significant effect on his environment. Parents, teachers, and peers may find him exasperating, and the behavioral style he acquires in turn may lead to the development of a conduct disorder or antisocial personality. If his parents and siblings are able to deal with him in a positive, adaptive manner, the outcome may be positive, but an active, aggressive, energetic style is likely to dominate his personality. In the same way, the biologically shy child is likely to remain shy. If raised in a stern environment or exposed to physical and emotional abuse, such a child may develop a very avoidant personality style. If a child like this is treated sensitively and manages to avoid being traumatized, he or she may show a very successful adaptation in life.

ADHD is interesting in that behavior characteristic of this cluster of syndromes frequently is changed significantly by the use of the appropriate medication—usually CNS stimulants (discussed in Chapter 17). In this case, the person's state is modulated by the medication. Without this tuning of the brain, the probability that the child with ADHD will sit still and pay attention in class is low. With medication, however, compliant behavior may be more likely than the disinhibited, disruptive, and distractible activity typical of these children. In contrast, behavioral treatment of ADHD is less frequently successful than is the pharmacological approach. It seems that the right type of learning is difficult to bring about—the temperament dominates the clinical picture, and experience, short of extremely intense or traumatic experience, has a limited effect. For those among the 65% of Kagan and associates' children who fall between the inhibited and uninhibited groups (discussed in the previous section), perhaps experience and learning play a greater role in determining basic personality orientation. Among members of this group, we hypothesize that psychotherapeutic interventions are more likely to be efficacious in changing personality than among those with extremes of temperament.

The Reciprocal Interaction of Temperament and Environment

Temperament, because it influences the probabilities of behaving in certain ways, can lead to a significant shaping of the environment. Thus, temperament can have a significant effect on one's learning history. A corollary is that temperament not only affects the kind of environment the person encounters, it also affects how and what a person learns from his or her experience. Distractability, for example, may lead one to overlook the details of certain transactions and may interfere with learning from those encounters. For the shy person, a single experience of interpersonal failure may provide an education that lasts for a lifetime. To a natural extrovert, the same sort of interpersonal failure may have little or no lasting effect.

Thomas and Chess (1977, 1980) looked at the reciprocal interaction between temperament and environment and were impressed with the importance of the *social* context. This led them to concern themselves with *goodness of fit* between child and environment:

> [This] goodness of fit results when the properties of the environment and its expectations and demands are in accord with the organism's own capacities, motivations, and style of behaving. When this *consonance* between organism and environment is present, optimal development in a progressive direction is possible. Conversely, poor fit involves discrepancies and *dissonances* between environmental opportunities and demands and the capacities and characteristics of the organism, so that distorted development and maladaptive functioning occur (Thomas & Chess, 1980, p. 90; emphasis in original)

These findings are consistent with the emphasis of Plomin and Daniels (1987) on environment.

An infant's temperament expresses itself in interaction with an environment that is first and foremost an interpersonal environment. The vagaries of "goodness of fit" therefore must be innumerable. It is an infant's caretakers who first experience their child's temperament and whose responses will influence how and in what way this temperament is brought into some sort of alignment with the demands of the environment. Even when the fit may not appear especially problematic, parents vary in their motivation and aptitude for helping a child who is constituted in a certain way to develop useful strategies or processes for bringing this constitution into an adaptive alignment with the specifics of the environment.

Consider the example of a constantly fussy baby. The relaxed mother with such an infant may be able to persist in attempts to soothe her child in the face of apparent failure without herself experiencing undue anxiety or distress. She may be creative and inventive in her efforts. Her infant's excitable temperament in this kind of dyadic context may became modified to a greater degree than when a similarly constituted infant is cared for by an anxious, helpless, and not particularly inventive caregiver. The relaxed mother may provide learning experiences for her infant that mitigate its fussiness via learning, whereas the anxious mother may provide learning that deepens or exacerbates expression of the temperamental variable.

Children who are temperamentally biased in one way or another may require more active engagement with caregivers to help compensate or correct for their innate dispositions. For example, one young boy has always seemed to generate chaos in his environment from early on, an apparent expression of his lively, inquisitive cognitive style. Lego models occupy strategic spots throughout his room. Science projects poke from shelves. His school backpack is stuffed with papers. He can wash his hands and forget to turn off the water. His parents first found themselves compensating for his innate and often delightful disarray. Subsequently, they deliberately set out to get him to establish certain organized habits, a project that required considerable effort and generated a shared feeling of guilt that their own excessive attentiveness may have led to his disarray. This concern was dispelled when his younger sister came along and seemed organized almost from birth; her temperament required less shaping. Different temperaments make different demands on caregivers, and different caregivers will show considerable variability in their aptitude and motivation in responding appropriately and adaptively to the child's temperament.

Temperament can be influenced to some degree by the child's developing capacity for reflective self awareness. Thus, for instance, a shy person can deliberately behave in ways that stretch her behavioral repertoire or at least minimize its influence. Presumably such learning across time can, in some cases, become stable enough that the temperamental influence recedes in large areas of behavioral functioning. Nonetheless, under stress, one might expect the basic temperament to be more visible in such people. The disorganized, distractible child can develop neural networks associated with organizational habits if given adequate support in doing so. The establishment and activation of these networks over time changes the likelihood of their subsequent activation. Thus, procedural learning may shape the expression of temperament.

Temperament and Psychopathology

The fit between child and environment is never perfect. Winnicott (1960) suggested that this is not a bad thing, because a hypothetical "perfect fit" between an infant and its caretakers (where "perfect" is defined as total maternal attunement and adaptive responsiveness to her infant's needs) would undermine a child's spontaneous exercise of its adaptive capability (apart from being impossible). Within limits, *imperfect fit* leads to the exercise of those capabilities providing much of the scaffold for subsequent personality development. Thus Winnicott was led to observe that what was necessary to support normal developmental processes was a "good enough" fit between an infant and his or her parents. There always will be some degree of mismatch, but in one way or another the child provokes certain kinds and intensities of reaction from the people around it, in response to its behavior, and the learning (neural plasticity) that occurs as a result of this experience serves to embellish or modify the basic temperamental style.

If fit is too flawed, normal developmental processes can be derailed or warped, with psychopathology as the yield. For example, Thomas and Chess found that for a "difficult" child, when the child is not well matched with the environment, there is an increased likelihood that the child will develop a behavior disorder. In one sample, 70% of the children they classified as difficult acquired "clinically evident behavior disorders (a mild reactive behavior disorder in most cases)" (1980, p. 74) by the age of 10 years.

Temperament can lead to psychopathology when a child has unhelpful or incompetent training experiences (bad fit). The shy child who is ridiculed or unsupported by the parents may go on to become pathologically shy, whereas another equally shy child who is supported and encouraged may develop an adaptive behavioral style. There are other ways in which temperament may contribute to psychopathology. For example, in some cases the constitutional imperative associated with a given temperament may be so pronounced that there is an increased likelihood of psychopathology. Temperament in such cases can be considered dynamically as leading to psychopathology by reducing behavioral plasticity.

Psychopathology also can result when an individual's temperament is somehow not adequately and constructively accommodated by his or her life structure. Thus a distractible person who becomes an accountant or air traffic controller may experience stresses that could lead to pathology. Similarly, a gregarious person who finds him- or herself working alone may suffer as a result. Life structures that don't conflict with pronounced temperamental variables are likely to be less pathogenic.

Finally, if a society is unable to provide appropriate niches that can accommodate people with varying temperaments, psychopathology can be the result. A border collie bred to walk great distances while herding sheep will develop neurotic symptoms if forced to live in an apartment in the city. Similarly, highly active children may become symptomatic in environments requiring long periods of sustained attention. Different societies are more or less successful in providing the variety of niches within which diverse temperaments can find expression.

TEMPERAMENT AND PSYCHOLOGICAL TREATMENT

Temperament has important implications in the clinical setting. Successful therapy is likely to maximize an individual's capacity to be aware of the influence of his or her temperament on behavior. Therapy is likely to involve helping patients stretch their behavior beyond limits previously established by temperament. Furthermore, good treatment is likely to flow with the current of stable temperamental variables and avoid attempts to change the relatively inflexible. Thus, we help patients to understand that they will probably continue to be shy, or disorganized, or avoidant, and so on, but that these variables will be less likely to determine behavior, so that the patient can establish new behavioral possibilities.

Assessing the respective roles of temperament and learning in producing specific personality configurations may permit one to make realistic projections regarding the kinds of change possible through psychotherapy (i.e., through learning), as opposed to the kinds of change that might ensue from pharmacological interventions (through neuromodulation). It may be that certain aspects of personality are extremely resistant to change because change would require a significant alteration of the biological substrate, something that we have no effective means of doing.

In autism, for example, some researchers maintain there is a cognitive disorder involving failure to develop a "theory of mind" (Frith, 1989; Happé et al., 1996). As a result, an autistic person is unable to formulate representations of what others might be experiencing. This presumably involves a neural anomaly that cannot be altered, and Happé and Frith (1992) were impressed by what they contend are parallels between the functioning of autistic persons and that of normal vervet monkeys in this regard. Whether the monkey analogy is apropos, autistic individuals are different from most people and the probability that any psychotherapy could "cure" an autistic person is slim. Nevertheless, the judicious use of medication, combined with carefully planned behavioral approaches, may have positive effects on the functioning of autistic individuals.

It seems likely that severe personality disorders involve some degree of neuropsychological variant of temperament. Although not clearly demonstrated, this hypothesis has tantalized researchers working with psychopathic personalities for many years (e.g., Hare, 1978; Lykken, 1957), and it may well be the case for other personality disorders as well. For example, such phenomena as impulsivity, or the "splitting" observed in borderline personality disorder, may reflect either neural developmental variants or frank neuropathology (Grigsby & Hartlaub, 1994). Such vagaries of neural organization may range from subtle to severe. Gardner, Lucas, and Cowdry (1987), for example, found more neurological soft signs among borderline persons than among "normal" control subjects. Although the significance of such soft signs is unclear, this result suggests that the search for a neural substrate for borderline personality is a reasonable endeavor.

It is essential that we learn the extent to which temperament sets limits on change. Some aspects of personality cannot be changed, some may be changed only by pharmacological means, and others may be affected by a wide range of environmental interventions or manipulations. Trying to change relatively immutable aspects of temperament is likely to be futile and frustrating. However, despite the difficulty inherent in the process, certain aspects of temperament's expression probably can be changed. So while there will be many cases in which psychotherapy cannot bring about "normal" functioning, therapy may enable an individual to function adaptively within the constraints imposed by biology and irreversible developmental history (Gollin, Stahl, & Morgan, 1988).

SUMMARY AND CONCLUSION

We began this chapter by arguing that it is useful to consider temperament as a complex set of emergent properties in accordance with the principles of dynamics that were explored in greater detail earlier in this book. Examining temperament from the point view of dynamics reminds us that temperament is a process variable; it influences behavior by affecting the probabilities associated with the activation of certain configurations of neural networks. Temperament is dynamic, and neither monolithic nor immutable in its expression. Even people with a pronounced temperament of one sort or another may behave in certain contexts in ways that don't reflect the presence of a given temperamental variable.

While temperament is likely to have a significant degree of heritability, environmental influence also plays a crucial role in determining how temperamental variables express themselves across time. Goodness of fit between caregivers and infants appears to have a special status in terms of the ultimate expression of temperament. Temperament can lead to psychopathology if it overshadows all environmental ministrations and compensatory efforts or if fit fails in certain ways. Temperament also may express itself in psychopathology if social structures or roles cannot be provided that allow a given temperament to gain expression. Finally we argued that a proper understanding of temperament is critical for realistic goal setting in psychotherapy and for conceptualizing the direction of change for a given patient.

11

MONKEY BUSINESS: COGNITION IN NONHUMAN PRIMATES

INTRODUCTION

We opened this book by arguing that the brain's organization can be understood only within an evolutionary context, in which its pattern-recognizing and pattern-generating activity is assumed to have been shaped by the pressures of natural selection. Subsequent chapters dealt with data and concepts regarding the anatomical, physiological, and neurodynamic organization of the brain. Our emphasis has been on how the brain appears spontaneously to maintain its activity in the vicinity of states of self-organizing criticality, characterized by a dynamic equilibrium between stability and openness to change. Self-organizing criticality thus plays a fundamental role in the brain's capacity to react to novel stimuli in ways that more often than not facilitate adaptation. All psychological phenomena—cognition, perception, consciousness, behavior—represent emergent properties of the brain's self-organizing activity.

In this chapter we move away from more basic neurobiology in order to discuss data gathered by primatologists concerning striking similarities in the behavioral and cognitive functioning of human beings and certain other primate species. Nonhuman primate behavior and cognition offer a window into certain fundamental psychological phenomena. Psychological phenomena in humans are emergent from physiological activity in specific environments, and the same holds true for other animals. We will be most concerned with primates, especially the great apes (Pongidae). From an evolutionary perspective, we are more closely related to these than any other animals. We share common ancestors as recently as several million years ago, and approximately 98.5% of human DNA is similar to that of chimpanzees and bonobos. Very striking also is the fact that evolution, although it has given humans a larger brain with a more developed prefrontal cortex, nevertheless has left ourselves and the great apes with a number of important emergent psychological capacities in common. We don't want to overemphasize the similarities, as there certainly are important differences among ourselves and other primates, but the fact that our own brains and those of these other species are so similar (compared with dogs or rats, say), and that cognitively and emotionally we seem more akin to apes than to any other species, is evidence of the significance of the brain in organizing behavior, cognition, and experience.

Although we will focus primarily on cognition, one theme running through this chapter is the *social* context for cognition—that is, how successful adaptation for primates is to a large degree dependent on successful *social* adaptation. Therefore, it comes as no surprise that observations of primate social structures reveal a high degree of complexity in the cognitive operations that some primates can bring to their participation in the group. Apes and humans behave in ways that suggest that they possess a highly differentiated view of the interpersonal field. Among the great apes, this view appears to include well-differentiated, internally represented models of self in relation to others. We also will review data that demonstrate the dynamic effect on emergent cognitive functioning that the acquisition of language appears to have on primate consciousness and representational operations. If taught language, apes are able to use it to communicate what is in their minds, as well as their understanding of another's mind. Language permits them further to fine-tune their capacity to represent experience in increasingly differentiated ways, and even to teach these new ways to offspring.

We want to make a few basic points. First, although primates generally have complex social structures and the capacity to navigate these complex social environments is essential for survival, our intention is not to review the vast literature on the significance of relationships and social structures for social and psychological development. Rather, we examine social behavior because of what it reveals about the cognitive capabilities of primates, ourselves included. Second, different primate species have widely varying cognitive and behavioral capacities. Although genetics imposes specific constraints on the psychological capacities of each species, the diversity existing with regard to specific variables, as well as the capacity for adaptive learning, also reflect genetic influences. For example, although each species has what might be considered a kind of a modal temperament, there also exists considerable intraspecies variability, as well as a considerable capacity for adaptive learning. Third, we will present data which strongly suggest that humans are not the only species with a capacity for reflective self-awareness. The data supporting the existence of self-awareness among the great apes are compelling and interesting. Not only are these animals able to represent themselves in their own minds, they also seem to be aware of themselves as individuals and can think about themselves. In addition, we will demonstrate that in association with reflective self-awareness, the great apes seem to have a *theory of mind*. That is, they are able to think about the thought processes of other individuals. This theory of mind hypothesis has been supported by experimental and observational data suggesting a fairly sophisticated ability to consider other animals' perspectives on events. For example, nonhuman primates are able to engage in complex kinds of deception that seem to involve a theory about what others are thinking.

We will present data that have engendered considerable debate concerning whether chimpanzees or other apes have a true capacity for language. We don't intend to enter that debate but will discuss evidence indicating that these animals learn to use symbols for communication and thereby acquire the ability to convey novel ideas spontaneously. Chimpanzees even have demonstrated the ability to perform categorization tasks that require an abstract understanding of linguistic concepts. Furthermore it appears that in conjunction with an enlarged capacity to use symbols, some primates seem to have developed what appears to be a capacity for such behaviors as fantasy play. Finally, some chimpanzees have found their newly acquired linguistic capabilities so valuable that their young acquire such abilities spontaneously, and language-capable animals have been observed actively teaching others to use language.

ATTACHMENT AND SEPARATION

The evidence is overwhelming that primates require secure attachments to caregivers for normal physiological, psychological, and social development. Hence, for any primate, and especially (in the context of the model we present) for any human primate, "adaptation" means successful adjustment to the set of psychosocial circumstances within which the animal finds itself. The unfolding of an individual person's development is mediated, to a significant degree, by the specific qualities, capacities, and vicissitudes of the relationships formed with primary attachment figures. These relationships are the medium within which basic behavioral and biological regulation is achieved. In addition, caregivers shape and prepare their children for some kind of adaptation within a given cultural context.

Primates, especially apes and humans, experience a relatively long period of childhood dependency—something that potentially has adverse consequences for survival among animal species. Research has established what seems intuitively so obvious: that empathic caregiving is essential for normal psychological and social development. Without appropriate care during the earliest months and years of life, considerable emotional distress and lifelong problems in social functioning result. Harry F. Harlow's experimental studies of the effects of extreme deprivation on infant rhesus monkeys (Harlow, 1958; also Harlow & Harlow, 1973) demonstrated the profound need of these animals for a nurturing mother. Young primates deprived of their mothers demonstrate such stereotyped behaviors as pacing, rocking, and self-huddling, as well as withdrawal from social contact, fearfulness, aggressive and assaultive behavior, lack of play, absence of self-grooming, and impaired sexual performance (Bramblett, 1994).

Separation from attachment figures is distressing for young primates and has long-lasting behavioral sequelae. For example, rhesus monkey infants separated from their mothers complain actively at first, and subsequently become very depressed, withdrawn, and despairing (Seay, Alexander, & Harlow, 1964). Even relatively brief periods of separation (6 days) in young monkeys produced behavioral effects that can be observed months later (Spencer-Booth & Hinde, 1971). Pratt and Sackett (1967) reported that monkeys deprived of varying degrees of social contact as infants developed long-lasting preferences for association with animals having a similar developmental history. Similar deleterious effects secondary to disruptions of attachment have been demonstrated for humans by Spitz (1945, 1946; also Spitz & Wolf, 1946), Bowlby (1969), and others.

DOMINANCE AND SOCIAL HIERARCHIES

Primates generally have complex social structures. For many primates—baboons and chimpanzees, for example—dominance and one's place in the hierarchy is of utmost importance. For others, like bonobos (sometimes called pygmy chimpanzees), dominance is less salient. Humans probably fall between chimpanzees and bonobos in this regard. Perhaps the most common cause of aggression in primate groups involves "the establishment and maintenance of dominance relationships" (Walters & Seyfarth, 1987, p. 307), although this varies by species. For some species, such as the howler monkey or the bonobo, the aggression involved in maintenance of the hierarchy is minimal and the society is relatively peaceful (although there are dominant individuals and/or mother–son pairs among bonobos). In contrast, chimps (for whom there are separate male and female hierarchies) place considerable emphasis on aggression in establishing each animal's place in the pecking order.

Extreme aggression is observed among hamadryas baboons (*Papio hamadryas*), which have one of the most rigidly structured and aggressively defended dominance systems. Among baboons, small groups are dominated by a single male "with an absolutely unspeakable disposition" (Bonner, 1980, p. 90). This male usually is accompanied by several females, of whom he is extremely possessive. According to Bonner, if one of the male's female companions strays, he will charge at her ferociously, perhaps biting or slapping her. Although not exactly sensitive with females, male baboons are even more vicious with rival males. Female baboons themselves are rather aggressive. They have their own hierarchy, and if challenged, the dominant female will defend her position and recruit the assistance of the dominant male in this effort.

Despite the fact that they may be highly competitive in establishing dominance, many apes also are capable of complex cooperative activity. It is interesting to compare baboons with chimpanzees, who live in larger, less rigidly structured social groups, and for whom dominance is a function not only of the aggressiveness of the males but also of their ability to form alliances (de Waal, 1982). For example, on occasion a male chimpanzee unable to wrest the dominant position from another will rely on one or more male co-conspirators, something a baboon never would do. In other cases, it has been observed that if the females in a chimpanzee group are not particularly fond of a male who seeks dominance, they may sabotage his efforts by supporting his competitors or simply by failing to show support for his cause.

There is good evidence that members of many primate species know their own status within the group, as well as that of other individuals (Seyfarth, 1981). In fact, juvenile primates frequently are granted status in accordance with the standing of their mothers in the group (Walters & Seyfarth, 1987). This suggests that others recognize both the mother's standing and the mother–juvenile relationship. In large groups of chimpanzees, as with humans, it may be difficult or impossible to specify a linear dominance hierarchy; rather, there seem to be subgroups of individuals varying in status (Bygott, 1979).

As a general rule, unless dominance is unclear, each individual seems to know his or her place in the community, and the society functions relatively smoothly. This does not mean that individuals slavishly adhere to a fixed hierarchy. Rather, the establishment of dominance and submission is a dynamic process that probably is ongoing, expressed in ways that range from subtle through blatant in nearly every interaction. Consequently, rank—at least among males—is relatively susceptible to change. The rank of males may vary considerably over time, with different males seeking the upper hand frequently; in contrast, female status tends to remain more constant over their adult lives (Walters & Seyfarth, 1987).

Expressions of chimpanzee dominance and submission frequently are ritualized, and relatively stereotyped dominance displays constitute a significant part of primate interaction. Nonetheless, many innovative behaviors have been observed among chimpanzees in service of their attempts to exert influence (e.g., Goodall, 1971, 1990). These ritualized expressions of hierarchical status and of dominance and submission are part of the self-organizing glue that binds primate societies together.

RECONCILIATION FOLLOWING CONFLICT

When dominance is not clearly established, group tensions may be high (as discussed in a recent book by ethologist Frans de Waal, 1996). When tempers flare over dominance, this leads to high levels of intragroup tension and there often are strong group pressures for rivals to resolve their differences. Thus, chimpanzees—and other primates also—have acquired elaborate means of patching things up. For this reason, primate hierarchies are characterized by diverse, ritualized behaviors, the purpose of which seems to be reconciliation. Several variations on conciliatory behavior were described by de Waal (1996), who noted that golden monkeys hold hands, chimpanzees kiss one another on the mouth, bonobos engage in sexual behavior, and tonkean macaques (*Macaca tonkeana*) smack their lips. Chimpanzees frequently reconcile their differences by means of social grooming.

These specific reconciliatory behaviors, although habitual, are not necessarily innate, but may be acquired via social learning. This was demonstrated in an experiment conducted by de Waal (1996) and his colleagues at the Wisconsin Primate Center, using stump-tailed and rhesus macaques. Stump-tails are a relatively tolerant but assertive species that places a high value on reconciliation. Rhesus monkeys, which are somewhat smaller than stump-tails, have a strict hierarchy and are much less likely than stump-tails to engage in reconciliatory behavior. De Waal and his associates put together a group of rhesus monkeys with a group of slightly older stump-tails for a period of 5 months. Over this time, the species increasingly interacted with one another; the rhesus monkeys gradually became somewhat less aggressive, and eventually were as likely to make up with one another after a fight as were the stump-tails. The rhesus monkeys maintained this behavioral change even after the stump-tails were removed and they were left to themselves—suggesting acquisition of a habit by procedural learning mechanisms. In this experiment, a change in the behavior of individual monkeys effected a change in the culture of the group.

HUMANS AND DOMINANCE

As with other primates, from birth onward human beings are preoccupied with making their own positions within their social context. School-age children establish informal group allegiances that can have clear-cut informal membership criteria and, perhaps more importantly, exclusionary criteria. Adolescents are notably preoccupied with establishing their status in the peer group and often are dominated by a dread of exclusion from their circle of friends. Children and adolescents can be ruthless with one another and quickly learn just where they stand in the pecking order. Adults also remain preoccupied to greater or lesser degrees with establishing their relative position within social structures. Being shunned, or losing one's status within the group, remains a central fear for most humans. Academics' status is determined by grants, publications, or becoming department chairs and deans. Yet, unless we think explicitly in terms of dominance interactions among people, we tend not to notice them. Sometimes these interactions are subtle, but more often we simply automatically and nonconsciously act out our respective roles. Similarly, it is unlikely that apes or monkeys give much deliberate thought to matters of dominance. Instead, dominance issues are implicit in behavior that is emergent from neural and social self-organizing dynamics.

Bion (1959), in his studies of groups, found considerable qualitative data regarding the apparent need of people in groups for a leader and concerning the processes involved in establishing rank. For humans, as well as chimpanzees, one's place in the hierarchy may change over time; achieving certain kinds of social status may have a disinhibiting effect on the use of aggression, or the exploitation of individuals with lower status. In general, males tend, overtly or subtly, to dominate females. Aggressive, narcissistic, often manipulative males attempt to dominate males who are less driven or who see themselves as something other than leaders. Complex systems of laws and social mores act to codify status assignments within a given society but also may serve to set some limits on genetically acquired tendencies to establish social hierarchies on the basis of physical power or status. These complex legal and moral codes, in conjunction with humans' inclination to seek alliances, can result in a complex and shifting pattern of dominance in more open and democratic societies, while rigid structure enforced by institutionalized means, often including violence, maintains the inflexible dominance hierarchies of authoritarian regimes.

REFLECTIVE SELF-AWARENESS IN THE GREAT APES

It seems unlikely that humans are the only species that possess reflective self-awareness, although some controversy exists among primatologists, ethologists, psychologists, and evolutionary biologists regarding whether and which species, besides humans, possess this capacity (e.g., Heyes, 1993), or whether any others do. Although it is thought possible that elephants or large marine mammals like whales and dolphins are aware of themselves as separate organisms, the question is difficult to answer for these species in large part because of the difficulties in devising a valid test of the hypothesis. How could one determine, for example, that a killer whale is able to reflect on itself? Research with the great apes, on the other hand, has yielded evidence suggesting that these animals experience a relatively refined capacity for self-awareness.

Self-representations and self-awareness may be useful adaptations, especially among animals whose cultures are characterized by complex social relationships and dominance hierarchies. In fact, some ethologists argue that self-representations and self-awareness may lie behind animals' comprehension of their own place in a dominance hierarchy (Essock-Vitale & Seyfarth, 1987; Seyfarth, 1981).

Chimpanzees were the first nonhuman primates for which fairly persuasive evidence of self-awareness was obtained, through the use of an experimental paradigm referred to as *mirror self-recognition* (MSR), a procedure devised by Gordon G. Gallup (1970). The rationale behind this approach is that many animals, when confronted with their own reflection in a mirror, respond as they would to a stranger of their own species and sex (Anderson, 1984). Gallup exposed four chimpanzees to a full-length mirror placed outside their cages for 8 hours a day over a 10-day period in order to get them used to looking at themselves. On the 11th day the animals were anesthetized and marked over one eye and on the opposite ear with an odorless nonirritating red dye. The mirror was removed, the animals were returned to their cages, and they were observed in order to determine how frequently they spontaneously touched either of the areas that had been marked. The mirror then was returned to its former position outside the enclosure.

All the chimpanzees tested with the mirror discovered spontaneously that they had been marked and seemed interested in examining the marks in the mirror. They used their reflection to allow them to touch the marks repeatedly, and often smelled and inspected their fingers visually after having done so. The amount of time spent in front of the mirror was four times greater than the time the apes spent looking in the mirror prior to the marking. A similar finding was reported for orangutans (Lethmate & Dücker, 1973).

Whether gorillas have self-awareness is unclear, although it has been argued that a failure to find evidence as robust as that for chimps reflects gorillas' different temperament. Nonetheless, Patterson and Cohn (1994) have provided other evidence of self-awareness in Koko, a lowland gorilla who has been trained in sign language (Patterson & Linden, 1981). At the age of about 3½ years, Koko began to engage spontaneously in "mirror-guided self-directed behaviors" (Patterson & Cohn, 1994, p. 273); among other things, "Koko would groom her face and underarms, pick at her teeth, and examine her tongue while studying her reflection. She would also comb her hair, make faces, and adorn herself with hats, wigs, and makeup in front of the mirror" (p. 274). Koko paid special attention to parts of her anatomy (e.g., her tongue) that she could not see without a mirror. Patterson and Cohn later found evidence of self-awareness using MSR when Koko was 19 years old; they noted that "during the marked session, the majority of Koko's initial self-grooming behaviors involved removing the paint from her brow" (1994, p. 278).

Drawing inferences based on observations of Koko may be complicated by the fact that she has a vocabulary of several hundred words in American Sign Language. As we will discuss later, some authors have argued that language may be necessary for consciousness; perhaps, because she could use language, Koko had an advantage over other gorillas in this regard. In any case, Koko's skill in using symbolic language provide intriguing evidence of self-awareness, as do her spontaneous responses to questions by means of sign language. For example, when asked who she is, Koko typically responds with something like "Koko," "me," or "gorilla." Asked to identify the gorilla she saw in the mirror, Koko's response, upon seeing her own teeth, was "me there Koko good teeth good." When asked how she is feeling, she responds with such comments as "fine Koko." In contrast, her response to the question, "Who is Mike?" (her gorilla companion) was "devil" and "bad," which Patterson and Cohn noted was typical of Koko's past spontaneous comments about Mike (1994, p. 280). Similar data were obtained regarding Chantek, an orangutan who also was taught language (Miles, 1994) and who demonstrated convincing evidence of self-awareness.

In addition to data obtained using the MSR protocol, other observations suggest that apes may be aware of themselves as individuals. For example, chimpanzees allowed to explore their images in a mirror spontaneously examine body parts that otherwise are invisible to them—the back, the face, and the inside of the mouth, for example. Female chimps have been seen turning around to inspect their genital swellings. Many apes have adorned themselves and examined the results in the mirror; Koko likes to put on lipstick. Although the data may be open to other interpretations (if B. F. Skinner were still around, he undoubtedly would have a bone to pick with this perspective), the evidence certainly suggests the possibility that when they look in the mirror, these animals know they are looking at themselves. Primates other than humans and apes show no signs of such behaviors suggesting self-awareness.

SELF-REPRESENTATIONS AND REFLECTIVE SELF-AWARENESS

Self-representations are distinct from the capacity to be aware of those representations as models of oneself. In other words, self-awareness is a function of an interaction between the representational schema we call the self on the one hand, and the system mediating awareness on the other. Animal research suggests that some kind of reflective self-awareness may be present in great apes but does not shed much light on the question of whether other animals without this reflective ability might possess representations of themselves. Perhaps only humans and apes have well-developed reflective self-awareness, but it seems reasonable that other species might have a capacity for some kind of self-representation (see de Waal, 1996; Vauclair, 1996).

Certainly among humans, relatively stable self-representations may serve to mark and maintain one's position in the pecking order. Thus at one extreme we see self-representations that reflect an aggressive sense of entitlement to all the resources and privileges the group and the society have to offer, while at the other extreme are self-schemas characterized by a deeply felt sense that one deserves little or nothing. Interestingly, it appears that many humans rise to the top of the hierarchy not because of any special talents or accomplishments but primarily because they believe they belong there. Politicians and plenty of celebrities who are famous for being famous come to mind.

ATTRIBUTIONS AND A THEORY OF MIND AMONG THE APES

If great apes have the capacity for reflective self-awareness, it raises the possibility that they are aware that other apes have minds, selves, desires, and thoughts of their own. As van Hooff (1994) put it, "there can be little doubt that the intelligence of nonhuman primates manifests itself primarily in the social realm. They know about social relations in a much more refined way than they know about their non-social environment" (p. 269).

For example, de Waal (1982) described a situation in a chimpanzee colony in which Luit, a male chimp involved in a dominance struggle with another male named Nikkie, appeared to recognize that his facial expression might betray his anxiety, something that would work against his striving to be in charge. With the support of two females, Luit had chased Nikkie into a tree. Shortly afterward, Nikkie began hooting at Luit from the tree. Sitting with his back to Nikkie, Luit was observed to have an "anxious-fearful" grin (a sign of submission) on his face, which he covered with his hand, pressing his lips together. According to de Waal (1982), "I saw the nervous grin appear on his face again and once more he used his fingers to press his lips together. The third time Luit finally succeeded in wiping the grin off his face; only then did he turn around. A little later he displayed at Nikkie as if nothing happened" (p. 133). Then, de Waal notes, with the help of one of the females, Luit again chased Nikkie into a tree.

This observation suggests that Luit was aware of his internal state and knew his state might be conveyed in his facial expression. He also seemed to know how he was likely to be perceived by his rival.

Chimpanzees appear to have a good idea what kinds of knowledge other animals can and cannot have in different situations. Povinelli (1994) described an experiment in which chimpanzee subjects observed two humans, "one of whom (the knower) would hide food under one of several cups, and one of whom (the guesser) would be outside the room during the hiding procedure. The subjects would see that the knower had food and was placing it in one of several cups, but a screen would prevent them from seeing exactly which cup held the food; they would also see that the guesser had left the room" (p. 289). Following this manipulation, the person designated as the "guesser" would return to the room, the screen would be removed, and both guesser and knower would point at different cups, "advising" the chimpanzee as to the location of the food. Clearly, the guesser would not have seen the food being hidden, and three of the four chimpanzees proved themselves consistently able to take the knower's advice over that of the guesser (Povinelli, Nelson, & Boysen, 1990). Rhesus monkeys, in contrast, were unable to perform this task (Povinelli, Parks, & Novak, 1991, 1992). In order to determine how the different species of primates fared on this problem compared with humans, the test also was administered to 3- and 4-year-old children. The 3-year-old was unable to perform accurately, whereas the 4-year-old not only was accurate but was consistently better than the chimpanzees (Povinelli & deBlois, 1992).

In another study, Povinelli, Nelson, and Boysen (1992) trained chimpanzees to be either an *informant,* who had knowledge of the location of food, or an *operator,* who lacked this knowledge but could operate a set of controls that would deliver a food reward to both participants. Subjects were trained in one or the other role until they could perform it without error; then the roles were switched. The investigators found that new learning was not required: the subjects who had been operators quickly demonstrated a grasp of their new role as informants, and the same was true of the informants-turned-operators. Thus, rather than simply responding to learning contingencies, the chimpanzees seemed to take others' perspectives and to adopt these for themselves when it was appropriate to do so.

Tactical Deception

If an animal is able to make judgments about another animal's mental state, it follows that the first animal might be able to use this capacity to manipulate the second animal's perceptions of a situation. We just saw something like this in the case of Luit and Nikkie (in the previous section), when Luit made a deliberate effort to conceal evidence of his anxiety in the context of a dominance struggle, but similar findings have been reported by primatologists in many other settings. Byrne and Whiten (1985) suggested the use of the term "tactical deception" to refer to behavior that is ostensibly genuine but that is actually intended to deceive another. They argued, following Dawkins and Krebs (1978), that communication might be shaped by natural selection in part for the manipulation of other individuals to the communicator's advantage, rather than simply for the transmission of truthful information.

Whiten and Byrne (1988) solicited accounts of deceptive behavior from primatologists around the world and discussed 13 different subcategories of deception, "grouped within the five major functional classes of *concealment, distraction, creating an image, manipulation of target using social tool,* and *deflection of target to fall guy*" (p. 234; emphasis in original). For example, one baboon who was being chased by another baboon suddenly adopted an alert posture, turning to watch the horizon in a manner typical of that species when a predator has been observed (p. 233), although no predators were in the vicinity.

In an example cited by de Waal of chimpanzees "creating an image" (1982, p. 48), a chimp named Yeroen hurt his hand while fighting with Nikkie (Luit's rival); de Wall and his associates observed that whenever Yeroen walked past Nikkie and for as long as Nikkie could possibly see him, Yeroen hobbled "pitifully," but once he was out of Nikkie's sight he resumed a normal gait. This behavior continued for nearly a full week. Whiten and Byrne (1988) also discussed an instance originally described by F. X. Plooij in which two chimpanzees attempted to outsmart one another. One chimp was alone, waiting to be fed some bananas. The fruit was in a metal box that was opened from a distance just as another chimpanzee appeared. The first animal abruptly closed the box, nonchalantly walked away, and sat down as though he had no interest in the box. The intruder left, but when he was out of sight of the first chimpanzee, hid behind a tree to observe the first chimp. Meanwhile, the first chimp, unaware of being observed, returned to the box and opened it. At that point, the second animal came over and helped himself to the bananas (Whiten & Byrne, 1988, p. 242). In this case, each animal attempted to deceive the other. Besides scheming, each animal must have had an idea what the other was thinking and wanting; in other words, they each demonstrated possession of a theory of mind.

It seems plausible that successful deception is one adaptive advantage of communication for animals that must compete with one another for scarce resources. Similar deceptive behavior has been reported among chimpanzee females and subordinate males, who may sneak away to have sex away from the group, unseen by the dominant male. Deceptive behavior certainly is ubiquitous among human beings, who have developed highly sophisticated manipulations. For our purposes, more compelling than the notion that deception has an evolutionary adaptive basis is the idea that the capacity to deceive reveals a complex representation of both self and other in a sustained, organized, and instrumental way across time.

Symbolic Language: Washoe Teaches Loulis to Talk

Since the first attempts to teach language to chimpanzees, the scientific community has been divided as to whether apes have the capacity for true language. The primary questions involved concern whether ape language reflects simple conditioning (Epstein, Lanza, & Skinner, 1980) and whether apes are capable of using human syntax (Chomsky, 1988). While not taking sides in this controversy, we are impressed with the ability of apes to communicate novel ideas and use symbols in novel ways.

Washoe, a wild female chimpanzee captured as an infant, was taught American Sign Language (ASL) by Beatrice T. Gardner and R. Allen Gardner (1971; also R. A. Gardner, B. T. Gardner, & van Cantfort, 1989). Washoe acquired the ability to use signs fluently, and signing became a routine part of her behavioral repertoire. She frequently was observed signing to herself when alone, often practiced new signs, and "read aloud" to herself from picture books by signing. On occasion, the signs she made indicated that she was thinking about performing some action, as when she signed "up hurry" then climbed a rope ladder.

Washoe taught her adopted son, Loulis, to use signs (Fouts, 1997; Fouts, Fouts, & van Cantfort, 1989). Fouts and his coworkers deliberately chose not to teach ASL to Loulis in order to ascertain whether he might learn to sign by observing Washoe. The researchers themselves used few signs in Loulis's presence and used spoken English or chimpanzee vocalizations to communicate with Washoe, who understood some English relatively well. By his 8th day with Washoe, Loulis already had learned the name of the man who brought breakfast, and shortly afterward he had learned the signs for *tickle, drink,* and *hug.* Over time, his use of ASL grew considerably. Learning mostly on his own, he observed his mother, and practiced by himself and with other adults. According to Fouts (1997) the large majority of his signing was spontaneous, not prompted by Washoe. Yet, once in a while, Washoe actively attempted to teach Loulis certain words. On at least one occasion, Washoe even took Loulis's hand and placed it in the proper position to make a specific sign (*food*). As Fouts (1997) pointed out, this was probably the first time one nonhuman taught another nonhuman to use a uniquely human language.

Austin, Sherman, and Vicki: Language and Complex Cognition

Austin and Sherman were male chimpanzees taught to use a keyboard for communication with one another and with their experimenters (Savage-

Rumbaugh & Lewin, 1994; Savage-Rumbaugh, Rumbaugh, & Boysen, 1978a, 1978b). In a fascinating series of studies, Savage-Rumbaugh and her associates showed that these two apes could use their symbolic language with remarkable facility to convey information and state their plans. As they describe the protocol in one such experiment, "we built six food sites in the chimps' rooms, each of which required a specific tool to gain access to the site—key, money, stick, straw, sponge, and wrench. We put food in one site at a time and introduced one tool at a time. Ultimately, we randomly selected a tool site to be baited, then displayed the tray of tools and encouraged the chimps to survey the situation and decide which tool they needed and how to request it" (Savage-Rumbaugh & Lewin, 1994, p. 80). Once Austin and Sherman had become facile in the use of this setup, the experimenters designed a study in which only one chimp had access to tools and only the other chimp had access to food. Almost immediately, the two chimpanzees understood what was expected of them, and the chimp with access to food began to request the appropriate tool from the other chimp.

This pair of animals was capable of using their language for a variety of purposes. They could announce their plans, then do what they had indicated that they would do (e.g., going to get food in another room; Savage-Rumbaugh et al., 1983). On one occasion Austin stated that he intended to make a funny face, which he proceeded to do. They could express preferences for foods, and for other items as well. Sherman, for example, acquired a colored plastic drinking glass of which he was rather fond, and he would insist, using the keyboard, that his drinks be presented in the glass.

Austin and Sherman also were capable of using abstract linguistic concepts. For example, taught symbols for the words "food" and "tool," they were required to perform tasks involving different degrees of abstraction. After learning the superordinate concepts (*food* and *tool*), both chimpanzees were able to indicate to which category each of a series of items (e.g., banana) belonged, missing only 1 item out of a total of 33 trials between the two chimps. A similar capacity for categorization was demonstrated by the chimpanzee Vicki, who was raised in a home as though she were a human child by Catherine and Keith J. Hayes (see K. J. Hayes & Nissen, 1971). Vicki could sort objects by color, shape, or size. She was able to sort a set of 40 pictures into 2 categories: either humans or nonhuman animals. It was noteworthy that Vicki put her own picture with those of the humans (K. J. Hayes & Nissen, 1971).

Koko Says What's on Her Mind

Investigations of primate language have turned up a number of other surprising behaviors. The gorilla Koko, for example, knows the signs that go with many English words, and has played at rhyming and making plays on words (Patterson & Linden, 1981). When upset, and sometimes when playing, she uses insults of her own invention. She is able to use sign language to indicate when she is afraid of something, and once referred to a past emotional state (anger) 3 days after an incident (Patterson & Cohn, 1994, p. 282). Like Washoe, she sometimes signs to herself when she is alone.

Primate Fantasy Play

Nonhuman primates trained in language, like children, have been observed engaging in fantasy play. According to Catherine Hayes (1951), the chimpanzee Vicki frequently pretended to play with an imaginary pulltoy. Similarly, Koko used a rubber snake to play at chasing one person around the room, pretending that the snake was biting him on the arm (Patterson & Linden, 1981, p. 136). Patterson and Linden wrote that "Koko spends a good deal of time talking to and playing games with her toys. This is a private pastime of hers, and she does not like to be watched when she is doing it. She seems to get embarrassed when she discovers someone observing her while engaged in such play, and she abruptly breaks off whatever she is doing. One day I noticed Koko signing *kiss* to her alligator puppet. When she saw that I was looking, she abruptly stopped signing and turned away" (1981, p. 137). Koko plays with dolls, to whom she signs. She also likes drawing, and while not "particularly artistic," she is able to "come up with some fair representations, especially if she is copying from a picture or model. She uses appropriate colors and gets objects in their correct places" (p. 137). Koko is not the only ape to try her hand at representational painting and drawing. Fouts (1997) reported that the chimpanzees Washoe, Dar, Tatu, and Moja all enjoyed their painting and took it seriously. Using ASL, they could explain what they had drawn, and all four gave titles to their works (one of Washoe's was titled "Electric Hot Red").

Tall Tales

Telling lies is apparently not the sole province of human beings. Just as they engage in tactical deception, some language-trained primates have been caught red-handed in falsehoods. For example, in her excitement, Koko bit someone lightly while playing chase with him. When Patterson asked Koko what she had done, Koko immediately replied "not teeth." Patterson told Koko that was a lie, to which Koko's response was "Bad again Koko bad again." The orangutan Chantek also was observed engaging in various kinds of verbal and nonverbal deceptive behavior (Miles, 1986, 1994).

Lying and nonverbal tactical deception may have adaptive significance, and both certainly are ubiquitous among human children and adults. Tactical deception is interesting in that it involves acting *as if* something were the case, when in fact the actor's own representation of reality is inconsistent with the image he or she is attempting to create. Primates who engage in deception thus are apparently not limited by their representations of things but have the capacity to imagine things as being other than they actually are. This capacity is apparent as well in their fantasy play—Koko chasing her human companion with a rubber snake, for example, or playing with her dolls.

LEARNING LANGUAGE PRODUCES BEHAVIOR CHANGE IN NONHUMAN PRIMATES

The use of language appears to have produced enduring changes in behavior and personality in some apes. Many animals have been observed signing to themselves much as young children talk to themselves, or perhaps in a way that is analogous to how adult humans often talk to themselves with inner speech. They are able to learn how to use signs from one another. Moreover, those who already have language sometimes actively attempt to instruct those who do not. Young chimpanzees possess the cognitive capacity to acquire language spontaneously, and language becomes an enduring part of their behavioral repertoire.

If a sufficient number of chimpanzees in a group could be taught ASL, it would be interesting to follow that group over time to see whether language became a significant part of their culture, and whether it was spontaneously taught to and acquired by young chimps and the language-naive. Would they, like primates in the lab, devise their own novel symbols for unnamed objects or concepts? The observations of Loulis suggests that they might. Would expansion of chimpanzees' capacity for communication have significant effects on individual behavior or on patterns of interindividual interaction? Would the use of sign language persist, or would it die out? Chimps in the lab seem to have recognized the advantages of a more highly differentiated means of communication than the one they use naturally; would that be sufficient incentive for them to maintain it in a group without human interference? Would a chimpanzee culture have what it takes to maintain such a language without it degenerating over time?

The brains of great apes apparently have a capacity for language despite the fact that there is no evidence of spontaneous development of standard symbolic languages among apes in the wild. The data presented above raise several interesting and important issues. First, language can be acquired by procedural learning among animals with no prior history of language use. As a consequence, their behavior is altered significantly. Second, they appear to recognize, at some level, the adaptive value of a language and attempt to use it not only with humans but with each other. Third, the acquisition of language seems also to change emergent cognitive abilities. This was demonstrated by the finding that many language-trained apes seem to acquire the ability to think in abstract categories. Finally, although one must be cautious in drawing inferences concerning humans from observations of nonhuman primates, the data may help to illuminate the relationships between cognition, language, and consciousness.

The chimpanzees Austin and Sherman (discussed above) provide a striking example of how, in association with the learning of language and with socialization in human mores, chimpanzee behavior may be changed significantly and seemingly permanently. Chimpanzees in the wild are cooperative in many respects and will share meat obtained in a hunt with one another (albeit somewhat reluctantly), but they don't typically share fruits or vegetables. Instead, they tend to turn their backs on other chimps while eating, and while all may be eating from the same food source, they consume their individual meals in private. In the process of training Austin and Sherman to communicate cooperatively to obtain food, (Savage-Rumbaugh and Lewin (1994) managed to encourage them to share food as well. Sherman, who was dominant, would be approached somewhat nervously by Austin, requesting a share of Sherman's food, even when no humans were visible. According to Savage-Rumbaugh and Lewin (1994, pp. 76–77), "Sherman would sometimes look away as if trying to ignore Austin, but Austin would persist and Sherman's face would begin to assume a guilty expression, as though he were aware of breaking a pact between them. Sherman would then hand over almost half of the food to Austin. The sharing was nearly always done quietly and calmly, and Sherman and Austin even began to look at each other while they ate." Over time, this process became more natural for them, and they even introduced their own innovations into the way food was shared.

SUMMARY AND CONCLUSION

What can we take from this discussion of the emotional, cognitive, and behavioral lives of nonhuman primates? First, the overall pattern of similarities and differences between and among various species of primates (including humans) demonstrates the effects of natural selection in shaping behaviors that are adaptive within a wide range of contexts. The extreme aggression of dominant male baboons and their rigid, authoritarian social structures presumably confer a survival advantage in the competitive world of the African savannah, where leopards and other dangerous predators are a constant threat.

Certain basic themes are apparent across species, although the precise manner in which they are manifested may show striking variability. Infantile dependence and attachment (and the kinds of social and psychological pathology resulting from its disruption) are nearly ubiquitous among primates. A depressed rhesus monkey abandoned by her mother reacts much like a human infant in the same situation. Early social deprivation profoundly affects future patterns of relationships for monkeys, and for humans as well. Dominance hierarchies are present across species, although that of the bonobo differs greatly from that of the baboon, the human, or the chimpanzee. Reconciliation is very important for the maintenance of harmonious relationships among chimpanzees, bonobos, stump-tailed macaques, and *Homo sapiens*.

From an evolutionary perspective, the way in which reflective self-awareness was favored by natural selection is not entirely clear, but for intelligent social animals it has certain advantages. One such benefit is the ability to understand one's place in the group, as well as the relative position of others. A second benefit is the (presumably) associated theory of mind that accompanies self-awareness. The ability to take another's perspective may contribute to smooth social interaction and enhanced survival in the group. For animals with a prolonged period of childhood dependency and associated strong emotional attachments, a theory of mind facilitates adults' ability to understand the needs of and to care for their young.

Self-awareness also provides a higher-level cognitive capacity that can permit behavior change. If one's behavior is more or less nonconscious and automatic, this may be advantageous insofar as it makes one's reaction to events rapid and—as a result of learning—adaptive. However, an idiosyncratic learning history may lead to the acquisition of maladaptive habitual behaviors as well. Ongoing learning itself may modify such habits, but awareness of self adds another dimension to personality. If one is able to monitor one's activity and to assess with some degree of accuracy its effectiveness, and if one has even a limited capacity consciously to regulate one's behavior, one has the ability to change. In other words, reflective self-awareness permits further refinement of an individual's adaptation to the environment.

The many cognitive and behavioral similarities among primate species also should give us some confidence, in drawing inferences regarding brain functioning and personality, that research using primates is unquestionably relevant for understanding human functioning. If the nervous systems of different species of monkeys show similar schemes of functional organization, it seems unlikely that the situation should change abruptly when we get to human beings. Some may quibble with the relevance of studies of rats and marine invertebrates for understanding people, but when species as diverse as rats and monkeys show certain similarities, the same ought logically to hold true for humans and apes.

The attempt to teach language to the great apes is important for several reasons. One involves the fact that, of primates, only the apes seem capable of learning symbolic language *and* only the apes appear to possess the capacity for self-awareness. At one time, Gazzaniga and LeDoux (1978) argued, on the basis of their studies of humans who had undergone "split-brain" surgery for control of epilepsy, that language may be a sine qua non for consciousness. What the ape studies suggest is that human-like language may not be necessary but that a capacity for complex symbolic communication may be associated with self-awareness.

Finally, the acquisition of language seems to have produced significant and enduring changes in the behavior and cognitive capacities of at least some of the primates who have learned to communicate with people. We saw, for example, cases of gorillas talking to themselves and engaging in fantasy play, of chimps learning to cooperate on complex instrumental tasks, and of adult chimps attempting to teach their children sign language. In these cases, the animals' use of one functional subcomponent of cognition (language) was expanded through training, and they acquired the ability to use language spontaneously, in novel ways. As a result, these animals end up with personalities that are perhaps strikingly different from those of wild-type animals of the same species.

12

Conscious and Nonconscious Functioning

INTRODUCTION

The purpose of this chapter is to examine consciousness and its relationship to nonconscious functioning, using data from cognitive neuroscience and experimental psychology. As in our discussion of state, we begin with the assumption that consciousness, like other psychological phenomena, is an emergent property of the activity of a heterarchically organized array of distributed neural networks, each with its own modular structure. Consciousness therefore is not a *thing* or a *structure*, but a constantly changing, ongoing set of processes. Our goal in this chapter is to examine the dynamic nature of consciousness and to explore some of the implications of its modular architecture.

A logical corollary of the theory that the brain has a modular distributed architecture is that vast amounts of processing, perceiving, and organizing of stimuli precede and occur in parallel with (and, most often, outside of) the emergence of any experience of consciousness. Data from cognitive neuroscience will be presented that support the hypothesis that there are multiple systems for the regulation of behavior and that these can be subdivided grossly into two major classes which are dissociable but which interact with one another. Nonconscious processing, by means of which most of the brain's work is conducted, involves the automatic selection of cognitive, perceptual, and behavioral routines that are appropriate for a given situation and that require little or no thought or conscious deliberation for their activation. Consciousness, on the other hand, allows the individual deliberate access to a broad range of neuropsychological phenomena but possesses a severely limited capacity. Among its other important capacities is that it enables one to recognize and respond to novelty. This deliberate conscious control system allows the individual to override the automatic behaviors generated by the first (nonconscious) system and provides a mechanism for the development of new and adaptive behavior.

In this chapter, we also will review data providing empirical support for the idea that most neural processing takes place outside of awareness. Conscious processing is inefficient and has significant limitations in terms of the quantity and nature of the contents it can hold at any given instant—hence the need for nonconscious processing. In addition, because of the computational costs associated with conscious processing, activities that can become automatized and performed nonconsciously are very likely to become so, to the distinct advantage of the individual. The vast amount of parallel processing that takes place in the brain, the hierarchical nature of this processing, and the limited capacity of working memory dictate that most psychological phenomena occur nonconsciously.

Although nonconscious processing is significantly more efficient than conscious processing, consciousness has certain advantages. It permits the monitoring and modification of unconscious routines, and hence facilitates the acquisition of adaptive behavior. In addition, because of its limited capacity and serial nature, consciousness provides a coherent structure to experience. Nonconscious functioning, on the other hand, permits contradictory or inconsistent processes to take place in parallel. Conscious and nonconscious processing work in tandem to allow for split-second nonconscious recognition and reaction to circumstances, followed shortly by the possibility of self-correction, fine-tuning, and inhibition of responses—a mixture of tendencies that has unique adaptive advantages.

Consciousness is further limited in that not everything we perceive *can* be experienced consciously. The architecture of the brain dictates what material can gain access to awareness and the circumstances under which this can occur. Thus, awareness of some neuropsychological phenomena (e.g., proprioceptive stimuli processed by the cerebellum) is permanently barred because of the way the brain is wired. Other psychological phenomena may have their access to awareness restricted due to a variety of physiological and pathological factors (such as brain injury, medications, or neuromodulation). For yet other phenomena, access to awareness may occur readily, but selectively as a function of a host of environmental and internal variables.

One interesting aspect of conscious processing is that it seems to be intolerant of ambiguity. Consciousness organizes the available data into organized coherent stories or explanations, even when this involves frank confabulation. The study of persons who have undergone resection of the corpus callosum for control of epilepsy has demonstrated the common oc-currence of a process essentially indistinguishable from the "defense mech-anism" of *rationalization*. Clinically and theoretically, this is important in-sofar as we seem rarely to know the actual reasons for the things we do but nevertheless automatically come up with reasons when we must explain what we have done. These reasons may be plausible, and may even be accu-rate, but such accuracy may be coincidental.

Finally, in this chapter we discuss the concept of a *representation*, which is an emergent model of some perceptual, motor, or cognitive pro-cess. A person can be conscious of something only insofar as he or she is able to form and attend to a representation of it. We emphasize that a representation, like all complex psychological phenomena, is best under-stood as a set of processes rather than as an entity or a set of discrete en-tities. Given the process nature of representing, at any given moment a person can have only a single complete representation of ongoing experi-ence (a representation that may of course vary greatly across and within individuals in terms of its adaptive value, complexity, and stability across time). There are different modes available to the brain for representing experience. Some representations, because of their organization, may be only marginally available to consciousness. Other representational pro-cesses are likely to have properties that make them more readily accessi-ble to awareness. We will present some interesting data concerning the vi-sual system which demonstrate that perceiving an external object utilizes the same neural pathways as when the same object is brought to mind through imagination.

FREUD AND THE RELATIONSHIP OF CONSCIOUSNESS TO NONCONSCIOUS PROCESSES

Sigmund Freud was among the first explorers of consciousness to attempt to bring a scientific sensibility (if not a scientific method) to his studies of consciousness (1895/1966). In spite of the limitations of the neurological knowledge available to him and the difficulty of applying the scientific method to psychology during his time, he made observations on the nature of conscious and nonconscious processing—and the relationship between the two—that in many instances anticipate the findings of cognitive neuro-science and cognitive psychology. Freud's observations led him to conclude that conscious experience, and the organization of consciousness from mo-ment to moment, could be understood only if unconscious processes were assumed.

Freud argued as follows:

The unconscious must be assumed to be the general basis of psychical life. The unconscious is the larger sphere, which includes within it the smaller sphere of the conscious. Everything conscious has an unconscious preliminary stage; whereas what is unconscious may remain at that stage and nevertheless claim to be regarded as having the full value of a psychical process. The unconscious is the true psychical reality; *in its innermost nature it is as much unknown to us as the reality of the external world, and it is as incompletely presented by the data of consciousness as is the external world by the communications of our sense organs.* (Freud, 1900, pp. 612–613; emphasis in original)

Historically, people have had difficulty accepting the notion of nonconscious organizing activity. One perhaps can understand a visceral rejection of the original Freudian notion of an unconscious seething with sexual and aggressive impulses, because to accept such an unconscious seemed to require accepting unsavory possibilities about human nature. But many people are uneasy even about the prospect of nonconscious processing which does not necessarily require one to embrace such distasteful contents.

Some theorists have opposed the idea of nonconscious (and even conscious) functioning. Thus, for half a century, strident advocates of behaviorism considered the study of both conscious and nonconscious processing to be intellectually disreputable. William James, whose own thinking anticipated many current psychological concepts, could not accept the idea of nonconscious processing. In recent years the winds of theorizing have shifted, as cognitive psychologists and neuroscientists increasingly have focused their attention on these fundamental psychological phenomena. There now are a number of models of the neural basis of consciousness (e.g., Baars, 1988, 1997; Baars & Newman, 1994; Bogen, 1995; Dennett, 1991; Dennett & Kinsbourne, 1992; Gazzaniga, 1995; Kinney et al., 1994; Libet, 1985; Newman, Baars, & Cho, 1997; Sperry, 1966). The different perspectives reflect considerable theoretical disagreement, as well as the immense conceptual and methodological difficulties inherent in investigating something as intangible as awareness. Yet, while there is considerable disagreement, all these models presume considerable complex nonconscious processing.

CONSCIOUSNESS IS AN EMERGENT PROCESS

There are tremendous conceptual difficulties associated with any attempt to discuss or study conscious and nonconscious processes. This should not be surprising, given that the nature of consciousness has perplexed philosophers, scientists, poets, physicians, psychologists, and others for thousands of years. As with the concept of *state*, the terms "consciousness" and "the unconscious" have diverse colloquial and technical meanings, creating a situation ripe for muddied discourse. Almost everyone has some understanding of what is meant by consciousness. Yet the meaning of unconscious is likely to be even more obscure and diverse, with many people equating "the unconscious" with their personal understanding of what constitutes the Freudian unconscious (typically understood as a place fraught with antisocial wishes or impulses).

Philosophers and scientists have struggled for centuries over the relationship of the mind to the body. Much of the confusion originates in dualism, or in attempts to understand the relationship of the mind to the brain as a linear one. Often, this confusion has expressed itself in a quest to locate the mind within the brain, perhaps in a specific structure. René Descartes, for example, proposed that the pineal body was the locus at which the mind and brain come together. The fact is that there is no such locus, and there can be no such place, for the mind is a dynamic emergent property of the complete pattern of nonlinear activity of the brain's modular architecture at each instant.

A tendency to objectify the idea of consciousness often leads to the formulation of questions about its nature that lose track of consciousness as an emergent process, something relatively insubstantial. Therefore, unless it is editorially too cumbersome, we will try to use the terms *conscious processing* and *nonconscious processing*. To speak of *processing* counters the inevitable tendency to reify "consciousness" and "nonconsciousness." Nonconscious processing refers to neural activity that occurs without awareness. Strictly speaking, we argue that there is no *conscious mind*; rather, conscious processing is an emergent property of the functioning of certain distributed brain systems. Consciousness usually entails awareness of a thing or of many things: perceptions, thoughts, images, ideas, our selves, and other such phenomena. The contents of consciousness are whatever representations—words, symbols, images, thoughts, and so on—are *explicitly present in one's mind* (whatever that means) at any given time.

The brain has a structure, although this structure changes considerably over the course of life, and subtly from moment to moment. Yet, while the brain's structure is not unimportant, it is the brain's dynamic processes that give minds their distinctive properties. In contrast to the brain, the mind has no structure, and it makes no sense to discuss it as though it did. Mind is an emergent property of complex transactions among the environment, hierarchically organized neurophysiological processes, and other physiological properties of the organism (e.g., endocrinological processes). Mind is not a substance, something with an existence apart from neural *processes*. All psychological processes necessarily have a neural substrate and cannot be separated from neural processes.

THE CONTENTS OF CONSCIOUSNESS

Conscious processing, because of it complexity and nonlinearity, can have markedly different manifestations across time. At one moment, intense conscious focus may be brought to bear on some environmental happening. In the next, one's focus may become more diffuse. This variability occurs in part because changes in the valence of internal and external environmental stimulation can have effects that ripple through the system, affecting the quality of conscious experience. Some stimuli demand our attention, others encourage it, whereas still others lead us to look away. Like the wind on waves, the world and our reactions to it steer our habitual thoughts, feelings, and perceptions.

A brief introspective look at what passes through one's mind, while it may not tell us much about how the brain and mind operate (Nisbett & Wilson, 1977), at least can demonstrate some of the character of the contents of conscious awareness (the highly motivated reader may want to re-read some "stream-of-consciousness" sections of James Joyce's *Ulysses*, e.g., Molly Bloom's final interior monologue, pp. 723–768 of the Random House edition, 1934/1946). As you read the words on this page, you silently articulate what you read, moving through the text in blocks of a word, a phrase, or a line, depending on how rapidly you read. Other information is processed simultaneously. Perhaps you find this material boring or hard to follow, in which case you may be more aware of your own inner speech than you are of the meaning of the words you read. Perhaps you are reading automatically without processing the meaning, in which case you might reach the end of a paragraph and realize you didn't attend to anything you read. Without really noticing, you perceive the font, the margins of the page, the weight of the book, and other peripheral stimuli in the room. If you really are paying attention to what you are reading, you are processing the text in a sequential manner and can handle only a limited amount of information at a time. If the ideas are at times complex or novel, you may need to reread some sections to understand them fully. You may be thinking about the meaning as you read, trying to picture what we are describing in your "mind's eye." In the background of awareness, you may be hearing a song, or a part of a song, playing repetitively in your mind. You may be daydreaming, plotting revenge for an insult that made you angry earlier in the day, or thinking of what to do about dinner.

BASIC ASPECTS OF CONSCIOUSNESS

Consciousness, although an interesting, important, and useful property, is not a sine qua non of minds. Most neuropsychological processing takes place outside awareness, and most of it is permanently and completely inaccessible to consciousness. In fact, a thought experiment among some philosophers who study consciousness is to argue whether it makes sense to consider the existence of such an organism as a *zombie,* a "human being who exhibits perfectly natural, alert, loquacious, vivacious behavior but is in fact not conscious at all, but rather some sort of automaton" (Dennett, 1991, p. 73). Despite the fact that nonconscious functioning dominates our lives, there is no "unconscious mind" per se, only neural processes that take place outside awareness, in association with which "mind" (an emergent property) is manifested.

The performance of complex nonconscious behaviors has been observed among some individuals who have complex partial seizures. Although much of the activity seen during these neurophysiological episodes is relatively simple (e.g., lip smacking, chewing, laughing), it may be much more complex. Forster and Liske (1963), for example, cited the case of a patient who worked in a shirt factory and who, during a seizure, continued to stack shirts as he did normally, although failing to sort them by size. Other complex partial seizure patients have continued activities begun prior to a seizure, including playing the piano, driving a car, or delivering newspapers (Falconer, 1954; Steegman & Winer, 1961). Since consciousness appears to be impaired during seizures of this sort, the occurrence of purposeful (albeit automatic) activity as an aspect of the ictal phenomena shows it is possible to interact with the environment nonconsciously.

Consciousness even occurs during sleep. Specifically, when we dream (i.e., during rapid eye movement, or REM, sleep), we are conscious of events, thoughts, and feelings within the dream. This must be the case, since we can think about events within the dream, remember the dream upon waking, and even recall, within a dream, that we dreamt something similar on a previous occasion. Moreover, we even may become aware, within a dream, that we are dreaming—a kind of metacognitive phenomenon referred to by C. E. Green as *lucid dreaming* (1968; also Green & McCreery, 1994; LaBerge et al., 1981; Laberge, Levitan, & Dement, 1986; van Eeden, 1913). During deep (non-REM) sleep, however, we are unconscious.

Wakefulness and consciousness may be doubly dissociated from one another. Not only is it possible to be asleep but conscious (as in a dream), it is possible to be unconscious but wakeful. In what is known as the *persistent vegetative state,* for example, which is associated with certain serious insults to the central nervous system, the individual demonstrates a more or less normal arousal and sleep–wake cycles, but no conscious functioning. According to the Multi-Society Task Force on Persistent Vegetative State (MSTFPVS, 1994), "the distinguishing feature of the vegetative state is an irregular but cyclic state of circadian sleeping and waking unaccompanied by any behaviorally detectable expression of self-awareness, specific recognition of external stimuli, or consistent evidence of attention or intention or learned responses" (p. 1500). Such patients may smile, grimace, cry, grunt, moan, shout, or startle. They may turn toward auditory or visual stimuli, and on occasion may even visually pursue moving objects (MSTFPVS, 1994).

Persons in a persistent vegetative state are not comatose. A person in a coma is neither wakeful nor conscious. The state likewise differs from the "locked-in" syndrome, in which, as a result of lesions at the level of the pons in the brainstem, an individual is wakeful, conscious, and able to perceive environmental stimuli but is almost completely paralyzed. Someone who is locked in may be able only to breathe and to move his or her eyes from side to side.

Consciousness traditionally has been attributed to the brain's cortex, but it is probable that the matter is rather more complex than that. While the cortex clearly plays a role in consciousness, as we will see later in this chapter, it appears likely that the reticular formation of the brainstem, the reticular nucleus of the thalamus, and the intralaminar nuclei of the thalamus are crucial nodes of a modular distributed network that mediates awareness (Baars, 1997; Baars & Newman, 1994; Crick, 1984; Crick & Koch, 1990; Kinney et al., 1994; Weiskrantz, 1997). While the evidence is somewhat sketchy, there are suggestive findings. For example, Kinney and her associates (1994) reported on the neuropathological examination of Karen Ann Quinlan's brain. Quinlan, who experienced a cardiopulmonary arrest at the age of 21, developed a persistent vegetative state and died 10 years later. In her brain, Kinney et al. found extensive bilateral lesions of the thalamus, with a relatively intact brainstem. There was some cortical damage, but it was thought to be insufficient to account for the severity of her neurological condition.

PATTERN RECOGNITION AND PATTERN GENERATION IN THE BRAIN

Brains and their associated minds are sophisticated tools for the recognition and generation of patterns. As cognitive psychology has so clearly demonstrated, they do not operate logically or rationally. Neither is their functioning characterized by the kind of algorithmic processes proposed by some theorists, nor by the logical thinking attributed to them by proponents of the so-called man-as-rational-actor school of thought. Brains and minds were not designed by an engineer but by millions of years of trial and error. Minds exist in the first place because they have evolutionary significance. If the brain is like a computer, as some propose, it is perhaps more akin to some Rube Goldberg invention than to a standard digital computer.

We are capable of recognizing an almost infinite variety of patterns, and our capacity to do this reflects the interaction of our genetic inheritance, our experience, and the brain's dynamics (Kelso, 1981, 1995; Kelso et al., 1992; McKenna et al., 1990; Thelen, Kelso, & Fogel, 1987; Thelen & Smith, 1994). Similarly, our behavior is the manifestation of complex patterns of neural activity. As Kelso put it, "the human brain is *fundamentally* a pattern-forming, self-organized system governed by nonlinear dynamical laws. Rather than compute, our brain 'dwells' (at least for short times) in metastable states: it is poised on the brink of instability where it can switch flexibly and quickly" from one to another pattern (1995, p. 26; emphasis in original).

If not for our ability to recognize and generate patterns, even such routine tasks as walking or greeting a familiar person would require considerable deliberate effort. In fact, most of the time these activities—and others that are more complex—are accomplished automatically, nonconsciously, and with a minimal amount of effort. This "spontaneous pattern formation is exactly what we mean by *self-organization:* the system organizes itself, but there is no 'self,' no agent inside the system doing the organizing" (Kelso, 1995, p. 8). While much conscious functioning consists of recognition and generation of patterns (perceptual, cognitive, and motor), most of this activity takes place entirely outside awareness.

REPRESENTATION AND REALITY

The mind represents experience in ways that facilitate adaptive action. Everything of which we can be conscious presumes the ability to represent, or to model, some aspect of internal or external reality. We typically experience our models of the world and ourselves as seamless syntheses of multiple, hierarchically organized, distributed representations. Thus, as Kinsbourne (1995) noted, "conscious contents are the products of preconscious processing. At any time they embody the state changes that have occurred. The processing is opaque to awareness" (p. 1321). We will try to limit our use of the term *representations* to refer to the models by which thoughts, images, fantasy, and reality currently is depicted in awareness, and not to *potential* representations such as memories of which we are not presently aware.

Scholars in different disciplines attribute a variety of meanings to the word "representation." For our purposes, it is heuristically useful to think of consciousness as the medium of representational activity. So what happens to representations that are not currently active? They remain as potentially emergent phenomena associated given the activation of specific neural networks. Hence they exist only probabilistically, and not as actual representations stored in some darkened filing room in the brain. From this perspective, there is no such thing as a nonconscious representation. A neural network that currently is not active cannot, by definition, have emergent repesentational activity.

There does exist, however, an abundance of nonconscious, self-organizing activity. We have seen that such activity is emergent from all sorts of complex systems. Nonrepresented phenomena can and do often have a decisive influence on a person's behavior or experience. Certain states represent one mode of organizing activity that may occur without any form of direct representation. Anxiety and other affects can influence behavior without being represented in consciousness. Procedural knowledge is another example of such nonconscious organizational activity. Many early patterns of relational behavior are likely to be established, and subsequently enacted procedurally, without the participation of consciousness.

Modes of Representation

The brain has a number of different ways in which it can represent experience. For example, Kosslyn (1994) distinguished between depictitive and propositional representations. The former consist of images. Recalling our discussion of modularity in the visual system, such a representation is composed of at least two subsystems—visual–spatial and object representation. On the other hand, a propositional representation (Pylyshyn, 1981) is a logical, pseudological, or linguistic means of modeling reality.

There are other types of representations. Auditory images model sound waves, while olfaction does a nice job of providing representations of volatile chemical compounds in our environment. Motor representations (Jeannerod, 1994) create a sensorimotor model of bodies as they move about in the world. As we discuss later in this chapter, either representations themselves, their activation, or their access to consciousness may be defective in certain types of neuropathology. Abstract ideas (e.g., liberty, justice, or evil) also must be represented in some way, and while they are less tangible than concrete images of objects, such concepts frequently are mediated to some extent by visual images such as the Statue of Liberty, the Arc de Triomphe, a blindfolded Justice holding her scales, or a swastika.

Many perceptual phenomena tend to remain in the background of awareness, although we *could* potentially be aware of them: the sensation of your body against the surface on which you are seated, the feel of your clothes against your skin, the weight of this book in your hands, the texture of the paper, the angle of your head and neck, the temperature of the room. Normally outside awareness, these perceptions can be represented consciously through the deliberate or automatic shifting of attention, or as a result of the occurrence of unusual sensations (e.g., the "numb and tingly" paresthesias you experience after having your legs crossed for too long) or urgent ones (like the need to drain your bladder). Other psychologically relevant processes—unconscious proprioception, for example—may have no access to consciousness at all. One need not be aware of a particular activated neural network in order for it to influence one's functioning. In fact, most of the time we are blissfully unaware of what is currently behind our activity.

Self-Representations

A self-representation is a *model* of oneself in the world, another modular piece of the complete self–world representation that dominates our functioning at any given time. As we later discuss in chapter 16 on the self, self-representations are complex, hierarchically ordered phenomena consisting of such relatively concrete experiences as a feeling of the extent of our bodies in space (e.g., Schilder, 1935), as well as abstract ideas about who we are, how we fit into our social environment, and how we might relate to some supreme being. Even apparently simple abilities as moving about in space or feeling that one *could* move about in space require some means of representing oneself within the context of a representational world. Thus, it seems that most animals with complex nervous systems must have some kind of self-representation, although animals of most species may have little or no ability to reflect on their self-image.

CONSCIOUSNESS, WORKING MEMORY, AND ATTENTION

Conceptually, it is a simple matter to confuse attention, consciousness, and working memory. We maintain that the working memory system essentially *is* consciousness. The contents of working memory *are* the contents of consciousness—sensory data, imagination, thoughts, and feelings. Without rehearsal or repetition, these contents remain in working memory for somewhere on the order of 10–20 seconds. The limited capacity of consciousness ensures that we can hold in mind only one complete representation of ourselves and the world at any given time. Attention, on the other hand, involves the focusing of awareness on certain conscious phenomena to the relative exclusion of others (much as the fovea of the eye deals with visual stimuli in the central few degrees of arc of our visual fields, while everything else is consigned to peripheral vision and hence a reduced level of scrutiny). Posner and his colleagues (Posner, DiGirolamo, & Fernandez-Duque, 1997; Posner & Peterson, 1990; Posner & Raichle, 1994) consider the three major functions of attention to be orienting to environmental stimuli, executive control (e.g., direction of attention), and maintenance of alertness.

Kinsbourne (1988, 1995; see also Dennett & Kinsbourne, 1992) holds that at each moment there is "a dominant focus of patterned neural activity that underlies the phenomenal experience of that moment" (1995, p. 1324), and that "whatever subset of currently active cell assemblies participate in this dominant focus determines what content is represented in awareness and is related to the self. . . . From moment to moment the composition of the dominant focus changes, as representations become bound to it while others break away" (1995, p. 1324). This neural activity is the basis of our consciousness of the world.

THE NEUROPSYCHOLOGICAL LIMITS
OF CONSCIOUS PROCESSING

In A. D. Baddeley's modular theory of working memory (1986, 1990, 1992), the *central executive* is a system responsible for processing all types of information in conscious awareness. From one perspective, the central executive can be considered to vary along any of at least three important dimensions, including the *speed, capacity,* and *control* of information processing. *Speed* refers to how quickly one processes information. Simple conscious reactions to stimuli seem to require a minimum of about 100 milliseconds (one-tenth of a second; Blumenthal, 1977), whereas nonconscious reactions may take anywhere from 1 to 25 milliseconds, 1 or 2 orders of magnitude faster. Across the population, individuals can be seen to vary, probably with a normal distribution, with respect to their speed of conscious processing. The speed at which processing takes place can be affected by certain disorders: major depression seems to slow processing speed considerably, for example. Hypomania actually may improve the efficiency of processing—hence its appeal to the hypomanic individual—while full-blown mania involves a rate and quality of processing that is pathological. A quickening of processing speed also may account, in part, for the psychological appeal of CNS stimulants such as cocaine or amphetamines.

Working memory (i.e., consciousness) has a limited capacity, and here too there is considerable variability in the normal population. *Capacity* in this case refers to the amount of information that can be processed consciously per unit of time. In his classic paper on short-term memory, Miller (1956) argued that the number of items one can hold in consciousness is somewhere between five and nine. Miller was concerned primarily with the kind of material one finds on memory tests: digits, words, nonsense syllables, and that sort of thing. The number of items is a function of both individual capacity and the nature and information content of the items themselves (Baddeley, 1986).

At best, we can be aware of only a handful of things at a given moment. An increase in autonomic (sympathetic) arousal or CNS stimulants may enhance the sensitivity and capacity of our working memory, but the effects are transient and not strikingly different than our ordinary functioning. When one considers the immense volume of processing that must take place in the brain on a continual basis and the extremely limited amount of material one can hold in working memory, it becomes apparent why we need parallel, distributed, modular subsystems to handle most of our functioning automatically and outside of awareness.

Finally, *control* of information processing refers to the ability to direct attention appropriately, to maintain attention on a task that requires sustained concentration without becoming distracted, and to shift attention flexibly as a situation demands. Attentional control relies heavily on the activity of the prefrontal cortex and related areas (Baddeley, 1992; Luria, 1980). Persons with injuries of the prefrontal cortex are especially likely to demonstrate varying degrees of deficit in their ability to regulate attention. The typical problems observed among these individuals include distractibility and perseveration.

COMPARISON OF CONSCIOUS AND NONCONSCIOUS PROCESSES

Baars (1988), summarizes several comparative characteristics of conscious and nonconscious processing. In general, compared with nonconscious processing, conscious processing is slow, inefficient, and effortful. A modular perceptual subsystem specialized to perform a discrete task (e.g., auditory verbal perception of consonants) does its work quickly and with few errors, but it can only perform a specific task and its contents always will involve stimuli within a specific modality. Consciousness, however, although slow and cumbersome, has access to an extremely wide range of contents, among and between which it may make associations. Unlike nonconscious processing, which is massively parallel, conscious processing generally is serial in nature—one conscious experience follows another. Thus a person can have only one coherent representation of reality (self and world) in awareness at any given time, and attention can be focused only on a circumscribed part of that representation.

Conscious contents also are limited in that they almost always make up a single coherent stream of experience, although in some pathological conditions (e.g., certain toxic psychoses, or severe dissociative disorders) this coherence may be lost transiently. In contrast, nonconscious processing operates under no such constraints, and contradictory perceptions or impulses may coexist outside of awareness. This distinction is clearly demonstrated in the split-brain syndrome. When a person has undergone surgical resection of the corpus callosum, the separated sides of the brain are capable of operating to some extent independently. Yet, despite this relative independence of the hemispheres, the verbal side of the brain may be quite adept at explaining even rather bizarre behavior initiated by the nonverbal hemisphere, in a way that is apparently consistent and coherent (Gazzaniga & LeDoux, 1978).

CONSCIOUSNESS AS A GLOBAL WORKSPACE

Baars (1988) uses a "global workspace" (GW) metaphor to describe the functioning of consciousness; the GW "is an information exchange that allows specialized unconscious processors in the nervous system to interact with each other. It is analogous to a blackboard in a classroom, or to a television broadcasting station in a human community. Many unconscious specialists can compete or cooperate for access to the [GW]. Once having gained access, they can broadcast information to all other specialized processors that can understand the message" (p. 74). According to this model, "conscious events are simply those that take place in the [GW]; everything else is unconscious" (p. 74). Routine tasks are farmed out to myriad distributed subsystems for nonconscious and automatic processing. Novel tasks and situations, in particular, as well as those that are ambiguous (Baars, 1988), may demand a more deliberate, conscious, and nonautomatized mode of functioning.

Baars discussed several important characteristics of consciousness, some of which we now consider briefly. First, consciousness is biased toward perceptual input. That is, perception is very compelling, and when a person is awake and alert, sensory stimulation will play a major role in determining the contents of his or her consciousness. We should add that, for humans, consciousness also has a strong linguistic bias, so much so that some authors (e.g., Gazzaniga & LeDoux, 1978) even have suggested that language may be a sine qua non of conscious awareness; however, more recently, Gazzaniga (1995) has argued instead that the consciousness of the verbal hemipshere and that of the nonverbal hemisphere are qualitatively different. Language (another modular system adding to the mix of consciousness in humans) brings about a qualitative change in the emergent properties of consciousness; consciousness with language is distinctly different than consciousness without it (Vygotsky, 1934/1986).

Baars (1988, 1997) noted that another important characteristic of consciousness is the existence of a lag time between the onset of nonconscious processing of various stimuli and conscious awareness of those stimuli. Libet, for example, discussed research findings suggesting that there is an interval of 0.5 to 1.0 seconds between the presentation of a stimulus (sensory stimuli from the environment, or even electrical stimulation of the cortex) and the conscious perception of that stimulus (Libet, 1964, 1973; Libet et al., 1964). Shorter intervals are required to elicit detection of a similar stimulus without awareness (Libet et al., 1991). In other work, Libet (1985) found evidence indicating that there may be a delay between the initiation of an action and awareness of an intention to act, suggesting that the conscious intention could be a post hoc phenomenon rather than the initiator of behavior.

THE NEUROBIOLOGY OF REPRESENTATIONS: IMAGERY AND PERCEPTION

At any given time, the brain synthesizes the various representational subsystems to form an apparently seamless and unitary representation of the world and of oneself in the world. There can be only one such complete representation emergent at any given time, although it is updated and modified continually as internal and external environments change. Attention may be directed primarily to certain features of this complete representation, so that we are less aware, and sometimes unaware, of certain aspects of our encounter with reality. This experience of the world and of ourselves is mediated by our "internal" representations. Unless one's brain has the capacity to represent something—percepts, images, thoughts, emotions, abstract concepts, sense of the position of one's body in space—one cannot be aware of it. Everything one is aware of experiencing must be something one can represent, but not all variables affecting one's behavior are necessarily conscious or even representable to consciousness.

A significant body of research supports the idea that perception and imagery involve the same neural substrate. In other words, the things we perceive and those things we imagine (what Aristotle described as "faint copies of sensations"), share the same parts of the brain and are characterized by similar neural and psychological processes (Kosslyn, 1980, 1994). Consequently, from the point of view of neurodynamics, there is no firm line of demarcation between our experience of inside and outside, fantasy and reality. Yet, somehow we manage, for the most part, to sort it all out.

VISUAL IMAGERY AND VISUAL PERCEPTION

The importance of visual imagery in cognition, and the relationship of visual imagery to perception, has generated a fair amount of controversy, although Kosslyn (1994) suggests that research conducted over the past 20 years has brought the matter near a resolution. We will not review the debate here, but the interested reader can refer to several sources for more detail (e.g., Farah, 1989; Goldenberg et al., 1989; Kosslyn, 1980, 1994; Pylyshyn, 1981). The basic issue concerns whether imagery is truly similar to perception or whether it is secondary to linguistic, propositional representations.

Many researchers argue that both images and percepts arise out of qualitatively similar matrices, and a substantial body of data now supports this idea (e.g., Farah, 1989; Goldenberg et al., 1989). For example, Farah et al. (1989) used event-related potentials to study the cerebral processing involved in generating visual images and found increased activation of the occipital cortex, with increased activity in the left temporo-occipital region also. This pattern differed from that observed when subjects performed nonimagery tasks (reading or listening to words without being asked to generate images, and proofreading) but is similar to what ordinarily is observed during actual perception of visual stimuli. In another study, Farah and Perronet (1989) found that the amplitude of evoked potentials in the occipital area was greater among subjects who reported more vivid visual imagery, suggesting more intense neural activity in that area of the cortex.

In one study using positron emission tomography (PET), which provides a measure of regional brain activity, Roland and Friberg (1985) had subjects inhale radioactively labeled xenon gas before imagining walking along a specific path through their neighborhood. The radioactive tracer was taken up by those areas of the brain that were most active during inhalation. The resulting PET scans were compared with data gathered while the same subjects were at rest with eyes closed to limit stimulation of the occipital area by visual input. The authors found that the use of mental imagery led to significant increases in blood flow in several areas of cortex concerned with the processing of visual information.

While these findings support the hypothesis that visual imagery and visual perception share similar neural pathways, other studies provide even more compelling evidence. For example, Tootell et al. (1982) examined the mapping of different areas of the retina onto the cortex of the primary visual area (V1). The central portion of the retina, known as the *fovea*, receives visual input from an area that covers about 2° to 3° of visual arc. That represents an area of visual space approximately 1–1½ inches wide at arm's length. A person's vision is most acute in this central region, and cells carrying information from the fovea project to a disproportionately large percentage of the cortical cells in area V1. The neurons dedicated to central (foveal) vision occupy the posterior portion of V1, while more forward parts of primary visual cortex are associated with the remainder of the visual field. Tootell et al. (1982; see Figure 12.1) trained a macaque to stare at a bull's-eye pattern, and while it did so they injected it with radioactively labeled 2-deoxyglucose. The radioactive compound was taken up by active neurons and was detectable for a short time afterward. When the distribution of radioactivity in the brain was studied, it was found that a bull's-eye pattern had been mapped distinctly onto area V1. The center of the target was represented at the most posterior portion of V1.

A related finding was reported by Kosslyn et al. (1993), who used PET to test the hypothesis that a similar pattern of metabolic activity (i.e., in the primary visual cortex) would be found when human subjects used visual

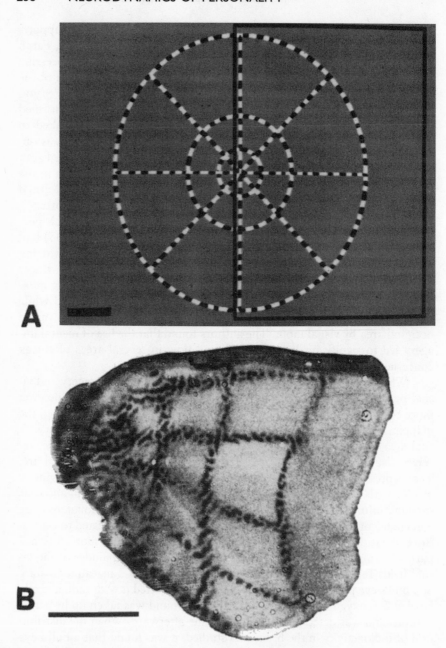

FIGURE 12.1. The photograph at the top (A) shows the visual stimulus to which a macaque was trained to attend and which stimulated the area of visual cortex shown below (B). The autoradiograph in Part B shows the pattern of activation of the visual cortex associated with looking at Part A. The darkened areas are cells which were active while the macaque was looking at the target and which took up the radioactively labeled 2-deoxyglucose. From Tootell et al. (1982, p. 903). Copyright 1982 by the American Association for the Advancement of Science. Reprinted by permission of the authors and the American Association for the Advancement of Science.

imagery rather than processing actual visual stimuli. Because PET provides resolution inferior to that of the technique used by Tootell et al. (1982), it was necessary to ask subjects to conjure up images that would activate larger, yet discrete, areas of V1. They therefore used two imagery conditions in which subjects with eyes shut were asked to (1) imagine uppercase letters of the alphabet and (2) actively judge such things as whether they contained any curved lines. In the first condition, subjects were asked to imagine the letters "at the smallest possible 'visible' size" (Kosslyn et al., 1993, p. 277). The purpose of this method was to confine the image to an area of visual space (and hence of visual cortex) roughly equivalent to that perceived by the fovea. In the second condition, subjects were asked to imagine that the letters were "at the largest possible 'nonoverflowing' size" (p. 277), thus activating extrafoveal areas of V1. The investigators found that imagining the small letters (which should have occupied only the foveal region of the topographically mapped area V1) led, as expected, to preferential activation of posterior V1, whereas imagining the largest possible letters led to activation of anterior V1 as well. The effect was similar to that observed in perception.

Despite the striking parallels between vision and visual imagery, there are differences in the processes involved in perception and image formation. Visual perception is, to a large extent, a bottom–up process (although Bruner, 1957, and others have shown that humans have a tendency to see what they expect to see, meaning it also operates from the top down). That is, visual stimuli create a percept via lower levels of the visual system hierarchy, through the eyes. Visual imagery, on the other hand, may be either bottom–up or top–down. If one looks at an object and then closes one's eyes and tries to maintain the image, the process initially is bottom–up, but it is maintained from the top down, as one uses the intention to hold a specific image in mind, along with the idea of the image (and possibly a verbal description of it), to refresh what is seen in the mind's eye. If, with eyes closed, one is asked to imagine a specific object that is not shown (say, in response to a question like "Is an Irish setter darker than a golden retriever?"), the images are created from the top down, utilizing connections that project from higher to lower levels of the visual hierarchy. In this case, the primary visual area (V1) may not be activated.

Kosslyn (1980, 1994) has argued that visual imagery may be represented via a quasi-spatial "visual buffer" which mediates both visual imagery and perception. By *buffer*, he means a subsystem specialized for transient storage and representation of visual material in working memory. The visual buffer comprises at least two subcomponents (Baddeley, 1990; Ungerleider, 1995) that code spatial location (in perception, location is mediated by the "dorsal stream," i.e., neural fibers running through the parietal and occipital cortex) and perceptual form or object recognition (mediated by the "ventral stream," which involves neurons running through the temporo-occipital cortex). Baddeley's (1986) "phonological loop" seems to be the analogous medium for auditory verbal images, and it seems logical that there are buffers for olfactory, somatesthetic and other images and sensory data. In general, sensory buffers appear to be mediated by areas of the cortex involved in processing specific modes of sensory input. Thus the occipital lobes are particularly active during mental imagery tasks (Farah et al., 1989).

If both imagery and perception are represented by means of identical perceptual buffers, then from a purely physiological perspective the difference between imagery and perception as experiences is somewhat indistinct. Moreover, we need only to consider the immediacy of the intense imagery that may be experienced in posttraumatic "flashbacks" to recognize that, in some cases, the distinction may be quite difficult to define. Yet, despite similarities in the way percepts and images are represented, most people have little difficulty discriminating between the two, with at least a reasonable degree of accuracy.[1]

There may be several reasons for the fact that fantasy and perception usually can be discriminated despite their qualitative similarities, but the primary one is that the representations characteristic of perception ordinarily are much more vivid than are those characteristic of imagery. This is because in perception the visual cortex is presented constantly with bottom–up visual stimulation, whereas in the case of imagery (unless you are a fantasy-prone person) the image must be conjured up by an individual either spontaneously or deliberately and under the direction of an intention (e.g., suppose you were told to imagine Elmer Fudd, with his hunting cap and shotgun, going after Daffy Duck).

Even when considerable effort is spent on the maintenance of an image, it tends to fade or change rapidly. Kosslyn (1994) suggested that, if imagery and perception use the same neural systems, this quick fading may be necessary in order rapidly and constantly to update what we actually see without interference from lingering afterimages. Thus, in the absence of sensory input, images tend to change rapidly. When we are awake, with eyes closed, the images become degraded and are contaminated by other imagery or cognitive processing. When we are asleep and dreaming, the images simply change rapidly; in contrast to perception, very little that we experience in a dream is stable, probably because there is no relatively constant environmental source of stimulation to permit the maintenance of a stable image.

What is true for vision—that imagery and perception appear to involve closely related processes and substrates—is likely to hold true for other sensory modalities. In perception, the ongoing and constantly evolving result

---

[1]Yet, some persons do have difficulty distinguishing the two. These "fantasy-prone" individuals (S. Wilson & Barber, 1983) are highly suggestible and have a great capacity for intense imagery involving multiple sensory modalities.

of this process is an emergent experience of the world, a composite synthesized by the distributed processing of the various sensory systems and accompanied by a running commentary by the verbal inner speech system. Essentially the same process is associated with imagery. The point is that *all* experience (of the self and of the world) represents the fusion of the operation of different sensory buffers and in its basic mechanisms perceptual experience is very similar to imagery (and fantasy).

Perceiving and imagining often work in tandem in interesting ways. Take the example of riding a bicycle along a familiar route. Obstacles, turns, variations in road surface, and the like all can be anticipated and internally represented prior to registering sensory input from the world. The internal and external blend and contribute to the emerging repesentation of the moment. Certain relational transactions seem to follow a similar pattern. One partner says something to another and anticipates the response before it appears or as it appears. Some of the seamless quality of much of lived experience may be partially emergent from the tendency to start to imagine nonconsciously, before external perception contributes its stimuli.

ATTRIBUTIONS ABOUT ONE'S OWN BEHAVIOR: RATIONALIZATION AND INTOLERANCE OF AMBIGUITY

People ordinarily believe they know the reasons for their actions. When asked why they did something, most people immediately have a rationale, whether or not they are willing to express it. In addition, people also seem to assume that others know why they do what they do. On both counts, they are mistaken. The data suggest that conscious processing is adept at providing rationales and explanations for behavior that frequently occurs for reasons that are completely opaque to these conscious processes.

For example, in their review of the literature on introspection, Nisbett and Wilson (1977) argued that there is little direct introspective access to most complex cognitive processing. They maintained that introspection is "based on a priori, implicit causal theories, or judgments about the extent to which a particular stimulus is a plausible cause of a given response. This suggests that though people may not be able to observe directly their cognitive processes, they will sometimes be able to report accurately about them" (p. 231). As Miller noted, "it is the *result* of thinking, not the process of thinking, that appears spontaneously in consciousness" (1962, p. 56; emphasis in original).

Evidence demonstrating the brain's capacity to generate erroneous but plausible *post hoc* rationales for behavior, irrespective of their accuracy, was reported by Gazzaniga and LeDoux (1978) in their work with corpus callosotomy patients. The corpus callosum, a fiber tract consisting of about

200 million neurons, connects homologous areas (i.e., essentially mirror-image areas) of the right and left hemispheres of the brain (see Figure 12.2). It consists of the *anterior commissure,* which connects the frontal lobes and part of the temporal lobes, the *body* of the corpus callosum, which connects the parietal lobes, and the *splenium* of the corpus callosum, which projects fibers from one occipital lobe to the other.

All or part of the corpus callosum may be resected surgically as a means of treating certain persons with medically intractable epilepsy (Bogen, Fisher, & Vogel, 1965; D. W. Roberts, 1991). This surgery, referred to as *callosotomy,* does not eliminate seizures but may reduce their frequency and severity, and it prevents the spread of a seizure from one hemisphere to the other. Callosotomy is an option for some persons whose seizures are frequent, severe, and uncontrollable, with no clearly localizable focus that might be resected. These people often have a lifelong history of

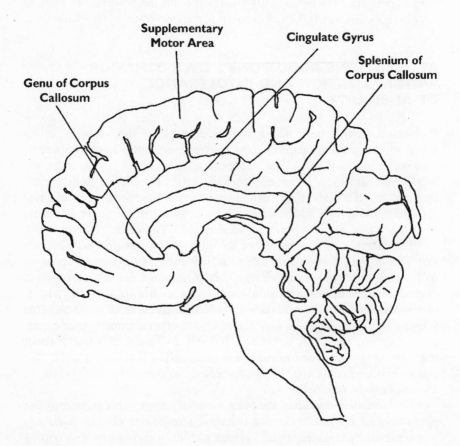

FIGURE 12.2. Sagittal (midline) view of the medial right hemisphere showing the corpus callosum, cingulate gyrus, and supplementary motor area (SMA).

epilepsy, frequently as a result of some developmental anomaly or child-hood neurological insult. Consequently, the assessment of persons who have undergone callosotomy must be interpreted cautiously, since it isn't possible to study the effects of the sectioning of the commissures in neuro-logically normal individuals unless our current ethical standards are sub-stantially altered, which doesn't seem imminent.

Callosotomy does not completely bisect the entire brain; it separates only the right and left cerebral hemispheres. Thus, many subcortical struc-tures are unaffected, so that both sides of the brain have access to emo-tional information and the level of arousal of both hemispheres is consis-tent. Moreover, many callosotomies are intentionally partial, leaving some commissural fibers intact. A complete callosotomy, however, totally abol-ishes the direct transmission of information from one hemisphere to the other. Early studies of persons who underwent callosotomy provided inter-esting data, but the significance of the findings was unclear (K. U. Smith & Akelaitis, 1942). Later work with the procedure, beginning in the 1960s in association with more sophisticated methods of assessment, yielded a num-ber of both subtle and dramatic findings.

The basic experiment is carried out as follows. Seated before a projec-tion screen, the subject is presented with a different picture in each visual field. The right visual field (which projects from both right and left eyes to the left hemisphere), for example, sees a chicken's foot, while the left field (which projects to the right hemisphere) sees a picture of a house covered with snow and a snowman in front. Following this, the subject is shown a set of eight pictures that includes a snow shovel, a chicken, and six unre-lated objects (e.g., toaster, hammer) and is asked to choose the objects that go with what he saw. If asked what he saw without these eight pictures present, the subject would reply verbally "a chicken foot" and nothing else, because the isolated left (verbal) hemisphere can speak only for itself and it saw only the chicken foot.

Gazzaniga and LeDoux (1978) presented stimuli of this sort to three callosotomy patients whose right hemispheres possessed varying degrees of language comprehension but who did not have the ability to speak. One subject, a 15-year-old boy identified as "P. S.," quickly responded by using his right hand to chose a picture of a chicken from a set of four different pictures. With his left hand, he chose a picture of a shovel from a set of four other pictures. According to the authors, "the subject was then asked, 'What did you see?' 'I saw a claw and I picked the chicken, and you have to clean out the chicken shed with a shovel" (p. 148). The response was im-mediate and plausible. If you didn't know the facts of the situation, you might take it at face value, assuming that this reflected the subject's reason-ing process. In fact, we know it was incorrect. Significantly, this was not a one-time occurrence; it happened repeatedly. Each verbal response con-veyed a sense of certainty; never was it presented as a guess. In other words, in this experiment the split-brain subject was conscious of his behavior but was unaware of its true origin; nevertheless he nonconsciously and automatically constructed an explanation for it. Gazzaniga refers to the left-hemisphere system that explains such behavior as "the interpreter" (1995, p. 1393).

A callosotomy subject is not always entirely pleased with this state of affairs, however. Gazzaniga (1985) reported that with another callosotomy patient ("J. W."), after this experiment was conducted for a few trials, "[J. W.] typically becomes agitated. The answer being offered by the left brain is at odds with what the right brain knows. The right brain knows why the hand is pointing to a particular card, and it is not taking the left brain's story lightly. It registers its disapproval through an emotional response. The patient is unhappy and the experiments are stopped" (p. 145). The patient then may be debriefed; the reasons for his behavior are explained to him, and the trials resume. Precisely the same situation ensues, despite the fact that he has just had his condition explained. The conscious knowledge has no effect whatsoever on this automatic, nonconscious process. It apparently cannot be deliberately controlled.

According to Gazzaniga's formulation, these findings reflect the brain's modular architecture at a relatively complex level of organization. The right hemisphere selects a picture, and the verbal mind takes note of this but is completely in the dark regarding the reasons for the mute hemisphere's choice. Because the "conscious verbal self comes to know the other selves through overt behavior," however, the verbal system glibly provides an immediate reason for the action (Gazzaniga & LeDoux, 1978). The verbal system essentially observes the individual's behavior and concocts a post hoc theory of what it was about. LeDoux & Gazzaniga (1981) suggested that the most interesting finding here is the way the left hemisphere readily interprets the behavior of the right brain as natural. This process is virtually indistinguishable from (and may be identical to) the process referred to as *rationalization*.

Why does this happen? The brain is such a complex system that it is impossible for us to know the reasons we do what we do. The verbal system, however, appears to have evolved a capacity to explain it all. Most of the time these explanations are plausible. It is not unusual, however, for such rationalizations to seem somewhat contrived. In some cases—those with paranoid schizophrenia, for example—the attributions that people make about the causes of their behavior are so bizarre that we consider them crazy. But whether one is schizophrenic or not, the underlying neural process associated with making attributions about one's behavior is fundamentally the same; the difference is in how far the explanations stray from the mainstream and whether the individual can evaluate them critically. At bottom is a cooking up of reasons for what one does, spontaneously, not necessarily based on any awareness of the real causes of one's activity, but often involving recognition of patterns learned in association with past experience.

NONCONSCIOUS FUNCTIONING: THE COGNITIVE UNCONSCIOUS

During the heyday of behaviorism, respectable scientists avoided talk of unconscious functioning at all costs. Times have changed, and both cognitive psychologists and cognitive neuroscientists have generally come to the conclusion, supported by a considerable amount of persuasive research, that most of our functioning takes place outside of awareness. Psychoanalysts should not be surprised by an emphasis on unconscious functioning, although they might be surprised to find themselves to some extent in agreement with most cognitive neuroscientists. There are, however, a number of important differences between traditional psychoanalytic and current neuroscientific understandings of nonconscious functioning. We will examine the neural perspective first, returning later in this chapter to what psychologists traditionally have considered to be the psychodynamic unconscious.

In a review of much of this research, Kihlstrom (1987) suggested the use of the term "cognitive unconscious," and argued that this realm of activity can be subdivided into unconscious, preconscious, and subconscious domains. Some processes "are inaccessible to introspection in principle under any circumstances" (p. 1450). For example, it is not possible for an individual to provide an explanation of how he or she discriminates similar consonant sounds. Similarly, we cannot gain introspective access to those neural processes that compel us to form attachments with other people. We simply do it, and this is such a fundamental aspect of our behavior that failure to form such attachments is viewed as indicative of severe psychopathology. Such phenomena as subliminal perception (as in *priming*, discussed in Chapter 5 and below) and implicit memory can be considered to be preconscious declarative knowledge, potentially having access to awareness but not reaching the threshold for representation in awareness. In hypnosis or dissociative states, the failure of certain representations to gain access to awareness may be considered a manifestation of *subconscious* phenomena. Kihlstrom considers this to reflect a failure actively to form links between self or object representations in working memory.

EXPERIMENTAL PSYCHOLOGY AND UNCONSCIOUS PERCEPTION

In an interesting program of research, Zajonc (1980; also Moreland & Zajonc, 1977, 1979) showed that an individual's preferences could be shaped by emotional influences of which he or she is completely unaware. In one set of studies, for example, English-speaking subjects were shown Japanese ideographs, to some of which they previously had been exposed briefly but which they did not recognize as familiar. Asked to rate the aesthetic appeal of the ideographs, they preferred those they had already seen even though they could not consciously distinguish them from those for which they were naive. In a similar study, Kunst-Wilson and Zajonc (1980) used a tachistoscope to present subjects with a series of randomly designed polygons for only 1 millisecond—much too short a duration for there to be any conscious awareness. Recognition of the polygons as previously seen was at the chance level (48%), yet of those polygons the subjects liked, 60% had been seen previously while 40% had not. This *mere exposure* effect has been supported in a number of other studies (Zajonc, 1980, 1984) and demonstrates the subtlety with which preferences can be unconsciously influenced.

Research on subliminal perception also has demonstrated that the autonomic nervous system may react to perceptual stimuli that never enter awareness. R. S. Lazarus and McCleary (1951) tachistoscopically exposed subjects to repeated presentations of randomized lists of 10 five-letter nonsense syllables (e.g., GEXAX), at speeds that varied from so fast as to be undetectable through slow enough to be seen easily. They then randomly conditioned subjects, pairing electrical shocks with randomly selected subsets of five of the syllables. During conditioning, the stimuli were exposed for a full second—sufficient time to make them readily recognizable. Following conditioning, subjects were again exposed to the stimuli in random order, at varying speeds, while skin conductance (a measure of autonomic activity) was recorded. At speeds too high to permit conscious perception, subjects showed a significant autonomic response to syllables which previously had been associated with the electrical shock.

This line of research came in for considerable criticism in the late 1950s and early 1960s (e.g., Goldiamond, 1958), and subsequently became unfashionable. Yet the early findings generally were robust, and a resurgence of interest in nonconscious processing and cognition led to refinement and development of the field (Bruner, 1992; Erdelyi, 1992; Greenwald, 1992; Kihlstrom, Barnhardt, and Tataryn, 1992; Merikle, 1992). In a brief review, Lewicki, Hiller, and Czyzewska concluded that not only are unconscious processes faster than conscious ones but they "are also structurally more sophisticated, in that they are capable of efficient processing of multidimensional and interactive relations between variables" (1992, p. 796).

IMPLICIT MEMORY, PRIMING, AND PROCEDURAL LEARNING

Explicit memory is the deliberate, conscious recollection of previously learned information or prior events (Schachter, 1987, 1992). If I recall the concept of explicit memory, that in itself is an explicit memory. Implicit memory, on the other hand, refers to a class of phenomena involving memory without awareness of having learned something. Experimentally, implicit memory is demonstrated by "changes in performance or behavior that are produced by prior experiences on tests that do not require any intentional or conscious recollection of those experiences" (Schachter, 1992, p. 244).

Priming, a classic example of implicit memory involving a type of learning that occurs outside of awareness, was discussed in Chapter 5 on the modularity of memory (Schachter, 1987, 1992). In the laboratory, the occurrence of priming is demonstrated by a researcher's attempt to determine whether prior experience with some unattended stimulus affects subsequent performance. Because they have a severe deficit in declarative memory, individuals with amnesia demonstrate little or no conscious (explicit) recall of events and information after the onset of the amnestic syndrome. However, Warrington and Weiskrantz (1973) found that priming is intact in amnesia (see also Graf, Squire, & Mandler, 1984). Priming effects can be seen in neurologically intact individuals as well as in those with amnesia, in response to stimuli of which the subject is either conscious or unconscious at the time of presentation. Priming demonstrates the operation of a mechanism by which behavior can be influenced by factors entirely outside awareness.

Recall of many procedurally learned processes takes place essentially nonconsciously. The use of one's native language as an adult, for example, is a complex activity that usually occurs with little effort (although one may be careful in one's choice of words). Even that judicious choice of words may reflect the operation of processes that are relatively automatic and unconscious. For some people such a cautious manner of speaking is so routine that it is a regular aspect of their character, an aspect which they rarely even notice.

AUTOMATIC AND NONCONSCIOUS RESPONSE TO NOVELTY

As a rule, our brains respond to novelty by activating the prefrontal cortex and its associated executive cognitive functions (planning, organization, and an active approach to problem solving, among others). It appears, however, that there may be a threshold below which one does not become aware of a novel stimulus, although it can be demonstrated that one has reacted to it. For example, Berns, Cohen, and Mintun (1997) found that people could be taught a complex sequence without demonstrating awareness that there was in fact a sequence. As they learned the sequence, the subjects' reaction times on the experimental task decreased significantly, although the subjects themselves were unaware of any improvement. After the subjects had learned the first sequence, it was changed. In response to the change, reaction times increased, then subsequently decreased again over time, once again showing a pattern that would be expected with learning. In contrast, when the subjects were presented with randomly sequenced stimuli, no learning was apparent.

By analyzing regional cerebral blood flow with PET, Berns et al. (1997) found that when subjects' expectations were violated (i.e., when the sequence changed), the left premotor (frontal) area showed increased activity, as did the left anterior cingulate gyrus, ventral striatum, and nucleus accumbens. The right dorsolateral prefrontal cortex and areas in the parietal and temporal lobes showed less activity. The above authors concluded that mechanisms involved in active maintenance of cognitive set, "like those responsive to novelty, can operate independently of awareness" (p. 1274).

BLINDSIGHT AND RELATED SYNDROMES

Sensory Perception without Awareness

Certain neurologically based visual disorders further demonstrate the dissociability of awareness and perception. For example, injuries to the visual cortex cause deficits of conscious visual preception (cortical blindness), producing a condition known as *blindsight* (Cowey & Stoerig, 1991; Weiskrantz, 1986; Weiskrantz et al., 1974). A cortically blind individual ordinarily is unaware of nearly all visual stimulation. He or she may be presented with a wide range of stimuli yet deny seeing them. However, if persuaded to guess at the location of a moving light, for example, or at the nature of a visual stimulus, the guess is likely to be fairly accurate. A patient with this syndrome may respond accurately to purely visual stimuli and be aware of the response but have no awareness of either the stimulus or the reason for the response. There is a dissociation between conscious vision, mediated by the cortex, and the nonconscious capacity to locate objects in visual space, processes that operate in tandem in the neurologically intact person. Caregivers and family members who observe spontaneous indications of blindsight, not understanding the phenomenon, sometimes believe the patient is feigning blindness.

There is some controversy concerning whether blindsight is mediated by subcortical pathways alone—specifically, the superior colliculus of the dorsal midbrain (Kentridge, Heywood, & Weiskrantz, 1997; Weiskrantz, 1995)— or whether it is due to preserved "islands" of the visual cortex (Gazzaniga, Fendrich, & Wessinger, 1994; Wessinger, Fendrich, & Gazzaniga, 1997). Blindsight has been demonstrated in monkeys in whom the entire area V1 has been resected (Rodman, Gross, & Albright, 1989); given the similarity of monkey and human visual systems, it seems likely that the cortex may not be necessary for the phenomenon to be observed. Baars (1997, p. 71) argues that area V1 "may be needed for spatial 'binding,' tying many visual areas into a single retinotopic display." In any event, while the precise details remain to be resolved, there is little controversy regarding the general relationship of blindsight to consciousness.

Blindsight apparently is not the only sensory phenomenon involving perception without awareness. Isolated cases of "blind touch" (Paillard, Michel, & Stelmach, 1983; Rossetti, Rode, & Boisson, 1995) and "deaf hearing" (F. Michel & Peronnet, 1980) have been reported. In the first, as a result of a left parietal lobe lesion, a patient was left with a deficit of conscious perception of touch to the right arm, regardless of the intensity of the stimulus. Despite this, while blindfolded she was able to point to the approximate location of the tactile stimulus with reasonably good accuracy (Paillard, Michel, & Stelmach, 1983).

Unilateral Spatial Neglect

Some individuals, as a result of lesions of the right hemisphere, demonstrate a syndrome variously known as *unilateral spatial neglect, hemispatial neglect,* or *hemi-inattention.* These persons tend to ignore, and often have no consciousness of, things to their left. Reports of neglect of the right side of space are rare, although neglect of the left is quite common. President Woodrow Wilson, for example, had many strokes both before and during his presidency, and in 1919, while still in office, he experienced a particularly disabling stroke that left him with a number of serious neurological problems, including hemispatial neglect (Weinstein, 1981). Aware of this deficit, Wilson's wife and his physician arranged Wilson's bed so that visitors to the president (including heads of state) could not stand in his left visual field, where they would have been ignored by the president. (Certainly this was not the only time when those close to a president tried to conceal his cognitive deficits.)

Some individuals with hemispatial neglect, although unconscious of stimuli on their left, nevertheless respond to some things on that side. They have no idea why they respond as they do and are prone to rationalize it. Marshall and Halligan (1988), for example, reported the case of a patient with hemispatial neglect who was shown line drawings of two houses that were identical, except that the left side of one of the houses was on fire while the other house was intact. The patient repeatedly described the drawings as identical, since she was unable to perceive the left side of either drawing. When asked to say which house she would prefer to live in, she always selected the house that was not on fire, failing to understand why one even would pose the question, since the two houses appeared the same (Weiskrantz, 1997).

Transient Reversal of Hemispatial Neglect and Anosognosia: Making the Unconscious Conscious

Several authors have demonstrated the relative reversibility of hemispatial neglect, using a method called *caloric testing*. Ordinarily used to evaluate vestibular functioning, this involves irrigation of the external ear canal with ice water (sometimes with warm water). In normal individuals, caloric testing initially induces a movement of the eyes toward the side being irrigated, followed by nystagmus (involuntary rhythmic movements of the eyes) to the opposite side (Adams, Victor, & Ropper, 1997).

Silberpfennig (1941) first noted that unilateral spatial neglect was temporarily alleviated by caloric irrigation, and similar findings have been reported by others (e.g., Bisiach, Rusconi, & Vallar, 1991; Cappa et al., 1987; Marshal & Maynard, 1983; Rubens, 1985; Storrie-Baker et al., 1997; Vallar et al., 1990, 1993). Bisiach et al. (1991), for example, discussed an 84-year-old woman who had sustained a right-hemisphere stroke and who subsequently denied that her left side was hemiplegic; in addition, "she insisted that her left upper limb—which she was able to touch and look at, if requested—was not hers but her mother's" (p. 1029). When interviewed prior to the caloric stimulation, the following dialogue ensued:

Ex: Whose arm is this?

Pt: It's not mine.

Ex: Whose is it?

Pt: It's my mother's.

Ex: How on earth does it happen to be here?

Pt: I don't know. I found it in my bed.

Ex: How long has it been there?

Pt: Since the first day. Feel, it's warmer than mine. The other day too, when the weather was colder, it was warmer than mine.

Ex: So where is *your* left arm?

Pt: (*Makes an indefinite gesture forwards.*) It's under there.

Up to this point, the patient clung steadfastly to her anosognosia, to the point that she maintained a delusional idea about her body image. Although alert, cooperative, and not obviously demented, she persistently confabulated in response to the examiner's questions about her situation. She was unconscious of her deficit, a potential representation of the left side of her body having no access to awareness. The patient's left ear then was irrigated with cold water and the conversation continued:

Ex: (*She asks the patient to show her left arm.*)

Pt: (*Points to her own left arm.*) Here it is.

Ex: (*Raises the patient's left arm.*) Is this arm yours?

Pt: Why, yes.

Ex: Where is your mother's arm?

Pt: (*Hesitates.*) It is somewhere about.

Ex: Where exactly?

Pt: I don't know. Perhaps here, under the bedclothes. (*She looks to her right, under the bedclothes.*)

Two hours after this experiment was concluded, the patient was again asked about her left arm and once more insisted that the arm attached to her shoulder was her mother's. The caloric testing was again conducted, following which she recognized the arm as her own. According to Bisiach et al. (1991), the test was conducted twice more, with similar results.

The mechanism by which caloric stimulation leads to a transient improvement in the patients' ability to represent reality accurately is unclear. Ramachandran et al. (1996) suggested first that the stimulation aroused the right hemisphere, causing the patient to pay attention to the left side. They also offered "a highly speculative conjecture" that the caloric induces a state akin to REM sleep during which disturbing material sometimes reaches awareness. Thus, "perhaps the vestibular stimulation partly activates the same circuitry that generates REM sleep, thereby allowing the patient to pull up unpleasant, disturbing facts about herself including her paralysis" (p. 51). This conjecture has no data to support it, but there have been findings that suggest a possible answer to the question.

Storrie-Baker et al. (1997) used caloric stimulation with an 83-year-old woman who had sustained a massive infarct of the right middle cerebral artery, with consequent left hemiplegia and severe unilateral neglect. Simultaneously, using EEG they measured the activation of the two hemispheres, finding an increase in activation in both hemispheres, especially the left, in association with caloric irrigation and diminution of neglect. This supported the hypothesis of Heilman (1979) and of Mesulam (1982) that the right hemisphere is dominant for regulating attention and that lesions causing neglect impair right-hemisphere arousal and the ability to focus attention on the left side.

Prosopagnosia: Conscious and Nonconscious Recognition of Faces

Focal injury of the brain may produce a variety of discrete cognitive or perceptual deficits (A. R. Damasio, 1990). In some cases, for example, it may be more difficult to recognize animals than manufactured objects

(Warrington & Shallice, 1984), or recognition of musical instruments may be defective while that of carpentry tools is preserved (H. Damasio & A. R. Damasio, 1989; A. R. Damasio, H. Damasio, & Tranel, 1989). These dissociations reflect the complex hierarchical modular organization of the brain.

Prosopagnosia, a severe impairment of the ability to recognize faces (Bodamer, 1947; A. R. Damasio, 1990; Farah, 1990; Hécaen & Angelergues, 1962; Moscovitch, Winocur, & Behrmann, 1997), is a disorder of this sort. It usually is observed in conjunction with bilateral lesions of the inferior temporal cortex (the fusiform gyrus; see A. R. Damasio, H. Damasio, & Van Hoesen, 1982; Gross & Sergent, 1992) but may occur with right-sided lesions of the same area (De Renzi et al., 1994). It can occur in isolation or as part of a more pervasive syndrome of impaired object recognition. A person with a deficit in the recognition of faces may be unable to identify faces but may remain able to recognize facial expressions, or to recognize an individual on the basis of his or her gait (A. R. Damasio, 1990; A. R. Damasio et al., 1982; Tranel, Damasio, & Damasio, 1988).

A person with face agnosia cannot identify faces, even very familiar ones such as those of famous persons or family members. Nevertheless, nonconscious recognition may occur despite impaired conscious recognition. Bauer (1984), for example, showed patients faces of famous persons and relatives, and with each face patients were asked to read names which may or may not have corresponded to the face shown. Although the patients could not consciously identify the faces, when a correct name was read skin conductance responses were greater than when incorrect names were read. (Skin conductance is a measure of autonomic response.) In a related study, Tranel and Damasio (1985) asked patients to study a group of familiar and unfamiliar faces and pick out those they recognized. Performance was at a chance level, but again skin conductance response was consistently greater for familiar faces.

In prosopagnosia, as with blindsight and related disorders, some systems in the brain recognize and respond to specific stimuli despite the fact that these stimuli have no access to consciousness. Thus, for certain basic reactions to occur, awareness of the nature of a stimulus is unnecessary. Again, this demonstrates the modularity of both the brain and the mind. It also illustrates the peculiar nature of consciousness, showing that many complex processes are entirely nonconscious and, indeed, may have no access to consciousness whatsoever, yet influence functioning. In prosopagnosia, emotional reactions to faces may remain intact, but the individual who cannot recognize faces has no conscious understanding of what produces such a reaction and is liable (as usually is the case) to rationalize such reactions quickly and spontaneously, all the while convinced of the validity of these contrived explanations.

VOLITION AND THE TIMING
OF PSYCHOLOGICAL EVENTS

Benjamin Libet has put considerable effort into understanding the sequential timing of neural and mental events, and especially the relationship between the neurophysiology and phenomenology of volition. Some of his work is relevant to material already discussed in this chapter, while some of it takes us beyond what we already have covered. His findings are controversial, and their interpretation, as well as the methods he employs, have been criticized by a number of neuroscientists. Despite this, there is an interesting logic to his results, and many are persuaded by what he seems to have uncovered.

Starting with his somewhat less controversial ideas, we will begin with Libet's "cerebral time-on" theory (1992), which proposes that "the transition, from an unconscious mental event to one that reaches awareness and is consciously experienced, can be a function of a sufficient increase in the duration (or 'time-on') of appropriate neural activities" (p. 264). Thus, for example, the tachistoscopically presented stimuli that frequently are used in this kind of research do not enter conscious awareness unless they are presented for a sufficient length of time. The brain perceives these stimuli, and may respond to them nonconsciously, but they do not reach the threshold required for them to enter awareness if they last for intervals as short as 20 milliseconds (see also Libet, 1989; Libet et al., 1991).

More controversial is Libet's work on volition, the status of which is somewhat less clear. Nevertheless, the findings have been consistent across a number of studies, and they seem reasonable given what we know of the brain's massively parallel, nonconscious processing. For the reader interested in the details of the debate, Libet's 1985 paper in the journal *Behavioral and Brain Sciences* may be a good start.

In short, neurophysiologists have identified what is called a *readiness potential* (RP), a scalp-recorded EEG phenomenon generated by the brain prior to the initiation of self-paced voluntary movements (Deecke, Grözinger, & Kornhuber, 1976; Gilden, Vaughan, & Costa, 1966). On average, this RP precedes a motor act by about 800 milliseconds, and Libet became interested in the temporal relationship between first awareness of the intention to act and the appearance of the RP.

The basic experimental design is discussed in Libet's 1985 paper. Subjects were asked to flex the wrist or the fingers of the right hand quickly, doing so whenever the urge should strike them (i.e., not in response to a stimulus). They also were told they could inhibit that urge if they chose to do so. During the experiment, Libet recorded the subjects' EEG, and an electromyogram (EMG) recorded activity in the appropriate flexor muscle. Subjects watched a revolving spot of light on a clock face on a cathode-ray tube; they were asked to move when they felt like it and to note the position of the rotating spot of light at that moment. EEG, EMG, and the clock face all were synchronized so that the initiation of movement, measured by the EMG, served as the point in time to which all other phenomena were referred, or "0-reference time."

Over a large series of trials, Libet found that the RP first was noted an average of 535 milliseconds prior to the onset of movement, as marked by the EMG. The average appearance of the intention to move as reported by subjects was about 190 milliseconds prior to the movement. Thus the readiness potential preceded the conscious intention to move by about 345 milliseconds—more than one-third of a second. In other words, some kind of widespread neural activity, indicated by the appearance of the RP, seems to have preceded any awareness of a desire to move.

The three major problems in interpreting these results are the meaning of the RP, the reliance on introspection, and the need of the subject to note accurately the position of the spot of light. All these issues are addressed by Libet in his 1985 article, his response to the commentary that follows it, and in previous work. Again, the interested reader should refer to these sources. Libet noted, however, that "the available evidence suggests that an RP precedes every voluntary act as well as the conscious awareness of the urge to perform each act" (1985, p. 535). Somewhat similar findings were reported by Ikeda et al. (1992) and by Romo and Schultz (1987). Both groups of authors found evidence of an RP originating in the supplementary motor area (SMA) significantly in advance of self-initiated movements. Assuming that Libet is correct, how are we to interpret these findings?

Libet argues that, because the readiness potential is apparent at least one-third of a second before awareness of an intention to move arises, "some neuronal activity associated with the eventual performance of the act has started well before any (recallable) conscious initiation or intervention is possible. This leads to the conclusion that cerebral initiation even of a spontaneous voluntary act of the kind studied here can and usually does begin *unconsciously*" (1985, p. 536; emphasis in original). His conclusion is that every conscious voluntary act is preceded by specific nonconscious processes that begin about one-half second before the act itself.

This seems plausible given what we already know about the brain, although further experimental confirmation is needed. The vast majority of processing occurs nonconsciously. Why should the formulation of an intention to act be any different? Are we to assume that consciousness is somehow favored in this regard? Why, indeed, should it be favored, especially when we consider how slowly and inefficiently (and with what limited capacity) consciousness operates compared with nonconscious processes? Should we assume that infants, before acting, formulate a conscious intention which itself initiates a motor act? Should we assume the same for nonhuman animals? If we do not make such assumptions, at what point in evolution, or in ontogeny, does this transition occur?

Libet's findings are consistent with those of the split-brain studies discussed earlier, leading us to assume that an intention to act arises nonconsciously (certainly there can be no argument about this nonconscious initiation when the left hand acts, apparently on its own, in a person who has undergone a callosotomy), followed by awareness of an intention, then by the act itself. The verbal, rationalizing faculty of the brain's left hemisphere immediately has an explanation for the act, even referring it back in time prior to the onset of the act. Recall the left hand choosing a snow shovel from several stimulus items in Gazzaniga's and LeDoux (1978) subject P. S. The left hemisphere immediately attributed this to the need for a shovel to clear chicken manure out of the coop. The left hemisphere essentially claimed ownership of an act with which in fact it had no involvement. Yet, it apparently experienced a sense of agency in the selection of a shovel.

Recall also that much of our behavior is habitual, occurring automatically and nonconsciously. If a conscious decision to act were required for everything we do, this would create a bottleneck making complex activity essentially impossible. If conscious volition is *not* necessary for behavior, what then is the purpose of having a sense of agency, a feeling of control? Is there in fact some conscious control over our activity? The answers are not entirely clear.

THE SENSE OF AGENCY AND THE BRAIN

Figure 12.2 shows the approximate location of the cingulate gyrus and the SMA (also called the medial premotor area) on the medial surface of the cerebral hemispheres. Lesions in these areas, and electrical stimulation of them in awake surgical patients, produce some interesting phenomena. A. R. Damasio and Van Hoesen (1983), for example, discussed a 35-year-old woman with an infarction of the left anterior cingulate gyrus, SMA, and medial motor area. On admission to the hospital, she was alert but mute, and only after several weeks did she regain spontaneous speech. One month after her stroke she had recovered sufficiently to describe her previous state of mind to the examiners. Although we can't really rely on her introspective report, it nevertheless is interesting.

Asked whether she had felt distress during the period of muteness, she replied that she had not and stated that she had not spoken "because she had 'nothing to say.' Her mind was 'empty.' Nothing 'mattered.' She apparently was able to follow our conversations even during the early period of the illness, but felt no 'will' to reply to our questions" (A. R. Damasio & Van Hoesen, 1983, pp. 98–99). After 9 more months, the patient felt she had recovered sufficiently that only "the volitional command of her leg and foot was distinctly defective, there being a delay in response to her express wish for movement" (p. 99). Interestingly, unilateral lesions confined to the supplementary motor area may produce a rather similar picture, with reduced spontaneity of movement (Laplane et al., 1977).

A different kind of syndrome was discussed by G. Goldberg, Mayer, and Toglia (1981), who reported that lesions of the medial frontal cortex may leave people feeling as though they are not initiating their own movements; instead, it feels as if someone else is responsible for the movement. A 63-year-old right-handed woman with a stroke in this region demonstrated uncontrollable motor perseveration with her right hand, in response to which the left hand would restrain the right arm and then complete the motor task begun by the perseverative hand. At times the rogue right hand interfered with the performance of tasks in which the left hand was engaged. At other times the right hand grasped some nearby object, and the patient would find herself unable "to release her grip voluntarily. She was unable consciously to inhibit the behavior although she was fully aware of it and was obviously frustrated by her inability to prevent it. She tended to restrain the movement of the right arm by holding it by her side with the more 'obedient' left arm" (G. Goldberg et al., 1991, p. 683). None of these movements was associated with any sense of agency or intention to move.

G. Goldberg and his associates also described a 76-year-old right-handed woman with a stroke in the same area who also showed motor perseveration with the right hand. The authors observed that when this patient made spontaneous, purposeful movements with the right hand, they seemed to have been initiated without any conscious volition. On one occasion, for example, the right hand picked up a pencil and started scribbling. "When her attention was directed to this activity, she reacted with dismay, immediately withdrew the pencil, and pulled the right hand to her side using the left hand. She then indicated that she had not herself initiated the original action of the right arm" (1991, p. 684). It was not unusual for the patient to demonstrate such behavior, to which she had strong negative emotional reactions. She was reported to have said, several times, that the right hand "will not do what I want it to do" (p. 685).

Two somewhat similar cases were reported by Banks and his colleagues (1989), and related findings have been reported by Talairach and associates (1973). This latter group stimulated the cingulate gyrus in epileptic patients and found the current elicited simple movements of the mouth, eyes, and both upper and lower extremities. When stimulation was done in the presence of certain objects, the patients responded with more complex behaviors during the period of stimulation. When the current was turned off, the behavior ceased. For example, presented with fruit, a patient might try to eat it, stopping only when the stimulation ended. In most cases, patients experienced this as though something beyond their control were being done to them. The movements did not feel self-initiated, yet they frequently rationalized the movements, providing incorrect explanations for why they had moved about.

When the human SMA is stimulated, two basic types of reaction are observed. At some sites, ongoing behavior ceases until the stimulation is turned off, and no new actions are initiated. When asked what they experienced, patients commonly report that their "will" to move was somehow disrupted, but they have no idea why. At other sites, electrical stimulation of the SMA may induce "vocalization and complex movement patterns" (A. R. Damasio & Van Hoesen, 1983, p. 103). Lesions of the dorsolateral prefrontal cortex (DLPC) also may be associated with an inability to initiate purposeful activity. Bilateral injuries of DLPC frequently are associated with apathy and an akinetic syndrome. These patients typically are unaware of their deficit (Luria, 1966, 1980).

These data are complex and defy easy interpretation. Although we do not yet understand the precise contribution of SMA, DPLC, and the cingulate cortex to voluntary behavior, it seems clear that lesions of certain areas of the medial cortex may produce a phenomenon that looks very much like a loss of "will" (i.e., volition or agency). Patients with such injuries appear to experience no intrinsic desire to do anything. Electrical stimulation of these same areas may produce either complete disruption and cessation of activity or involuntary behavior of varying degrees of complexity. In either case, patients report that they experience their own sense of agency as having been disturbed, declaring that some external force caused their activity or inactivity. In some cases, patients with lesions of the medial frontal cortex can engage in activity that feels to them as though it has an alien cause, despite the fact that they initiate the behavior themselves. Consistent with Libet's research, the conscious phenomenon of feeling like the agent behind one's actions does not appear to be the primary instigator of behavior in these reports.

The "readiness potential" observed prior to the conscious initiation of an action seems to have its origin in the SMA. The SMA, cingulate gyrus, and DLPC appear to be nodes in a distributed network mediating voluntary behavior. However, despite the fact that they play a central role in providing people with a sense of agency, the cingulate gyrus and SMA should not be thought of as a "volition center." Instead, they work in concert in a distributed network.

THE EXTENT AND EXERCISE OF VOLUNTARY CONTROL

How much control do we have over our behavior? A precise answer is difficult to give but there clearly are significant limits to deliberate conscious control. Consciousness is useful in novel or dangerous situations, when habit, for some reason, will not suffice, but most of the time we behave largely routinely and consciousness is engaged primarily in monitoring the situation. Unfortunately, only in recent years has the study of consciousness become fair game for neuroscientists and psychologists, so much is as yet unclear. Interestingly, current thinking has been strongly influenced by the writings of William James (1890), who seems to have been ahead of his time in many ways. James developed what he called the *ideomotor theory*. According to this way of thinking, conscious goals have an intrinsically impulsive quality about them. If they are unopposed by competing goals or intentions, we will engage spontaneously in the behavior suggested by the representation of that goal. Actions occur because inhibitions against them are absent. James, however, disagreed with the notion that unconscious functioning played a significant role in human psychology. In retrospect, we now see that his position vis-à-vis nonconscious processing was untenable. Yet, there remains much that is useful in James's theorizing, and Baars (1988, 1997) has dusted off and refurbished James's theory in the light of neuroscience and cognitive psychology.

Baars's model of voluntary activity has five basic hypotheses: (1) "all actions are initiated by relatively simple, momentary images of the goal"; (2) "competing events may drive the goal-image from consciousness"; (3) "most detailed information processing is unconscious and . . . executive processes have no routine access to the details of effector control"; (4) "the moment of willingness to execute the action *may* be conscious, especially when the time to execute it is nonroutine" (emphasis added); and (5) the image of the goal tends "to execute in the absence of any effective competition 'by default'" (1988, p. 260). Recognizing the hierarchical organization of the brain and behavior, Baars notes that each of these goals may have subgoals that are necessary for the execution of the primary objective.

OF WHAT VALUE IS CONSCIOUSNESS?

If the majority of neuropsychological functioning takes place outside of awareness and if zombies are indeed capable of engaging in all kinds of complex activity, of what value is consciousness? Is it just psychological fluff, the unnecessary epiphenomenon of neural processing? From an evolutionary perspective, it must have some utility, since mammals generally appear to be conscious, and some—the great apes in particular—have reflective self-awareness. If consciousness and self-awareness are conserved across species, this suggests that possession of these capacities confers an adaptive advantage, that species thus endowed were favored by natural selection. Of course, it also is possible that consciousness and self-awareness are spandrels (D. M. Buss et al., 1998), accidental by-products of the evolutionary process.

Unfortunately, it isn't easy to second-guess evolution, to discern the reason or reasons that consciousness and self-reflection evolved. For all we know, consciousness was a by-product of some other innovation, albeit an interesting and important by-product. It is less difficult, however, to examine some of the ways in which consciousness can be useful. While we could speculate about any number of these, we suggest that the following three "functions" of consciousness stand out among the others.

First, in novel or unfamiliar situations, routine, rapidly executed behavior may be inappropriate. According to Shallice (1988), human behavior is an emergent property of the functioning of two control systems—one that is slow, limited in capacity, and inefficient, but able to monitor and modify the details of functioning (consciousness), and one that is fast and efficient, with enormous capacity, but able to perform only automatically, and unable to alter its own activity (nonconscious functioning). The activation of the system regulating deliberate, conscious control permits one to analyze a situation and consider possibilities for action other than those to which one habitually may be disposed.

Second, in situations in which one must resist temptation, consciousness may be needed to override habitual modes of behaving ("veto" power; Baars, 1988). This is problematic when you are not aware of engaging in the behavior in question because it occurs automatically and nonconsciously. If goal images are intrinsically "impulsive," as William James (1890) suggested, it may be necessary to formulate competing goals by deliberate, conscious effort and actively to inhibit the performance of acts that you might want to veto.

Third, when performing a complex, nonroutine action (such as learning a new motor behavior), consciousness is important for monitoring the process of the activity and for evaluating the result. Although conscious attention may interfere with smooth performance of automatic tasks, it permits one to compare one's performance with an image of how the activity should go and to make whatever adjustments are necessary. Once an action has become overlearned and automatic, consciousness may be required in the initial phases of establishing a goal and evaluating the situation, and in the end, when assessing the outcome, but the processes in between are parceled out to more efficient automatic processing units.

Dennett (1991, p. 251) summarized the problem of consciousness and volition as follows:

> Although we are occasionally conscious of performing elaborate practical reasoning, leading to a conclusion about what, all things considered, we ought to do, followed by a conscious decision to do that very thing, and culminating finally in actually doing it, these are relatively rare experiences. Most of our intentional actions are performed without any such preamble, and a good thing, too, since there wouldn't be time. The standard trap is to suppose that the relatively rare cases of conscious practical reasoning are a good model for the rest, the cases in which our intentional actions emerge from processes into which

we have no access. Our actions generally satisfy us; we recognize that they are in the main coherent, and that they make appropriate, well-timed contributions to our projects as we understand them.

In short, we don't have any great degree of conscious control over our behavior. On the contrary. Not only is our control limited, but so is our insight: we have limited awareness of why we do the things we do. In fact, we *cannot* have accurate insight into our motivations; most of the time, we just go along with the plausible rationalizations, consistent with our belief systems, offered up by the verbal left hemisphere.

THE PSYCHODYNAMIC UNCONSCIOUS

For Sigmund Freud, the unconscious was a "psychodynamic" unconscious. As he originally saw it, the contents of the unconscious were dominated by impulses, wishes, and ideas that had been repudiated by consciousness and that continued in an ongoing way to press for representation. Paradoxically, in this model of the relationship of nonconscious to conscious processing, consciousness was accorded a certain enhanced status that may have continued the historical tradition of exaggerating its importance.

Gradually, Freud came to believe that the domain of nonconscious processing was much larger than the dynamic unconscious as he had originally conceived of it. It included an array of nonconscious organizing and adaptive processes and proclivities that could not exist within the original dynamic unconscious. His observations subsequently led him to reconsider the topography of the mind, giving much greater status to these nonconscious organizational processes and further diminishing the significance of consciousness as a factor in psychological functioning.

As we have seen, the majority of human behavior is determined by nonconscious processes, but what is traditionally thought of as a "psychodynamic" unconscious is only a small subset of these nonconscious operations. Behavior often is said to be "unconsciously motivated," and many early psychoanalytic ideas involved the assumption that there was a dynamic energetic equilibrium between conscious and unconscious minds. At one time, for example, there was considerable debate over whether "repression" occurred only once and thereafter was maintained automatically or required constant psychological vigilance and activity. The concept of "resistance" has had a similarly difficult history. Do patients in psychotherapy actively resist becoming aware of certain phenomena? Do they actively resist changing their behavior? Or, as the cognitive neuroscience model of nonconscious functioning suggests, are many "resistant" patients simply behaving habitually, automatically, and nonconsciously?

To a certain extent, early psychoanalytic formulations were problematic because they raised the specter of a homunculus, a "ghost in the machine," a privileged observer within the mind who could observe forbidden thoughts, impulses, or feelings and not be contaminated by them, who could avoid conveying any awareness of these forbidden contents to consciousness. These conceptual difficulties are eliminated by the adoption of a neuroscientific perspective on personality.

The brain is modified by experience. Attitudes, behaviors, patterns of emotional reactivity, and styles of interpersonal interaction all become routine over time, and all are initiated and maintained automatically and nonconsciously. They are mediated by neural networks, the probability of activation of which is a function of experience, the individual's current state, and the status of the environment. At times, especially in novel situations or other circumstances demanding a deliberate and conscious response, limited aspects of this habitual mode of behaving may become more susceptible to voluntary influence.

Consider the concept of resistance, for example. Assume that an individual tends to engage repetitively in some self-destructive behavior. He tends not to discuss it in his therapy. His therapist has (many times) interpreted his apparent unwillingness to discuss the behavior as indicative of resistance. When the therapist raises these issues, the patient feels criticized, becomes somewhat irritable, and eventually succeeds in diverting the flow of the conversation. How can we understand this?

Such a patient's self-destructive behavior may be an activity that was procedurally learned, that has a high probability of occurrence when the patient is in certain states (e.g., when depressed and lonely). If pleasurable gratification is associated with the behavior, this may increase the likelihood that he will engage in it, and decrease the likelihood that he will be inclined to give it up. No deliberate, conscious decision is required to engage in the behavior and, in fact, under the right circumstances, it is the easiest thing for him to do. Like nearly all automatic, nonconscious behavior, it is thoroughly rationalized, and the rationalization (which itself is automatic and nonconscious) is likely to be plausible.

When the therapist interprets the patient's behavior, her verbal assertion has no effect on his procedurally learned activity. With repetition, the interpretation may become part of his declarative memory ("My therapist says I'm trying to blah blah blah ... "), independent of the procedural learning system. The patient may avoid discussion of the issue because of a procedurally learned tendency to avoid interpersonal unpleasantness (his irritability and feeling of being criticized), and at times he even may have a bit of conscious awareness of doing so, but for the most part this tendency is mediated by more or less automatically activated neural networks.

For this patient to behave differently would require activation of a different set of neural networks, the activation of which has a low order of probability. This would involve some degree of deliberate, effortful activity, which in turn would require awareness of what ordinarily is an automatically performed behavior. Thus, "resistance" is primarily a manifestation of neural dynamics and their resulting behavioral inertia. One tends to do what one habitually does, not necessarily deliberately to avoid anything (although avoidance of displeasure may have been the genesis of a procedurally learned character trait), but because it has become the easiest (automatic) thing to do in a given situation.

SUMMARY AND CONCLUSION

Consciousness has severely limited speed and capacity. Conscious access to the details of psychological processes is negligible. Instead, consciousness involves awareness of *representations,* models of reality. Our ordinary waking consciousness is concerned with an integrated, multimodal, constantly shifting and evolving representation of ourselves and of the world. Nonconscious functioning is massively parallel, automatic, and extremely efficient. Some of what is unconscious is forever denied access to awareness (e.g., the perception of pheromones). Other processes (such as procedurally learned behavior) are unobserved by consciousness because they have become automatic with repeated practice and their monitoring has become increasingly difficult as a consequence.

Some potential representations are unconscious because the probability of their activation is low given the state of the individual and the status of the environment. These should not be thought of as "contents" of the unconscious. Rather, they are neural networks, currently inactive, that may be activated given the proper circumstances. Even when activated, such networks may not involve conscious representations but still may affect behavior in ways that are inaccessible to awareness.

Consciousness rarely has access to the actual causes of our behavior, although it is capable of creating a plausible and adaptive model of reality that is good enough for most purposes and that seems to have been good enough for natural selection. Although conscious control of our psychological activity is limited at best, by bringing certain phenomena into awareness we have the capacity to monitor and modify that activity in ways that work to our advantage.

13

MODULARITY, DYNAMICS, AND FUNCTIONAL SYSTEMS

INTRODUCTION

Although the brain is composed of a large number of relatively independent modules, it possesses a remarkable capacity for synthesis. Consequently, all human activity reflects an integration of many systems acting in concert to produce specific behaviors, through countless variable means. This synthetic activity is a reflection of the brain's spontaneous self-organization. The brain, as Rössler and Hudson (1990) argue, is a "giant dynamic system" that spontaneously maintains itself in the vicinity of states of self-organizing criticality. Human psychological activity is coherent in large measure as a result of this self-organization.

In this chapter, we examine the brain's self-organizing activity as it is expressed in various complex functions, especially the so-called *ego functions*, a term often used in psychoanalysis and psychiatry to refer to certain basic, adaptive, cognitive–perceptual abilities such as judgment, impulse control, and the ability to distinguish what is really happening from what one is only imagining (reality testing), among others. We are especially interested in the processes associated with reality testing, and hope to demonstrate its modular underpinnings, as well as the complex dynamic factors that contribute to this cognitive–perceptual capacity.

THE FREUDIAN EGO

Sigmund Freud talked about what he called *the ego* in diverse and occasionally contradictory ways. In his early writings, he used the term loosely and nontheoretically to refer to the "self" or "*das ich*" ("the I"). Many of the mental processes which came to be subsumed under the term *ego* in Freud's later model of the mind were initially thought to belong to what he called the "preconscious mind," and therefore they were considered to be observable by consciousness, if one made the effort. Gradually, Freud became aware that many adaptive processes functioned nonconsciously, a realization which led him to use the term *ego* in a different, more formal and theoretical sense. The ego became a system of *processes* that evolved to ensure the individual's self-preservation, and there was no associated presumption that these processes were accessible to conscious introspection. According to this way of thinking, these processes took place at the intersection between the neonate's emerging needs and tensions (as embodied in the "id"), on the one hand, and the environment, on the other. They were shaped to a large extent by learning.

When Freud used the term ego, often he was careful to note that the concept was merely an abstraction used to refer to certain mental processes which revealed the effects of learning and adaptation; he argued that the ego should not be construed as an entity but only as a theoretical construct (1923, p.7). Sometimes, however, Freud described the ego as a "structure" or an "agency," thereby contributing to the common practice of reifying the construct in ways that Freud himself had warned against. Hence Freud, and subsequently others, came to describe the ego as a psychological structure, having certain characteristics, and possessing a set of discrete functions.

As a result of this legacy, we have inherited a long list of specific *ego functions*. Among these are consciousness, sensory perception, memory, the awareness and expression of affect, thinking, control of motor behavior, language, reality testing, defense mechanisms (themselves a variegated lot of processes), integration or synthesis, and regression (Arlow & Brenner, 1964). Others have proposed their own more or less extensive lists of ego functions (e.g., Beres, 1956; S. Freud, 1940; A. Freud, 1966; Hartmann, 1950).

Freud's description of the ego as a set of *processes* is consistent with the model of the mind we have been outlining, while the ego as *structure* represents a reification that is at odds with both logic and findings from the neurosciences. We are concerned that both the reification of the concept and the inclusion of so many capacities in the domain of the *ego* has led to considerable theoretical confusion.

EGO FUNCTIONS AS EMERGENT PROCESSES

One problem with the common understanding of ego functions is that "functions" are *functional systems,* complex forms of self-organizing psychological activity having a modular architecture, comprising many component processes (Luria, 1973, 1980). This modular nature of behavior is characteristic of both simple and complex activity. As was the case for consciousness, state, and other personality processes we have discussed, we believe ego functions can be analyzed usefully in terms of dynamics and modularity. The dynamic point of view makes it plain that ego functions are neither static nor monolithic. An ego function is not something that a person either does or does not possess. Instead, the term ego function is an abstractive referring to processes that are emergent from the nonlinear interaction of an array of internal and environmental systems. The moment-to-moment emergence of a given ego function is dependent upon a wide array of influences: learning history, state, temperament, endocrine status, physiological variables, and environment, among others.

Furthermore, ego functioning is characterized by fluctuations and bifurcations. Thus, the manifestations of any given ego function show variability across time, and this variability can be graphically depicted by the use of a phase portrait that reflects the wide variety of influences on any emergent ego function. State and temperament are especially likely to be important contributors to the current expression of a given ego function. So, for example, a child who typically has reasonably good affect regulation is likely to be less able to regulate affect when she is in a state of fatigue or illness, and she may require help from her parents to control her affect and to reestablish autonomous affect regulation.

Temperament also can influence ego functioning. Take the example of the so-called difficult-to-soothe baby. It is hard for such a child to acquire an adaptive capacity for self-regulation, and the caregiver's ability to provide soothing experiences is likely to affect the development of the child's own capacity to establish self-regulation. Even when children who were initially "difficult to soothe" acquire reasonably reliable affect regulation, they may be more likely to be vulnerable to irritability and loss of control when under stress, a characteristic that may persist into adulthood.

Many ego functions operate nonconsciously to the degree that they might be said to be genetically "hard-wired," or they have become habitual through repetition and procedural learning. Consciousness may or may not be required in association with certain kinds of ego processes. Consider, for example, a child who becomes overstimulated and loses control over his affect or behavior. Through previous experience, he may have learned (with the help of his parents) that it is useful to withdraw to his room to get reorganized and thus effecting a change of state. When he experiences himself as "melting down," he may spontaneously seek a voluntary timeout. We see this as the activity of an adaptive self-regulating function that has been procedurally learned, becoming habitual (as determined by the child's state).

CAREGIVERS AND THE DEVELOPMENT
OF THE CAPACITY FOR AUTOMATIC,
ADAPTIVE BEHAVIOR

Capacities that fall under the rubric of ego functions, like most manifestations of personality, develop within the context of relationships with primary caregivers. Thus they are processes that have a biological basis but that also are shaped by learning as a result of interactions with others during early life. A young child's caregivers provide the relational context essential for the full development of basic regulatory processes. This prevents the infant from being overwhelmed by environmental stimuli, and also helps the infant reestablish equilibrium if it is perturbed by endogenously arising stimuli such as hunger or pain. The attuned caregiver thus adjusts the environment to the needs of the child to some degree, providing a buffer between the infant and the environment, modeling certain basic adaptive functions, and providing requisite physiological and psychological supplies. Caregivers use their adaptive capabilities, "lending" them to the infant, and hence providing functions the infant cannot as yet assume for itself.

Each time parents (or some other caregiver) lend their capacity for adaptive activity to an infant, the infant learns something. So, for example, a mother recognizes her child's distress as indicative of hunger and acts to meet this need. Across time the child experiences again and again the emergence of hunger and its resolution in transaction with the primary caregiver. In this way, procedural memories are established that permit the child to behave in an adaptive manner. Gradually, through establishment of procedural knowledge, and development of the child's own cognitive and motor abilities, the ego function first provided by the mother becomes a process that the child is able to perform independently and more or less automatically.

Each stage of life is accompanied by new demands and pressures that call for the development of skills (or ego functions) that previous stages may not have demanded. For example, as children become old enough to attend school, they are expected to focus their attention in a sustained way and to participate in group activities that may require self-control and the capacity to defer immediate self-gratification to the needs of the group. Although some children come to school with an already well-established capacity for organizing their time and knowing how to work, many children require significant and ongoing adult support to establish the capacity to engage in certain structured tasks. The processes associated with doing something like homework are acquired via procedural learning, through protracted dyadic transactions with parents, as well as through identifying with the parent's capacity to do work. Many skills necessary for participating in the culture require these sorts of training experiences, and individuals vary in both their capacity to acquire these lessons and in the quality of their training. Some of what appears to be pathological adjustment may in fact be related to failure to learn certain processes during an appropriate developmental period, perhaps due to lack of opportunity.

THE MODULAR ARCHITECTURE OF EGO FUNCTIONS: REALITY TESTING

In this section, our intention is to analyze a specific ego function—reality testing—and to show that it is best understood as a hierarchically organized, modular functional system, composed of very basic, as well as more complex, perceptual and cognitive abilities. We illustrate functional modularity by studying persons with various kinds of neuropathology, because such disorders may create discrete perturbations of various aspects of functioning revealing the modular architecture of complex psychological phenomena. One's grasp of reality may be affected in different ways as a result of different kinds of lesion in different areas of the brain (Grigsby et al., 1991).

M. K. Johnson and Raye (1981) made a useful distinction between the concepts of reality testing and reality monitoring. From their point of view, reality testing "generally refers to the process of distinguishing a present perception from a present act of imagination or act of remembering"; reality monitoring, on the other hand, "refers to the process of distinguishing a *past* perception from a *past* act of imagination, both of which resulted in memories" (p. 67; emphasis in original). We will consider both of these processes, but for simplicity and consistency with most of the literature on the subject we will use the term *reality testing*.

REALITY—AND REALITY TESTING AND REPRESENTATION

Defining "reality" is a tricky proposition. In some respects our philosophical position is what Walter J. Freeman referred to as "a form of *epistemological solipsism*" that "isolates brains from the world" (1995, p. 2; emphasis in original), as distinct from metaphysical solipsism, "according to which everything that exists is the projection of a brain." All we can know—of the world and of ourselves—is a function of representations (images and ideas) created by our brains, and those, for all intents and purposes, *are* our reality. If our representations diverge too much from those of our society or the people around us, we either keep them to ourselves, assume the social mantle of a crackpot, or run the risk of getting into legal or psychiatric trouble.

The concept of reality testing ordinarily rests on the assumption that there is an objective external reality in comparison with which we evaluate our perceptions. Reality testing thus is generally described as the ability to discriminate what is real from what is not real, especially in the realm of thought and perception. More precisely, it involves the capacity to assess the validity of one's mental representations of the world and of oneself. We don't take issue with the existence of some reality outside ourselves, but we do hold that at best we are only able to form a reasonably good working model of that reality. Despite their flaws, for most people, most of the time, these models do an adequate job.

The adequacy of these models is important; if an organism is to succeed in its environment, it must perceive that environment accurately enough to permit adaptive responses in an almost unimaginable variety of situations. While reality testing as traditionally conceived must occur constantly, like the vast majority of perceptual and cognitive functioning, most of the time it takes place automatically, outside awareness. In fact, it may be more accurate to say that we use reality testing only when our perceptions depart markedly from our expectations (i.e., reality *testing* may be a relatively infrequent occurrence for most people whose capacity to represent the world and themselves is intact). But when the functional systems by which we model the world are disrupted, or if we find it difficult to assess the accuracy of those models, the ability to perceive reality, or the feeling of reality, may be defective. As is true of other cognitive functions which lose their overlearned, automatic character following neurologic insult, the process of reality testing may not only change but it becomes less automatic, less efficient, and more conscious and effortful.

Because it is a dynamic functional system with a modular architecture, reality testing is influenced in a nonlinear way by a multitude of variables. For one thing, processes associated with representing the self in relation to the world, like other psychological processes, are heavily influenced by interpersonal experience. For example, when confronted with novel or unfamiliar circumstances, children are liable to check their parents' reaction to the situation, presumably to establish how the circumstance should be represented and to learn what the parents consider the appropriate response.

Representations of the world may be influenced by temperament, state, and the environment. An innately shy person, for example, is likely to view interpersonal situations very differently than would an extrovert. Similarly, the "difficult-to-soothe" child is likely to perceive a more abrupt, disjointed, and annoying world than the relaxed child. State also may strongly affect representational activity. Someone who is fatigued may represent experience with less acuity and may miss nuances in interpersonal situations that could be perceived from the vantage point of a different state. In like manner, intense affects often disrupt representational activity and undermine reality testing in ways consistent with the state. Thus, angry people may see affront and deliberate provocation everywhere they go. The press of inner needs also can affect representation. Thus a hungry person sees and represents the world in terms of food, whereas a sexually aroused person perceives others in ways heavily influenced by that arousal.

A host of other factors can also undermine representation and reality testing. Egocentrism can have a significant effect on reality testing because it leads to representations of reality that overestimate the degree to which an experience is about the self or overestimate the importance of the self in an experience. Disruption of social ties or lack of familiarity with local customs—as in a foreign culture—may lead to misperception or misconstruing of events. The same holds true for over- or understimulation.

THE MODULAR ARCHITECTURE OF REALITY TESTING

We now discuss case material and research, disentangling several of the component processes of reality testing to demonstrate that this functional system is quite complex. While certain syndromes we discuss below are rare (e.g., reduplicative paramnesia), others are observed frequently. Despite the rarity of some of these syndromes, the fact that they *can* occur demonstrates something about different aspects of the modular nature of psychological functioning and, in this case, of the process of evaluating the accuracy of our representations of self and world. In the material that follows, we cover a number of different disorders that disrupt various levels of the functional hierarchy, beginning with more basic aspects of perception, then moving on to examine cognitive and affective contributors to reality testing.

Disorders of Perception

The "accuracy" with which one perceives events is a fundamental aspect of reality testing. As discussed previously, the various perceptual systems are extremely complex functional systems that may be disturbed in diverse ways by injury to neuronal groups at different levels of integration. Thus, certain perceptual disturbances may literally affect one's ability to perceive what is in front of oneself. These are disturbances of the ability to represent the world. For example, persons with visual object agnosia can see a common object presented to them but cannot identify or even recognize the object as something previously seen (Farah, 1990; Hécaen & Albert, 1978). This is not a deficit of simple sensation or intellectual functioning, nor is it a problem in finding the right word for the object (i.e., a language disorder). Instead, in visual object agnosia, perception is no longer immediately, intuitively accurate. A patient with visual agnosia is liable to experience some reorganization of this functional system—spontaneously and non-consciously—which leads him or her to try to deduce the nature of the object from certain basic features. This was illustrated by the patient discussed by Hécaen and Albert (1978, p. 195) who misidentified a bicycle as "a pole with two wheels, one in front, one in back" and who called a pen and a cigar "cylindrical sticks of variable length." The patient could, however, identify objects immediately upon touch, showing that this was not a problem with language or knowledge of objects, but of visual recognition.

The passive quality of perception observed in association with many prefrontal lesions (and part of what is known as a *dysexecutive syndrome*) also may produce profound disturbances of the ability to grasp what is happening in the world (Luria, 1980). Let's examine what happens when a person with such a lesion is asked to look at a complex photograph and explain what is happening. Commonly we observe that rather than analyzing the picture actively, he or she is likely, with little deliberate thought, to pick out one detail and generalize from that detail to explain what is happening in the picture. Luria described the response of some patients who were shown a picture of a man who had fallen through the ice on a frozen pond. People were running to rescue the man. A sign by the pond read "Danger," while the silhouette of a city appeared in the background. Many of Luria's patients with prefrontal lesions failed to examine the picture actively. Instead they responded passively and often bizarrely. For example, one patient interpreted the picture "as showing 'high voltage lines' or 'wet paint' or 'wild animals' (because of the 'Danger' sign) or 'war' (because of the people running) or 'the Kremlin' (because of the outline of the city with the spires in the background)" (1980, p. 334). Thus reality testing in novel or complex situations requires an active ability to figure out what is happening, and it may be impaired if one's typical perceptual style is extremely passive.

Disorders of Complex Somatesthetic Perception

Several disorders of somatic perception involve circumscribed impairment of the representation of both the environment and the self. For example, Shapiro, Fink, and Bender (1952) described a syndrome called *exosomesthesia*, which they viewed as a pathological extension of the body schema. They reported on a patient who often localized tactile stimulation of his hand to objects in extrapersonal space, rather than to his hand, despite the presence of conflicting visual information. Many times the patient stated that it was the bed or the table that had been touched, not his hand. When the examiner asked how he could feel the bed being touched with a pin, the patient "would become tense, avoid the question, and insist, 'you touched the bed, not me' " (Shapiro et al., 1952, p. 483). In addition to the disturbance of body image that appears in exosomesthesia, it is interesting that these patients are unable to reconcile conflicting perceptual data obtained from different sensory systems (vision and somatesthesis in the case of Shapiro and colleagues' patient).

Bizarre somatic sensations also may be induced by factors other than brain lesions. This phenomenon is interesting in that one's representation of the body, which ordinarily seems stable, may be perturbed in extreme ways by the presence of atypical sensation. Lackner (1988), for example, investigated the effect of unusual sensory input on topographically organized somatosensory maps. Because previous research had shown that vibratory stimuli applied to a muscle appears to alter the proprioceptive information on which the brain acts, Lackner held a vibrator against a subject's biceps and physically restrained the forearm to prevent movement. This made the patient feel as though the arm was extended more than was actually the case. When Lackner had a subject hold his nose between his fingers while the biceps was vibrated, the person described a vivid sensation of his nose growing much longer (as the arm felt as if it was extended). For some subjects, the same kind of stimulation produced a sensation of their fingers (rather than the nose) being longer. This technique induced many other unusual kinds of sensation in Lackner's subjects.

Mnestic Disturbances

Sigmund Freud proposed that memory is an important component of reality testing. He argued that to distinguish ideas from reality, one must compare the idea "with the memory traces of reality" (1911/1957, p. 16). Amnestic syndromes, especially those characterized by confabulation, present several different pictures of impaired reality testing. Confabulation, which involves an uncritical and erroneous "recall" of inappropriate representations masquerading as memory traces, may include significant distortions of reality to which the patient clings resolutely although usually transiently.

Something similar to a circumscribed form of confabulation occurs in the syndrome of *reduplicative paramnesia* (Benson, Gardner, & Meadows, 1976; Pick, 1903; Weinstein & Kahn, 1955), in which, although otherwise well oriented, an individual tenaciously maintains a faulty orientation for person, place, or time. This occurs despite the unreasonableness of the person's belief and in the face of ample evidence to the contrary. Patients who experience reduplicative paramnesia may report incorrectly that they have four arms, or that they knew someone in their present life at an earlier time, or that there are two people who are almost exactly alike (say, their mother and someone almost identical to her), when in fact there is only one.

A more subtle failure of the process of reality testing (or, more precisely, of reality *monitoring*) may occur as a consequence of severe memory impairment. For example, a 24-year-old man had sustained a moderately severe closed head trauma 18 months previously. Both the patient and his family reported that he frequently believed events had happened when in fact he had only thought about them. For example, he erroneously thought he had made plans to get together with two friends, and he became angry when neither showed up. He then refused to believe that he had never discussed the plan with them. Similar incidents occurred on other occasions. He was capable of discriminating thoughts from reality at the time he had the thoughts (i.e., reality *testing* was intact), but the capacity to distinguish them in retrospect (reality *monitoring*) was defective. M. K. Johnson and Raye (1981, p. 68) assert that "fairly extreme errors about the origin of memories are probably more common than reality testing failures such as hallucinations" and suggest that problems of this kind may be even more resistant to correction than are misperceptions.

Rationalization

Different people's perceptions of the same phenomena are normally quite variable, a manifestation of the fact that the diverse representations of the world created by human perceptual systems involve a certain amount of idiosyncratic interpretation of what actually happens—epistemological solipsism again. More precisely, the human brain creates models of the environment, as well as detailed images of oneself and one's inner state as one engages in transactions with the world. For humans, as biological systems in which competitive natural selection processes shape the perceptual system, it is too much to expect that representation can be perfect. Instead, they usually are good enough to get by with.

Everyone experiences the world through the medium of his or her own representations, to which each individual gives a unique set of interpretations. We are all "spin doctors." Our representations and explanations of events are influenced by what seems to be the ubiquitous tendency of humans to explain themselves and their experience, a tendency that we have discussed in other contexts. Research in the area of attribution theory and cognitive dissonance strongly suggests this compulsion to explain may be observed much, if not all, of the time (Brehm & Cohen, 1962; Festinger, 1957; Festinger & Carlsmith, 1959; E. E. Jones et al., 1972; Zimbardo & Ebbesen, 1969).

We already have discussed the provocative studies with commissurotomy patients reported by Gazzaniga and his associates (Gazzaniga, Wilson, & LeDoux, 1977; Gazzaniga & LeDoux, 1978; Gazzaniga, 1985), suggesting that rationalization (or attribution) may be central to the functioning of the conscious verbal mind. Their research illustrated a curious but possibly adaptive form of impaired reality testing, in that the verbal mind (i.e., the left cerebral hemisphere, which also mediates use of the right hand) of their subjects had no idea why the left hand had done certain things, yet it confidently explained the left hand's actions as if it really knew the facts.

The left hemisphere, although disconnected from the experience of the right hemisphere, offers seemingly reasonable explanations for the actions of the silent half-brain and its left hand. The explanations are so plausible that we would probably accept them at face value and consider that the commissurotomized patient had made an adequate appraisal of reality if we did not know what actually led to the behavior of the left hand. Nevertheless, we know that in reality these explanations were wrong. In contrast, a patient with paranoid schizophrenia might inform us that he really hasn't put on weight but that a shadowy group of conspirators comes into his house every night and takes his clothes, leaving an identical-looking but slightly smaller set of clothing in their place. We feel justified in immediately dismissing this as a crazy idea and feel no need to seek evidence that either confirms or disconfirms his claim.

Because psychotic explanations are bizarre, unreasonable, and incompatible with our own ideas about the world, we are less likely to take seriously the rationalizations of the left brain of the person with schizophrenia than we are the explanations of a nonpsychotic but commissurotomized patient. Yet, if we consider whether their explanations are accurate or not, we should agree that reality testing is impaired for both individuals. When we examine the data more carefully, however, we find that the *process* of reality testing may be functionally independent of the content upon which it is operating. Neither the split-brain patient nor the patient with schizophrenia questions the accuracy of his thinking. The assessment of reality testing in these cases becomes a judgment, made (automatically and nonconsciously) by an observer (with his or her own idiosyncratic representations of reality), about the likelihood of certain explanations for events, thoughts, and feelings.

While it sometimes is argued that rationalization represents an attempt to protect oneself from devastating emotional reactions, the proclivity of the verbal hemisphere to explain events appears obvious. Furthermore, whether or not rationalization can be considered in any given case to be psychologically motivated, it clearly has a neural basis, and the brain's capacity for rationalization allows attributions to be made nonconsciously, with no deliberate action or effort. When cognitive capacity is limited, or is severely compromised by neurological disorder, we are likely to see rationalizations which grossly distort reality. Thus, impairment in reasoning ability and the capacity for abstraction may adversely affect the accuracy of representations of self and the world.

Reflective Awareness and Denial of Illness

Neurological disorders often are accompanied by a dramatic lack of insight into one's deficits—a limited capacity for critical evaluation of the appropriateness of one's activity. In such cases there is a lack of reflective awareness (Rapaport, 1951), an aspect of what Duval and Wicklund (1972) called objective self awareness—the consciousness of being conscious, or the awareness of one's cognitive and behavioral activity. Significant pathology of the prefrontal cortex is known to affect this aspect of psychological functioning. Reflective awareness also is defective, for example, in the syndrome of *anosognosia,* or denial of illness (Babinski, 1914; Weinstein & Kahn, 1955).

Among some patients, the denial of hemiplegia and other severe deficits, including visual field defects, incontinence, and amnesic or cognitive deficits, may be extreme. For example, Nathanson, Bergman, and Gordon (1952) described a group of patients who denied not only their hemiplegia but the existence of their affected extremity (recall the patient described in Chapter 12 who underwent caloric testing and became aware of her paralysis). Denial occurred even when they were visually confronted with the attachment of the extremity to their bodies. Such disturbances, commonly observed by professionals who work with stroke patients, often are associated with *hemiautotopagnosia,* a disturbance of the body image restricted to one side of the body.

Similarly, a patient of Weinstein and Kahn (1950) denied her urinary incontinence, yet while being interviewed the woman urinated in her bed. At first she denied having done so, then under repeated questioning blamed the problem on the dampness outside, and finally said it was the examiner who had wet the bed (p. 775). The authors reported that they had found this syndrome frequently to be associated with confabulation and disorientation, and noted that euphoria was present in more than half their sample as well.

Euphoria Following Frontal Lobe Injury

The euphoria associated with certain brain lesions can have significant effects on an individual's perception of things. As discussed earlier, lesions of the prefrontal cortex may affect individuals' ability to evaluate ongoing behavior critically and accurately. The consequent lack of insight into oneself contributes to problems with reality testing. A state-related factor which may affect the accuracy of reality testing is the euphoria that commonly accompanies lesions of the prefrontal cortex. It is common to see seriously impaired but euphoric patients who unrealistically maintain that they have no problems. When events disturb their emotional equilibrium, they may become transiently irritable, but the disruption tends to be short lived, and later is perceived as being of little consequence. The sense of euphoria softens the hard edges of reality and results in a failure to take things seriously.

Euphoria also may be associated with a failure to learn from experience, a common phenomenon among persons with prefrontal lesions. This problem calls to mind Luria's (1980, p. 253) description of dogs whose frontal lobes have been excised and which seem to have lost the capacity to "correctly assess the meaning of reinforcement." Particularly noteworthy among many euphoric human patients with prefrontal lesions is a "lack of marked emotional conflicts" (Luria, 1980, p. 256). Clearly such lesions may affect one's adaptation to reality, as well as one's ability to assess the environment.

SENSE OF REALITY AND REALITY TESTING

The *sense of reality* refers to the feeling that things are real. Most of the time we experience this automatically and implicitly. On occasion, however, the feeling that things are real may be impaired. *Depersonalization* and *derealization* are probably the most common disturbances of the sense of reality. These terms refer, respectively, to feelings of unreality and estrangement, a sense that oneself or the world is somehow strange or alien: in depersonalization, one's self feels unreal; in derealization, the world seems strange and unreal. An individual who is experiencing such feelings of unreality is not necessarily delusional, and the ability to discriminate reality may well be intact despite a disturbance in one's sense about the reality of the situation. Although depersonalization and derealization may occur independently of one another, ordinarily both are present. Other related disorders of reality sense include the following: *déjà vu*, in which one has an uncanny sense of familiarity about an event, as though it had happened exactly the same way at some time in the past; *jamais vu*, in which something that is familiar is experienced as completely unknown and unfamiliar; and occasional experiences of things being almost too real.

Depersonalization and derealization may occur as a result of or in association with such conditions as depression, vertigo, neurotoxicity, use of hallucinogens, sensory deprivation, sensory overload, alcohol intoxication, meditation, posttraumatic stress disorder (PTSD), complex partial seizures, schizophrenia, and electrical stimulation of the temporal cortex (Ackner, 1954; Cattell, 1966; Devinsky et al., 1989; Grigsby & Johnston, 1989; Mayer-Gross, 1935; Noyes & Kletti, 1976; Penfield & Rasmussen, 1955; Shorvon, 1945/46). The incidence in the general population is relatively high (Dixon, 1963; W. Roberts, 1960).

While the defining characteristic of the syndrome is a feeling of unreality, other manifestations of depersonalization and derealization are protean. Associated features include lightheadedness, a blunting of affect, ruminations, anxiety, perceptual anomalies (e.g., *micropsia* and *macropsia* in which things look either small and far away in the former or very large and close-up in the latter), a disturbed sense of time, agoraphobia, and fear that one is going crazy (Dixon, 1963; W. Roberts, 1960; Roth, 1959; Shorvon, 1945/46). Individuals who complain of feelings of unreality frequently report subjectively impaired memory and concentration, and may describe their experience as dream-like. A feeling that one is outside oneself, watching one's own mechanical actions and thoughts as if from a distance, is common. One patient volunteered that during a motor vehicle accident in which she had been injured, she had had "one of those funky out-of-body experiences."

Schilder (1935) noted a relationship between feelings of unreality and disorders of the body image. He described a patient with a left hemiparesis who felt that her whole body no longer existed, that it was rotting away. The objects and people around her also appeared changed and strange. In cases like this, feelings of unreality accompany deficits in reality testing, but more often depersonalization and derealization occur independently of problems in reality testing; insight remains intact. When depersonalization occurs in the presence of an impaired ability to monitor and evaluate critically one's experience and behavior, reality testing also may be defective.

The variety of etiologies for depersonalization and derealization is quite interesting, and suggests that despite the phenomenological similarity from one case to another, there may be a number of different unreality syndromes. Wilbur, for example, a 29-year-old man with complex partial seizures associated with a right medial temporal lobe focus and hippocampal gliosis, reported that his seizures always began with several seconds of a sensation of *déjà vu*, followed by 1 or 2 minutes of depersonalization and derealization, peculiar smells, and other phenomena typical of temporal lobe seizures. This is consistent with reports by awake seizure surgery patients that they sometimes experience strong feelings of *déjà vu*, depersonalization, derealization, and other distortions of the sense of reality in response to electrical stimulation of their brains (Penfield & Rasmussen, 1955).

However, the experiences of epileptics differ somewhat from the reports of Susan, a 32-year-old homemaker, and Mary, a 34-year-old registered nurse, both of whom experienced extreme feelings of depersonalization and derealization in association with episodes of vertigo accompanying Ménière's disease (an inner ear disorder characterized by episodes of vertigo, progressive hearing loss, a sensation of fullness in the ear, and tinnitus). In their cases, the perceptual disturbance was considerably more bizarre than the feeling of unreality described above by Wilbur (Grigsby & Johnston, 1989). There is an area of the superior posterior temporal lobe that has been found to be responsive to vestibular stimulation (Adams & Victor, 1989), and hence the depersonalization Susan and Mary experienced also may have had its genesis in the temporal cortex and may have differed from that reported by Wilbur as a result of the additional abnormal vestibular input (a dynamic disorder, perhaps), or because of recruitment of other areas of the brain in a widely distributed network.

The existence of a temporal lobe focus is less clear in the case of persons who have sustained minor head trauma with no loss of consciousness (Grigsby & Kaye, 1993). These individuals commonly have minor cognitive sequelae and no objectively demonstrable temporal lobe pathology. The same holds true for other cases of a disturbed sense of reality in the context of intact reality testing. Castillo (1990), for example, presented interview data from six persons who meditated regularly and who had experienced depersonalization/derealization.

SUMMARY AND CONCLUSION

To illustrate a distributed modular approach to understanding personality functions, we examined several disturbances of reality testing that may occur as sequelae of neurological insult. Our analysis suggests that the construction of realistic representations of the world is the emergent property of a complex functional system that may be disrupted by lesions in a number of areas of the brain. There is no one-to-one correspondence between the locus of a lesion and the type of disturbance observed. Instead, various types and locations of neuropathology may differentially affect this functional system. The resulting syndromes differ in severity, extent, and level of the hierarchy—some involving more global impairment of the ability accurately to represent the self–environment system, whereas others are more circumscribed in their effects.

Disturbances of affect, memory, thinking, body schema, reality sense, reflexive awareness, and certain aspects of perception all may disrupt reality testing in specific ways. Each of these functional systems itself is composed of a complex heterarchy of modules, which likewise may be differentially affected by various lesions. In each syndrome, to understand what is happening, we must look closely at the various *types* of deficits which present themselves. That is, we must examine the process of these failures, the aspects of the function which remain intact, and the nature of an individual's deliberate, spontaneous, and nonconscious attempts to compensate for the compromised functioning. All this must be done in the light of specific environmental constraints upon the exercise of the function.

Our discussion has implicated several factors in disturbed reality testing, including the following:

1. Disturbed perceptual functioning affects the ability to form adequate representations of the environment in a clear-cut, elementary way. One simply may be unable to perceive the environment accurately (e.g., visual agnosia).

2. An active perceptual style (in contrast to the passivity often observed among patients with prefrontal cortex lesions) is necessary to make sense of perception at the level of attribution of meaning in novel or complex situations.

3. Intact perceptual input across the different modalities, linked by reentrant signaling, permits the formation of an integrated representation of the world and the self.

4. If one is to engage in adaptive behavior, one's representations of the world and the self must be reasonably accurate. If we assume an intact basic perceptual apparatus, problems with reality sense and testing are likely to be a function of failures of integration at higher levels of organization.

5. The feeling that things (and oneself) are real gives one confidence in one's experience. This sense of things as real may be intact (or sometimes exaggerated) even in paranoid schizophrenia. On the other hand, feelings of depersonalization and derealization in otherwise normal persons may cause them to question their sanity and to doubt the accuracy of their perceptions.

6. Mnestic disorders involving confabulation lead to serious disruption of one's grasp of current environmental conditions (e.g., disorientation) and of past events. Less severe failures of episodic memory obviously may affect recall of prior occurrences or reality monitoring and thus may lead to failures to act in an adaptive manner.

7. Reflective awareness, the ability to evaluate oneself, one's activity, and one's experience critically and accurately, is impaired in many neurological disorders, especially those involving the prefrontal cortex.

8. An individual's state significantly affects the accuracy with which the self and the world are perceived.

The preceding analysis of reality testing seems to us consistent with the position that there is no such *thing* as the ego and that so-called ego functions are actually complex, dynamic, functional systems, emergent properties of widely distributed neural networks. Therefore, it may be somewhat misleading to use such broad, all-inclusive concepts as *ego* or *reality testing*. The terms encompass so many different phenomena that we believe it may be more useful to attempt to examine them individually, considering them in terms of their constituent modular subcomponents.

14

REGULATION
OF BEHAVIOR

INTRODUCTION

We have worked our way from neurobiology and dynamics toward the emergence of human psychological activity, examining some basic aspects of neurodynamics in an attempt to show how one's state, environment, and past experience presumably affect the probability of activation of specific neural networks. An important focus of our discussion so far has been the vast amount of nonconscious processing that constitutes the basic ground from which psychological phenomena emerge. The overwhelming volume of nonconscious processing does not minimize the significance of the capacity to behave with conscious intention or purpose. However much we may be limited by biological factors that are beyond introspection, we human beings nevertheless possess a capacity for voluntary behavior. Although much purposeful activity does not require the participation of consciousness, people can, and do, engage in deliberate, conscious, goal-directed behavior.

The human ability to regulate behavior emerges out of the interaction between the nonconscious activation of behavioral schemas (neural networks, in other words), on the one hand, and the capacity to monitor and reflect on this nonconsciously activated behavior, and to inhibit, adjust, or change it if such a course seems appropriate (easier said than done, of course), on the other. Thus, roughly speaking, there exist two complex modular neural systems, one characterized by habit, automaticity, and nonconscious processing, and another that mediates deliberate efforts to control our actions. We previously discussed evidence that most behavior is

279

activated nonconsciously and noted that the demands of adaptation, and the limitations of conscious processing, necessitate that most neural activity *must* occur outside awareness. On the psychological level, these nonconscious organizing tendencies can be thought of as habits, mediated at the level of neural networks, and having associated (and constantly changing) probabilities of activation.

In focusing on the mind's emergent capacity to fine-tune these nonconscious, automatic, habitual behaviors, to make necessary adjustments, and to undertake goal-directed behavior, this chapter introduces a neuropsychological perspective on the human capacity to behave purposefully. We will consider evidence that strongly implicates the involvement of the prefrontal cortex in neural processes associated with encountering novelty and with the deliberate conscious control of behavior.

DIFFERENT LEVELS OF ANALYSIS: BEHAVIOR, SCHEMAS, ATTRACTORS, AND NEURAL NETWORKS

Before beginning our analysis of how the two regulatory systems interact, we must first deal with the language that is used to describe these phenomena. Specifically, the terms *behavior, schema, attractor,* and *neural network* are taken from different levels of analysis (behavioral, psychological, dynamic, and neural, respectively), but they nevertheless represent phenomena that are essentially similar in many important details. Although there certainly may be important differences in meaning among these terms, we believe they may fruitfully be used somewhat interchangeably if we do not inadvertently confuse levels of analysis and if we clearly delineate their relationships with one another.

The most concrete of these terms is *behavior,* which for the moment we will define as any psychological activity that can be observed by another person or some kind of event recorder. Behavior is mediated by the activity of the CNS, and discrete behaviors are mediated by relatively discrete neural networks. Not all neural networks necessarily mediate a behavior, but behavior cannot exist without supporting neural activity. Thus the terms *behavior* and *neural networks,* although indicating phenomena on different levels of analysis (behavior and neurophysiology are of different logical types), permit us to discuss the same thing in two different ways. Importantly, the conceptual links between the two should be logically consistent, and theories devised at each level should also be consistent. If the conclusions of a behavioral theory are at odds with the conclusions suggested by a neurophysiological theory, one of the two is a less accurate representation of the phenomena, and we must either conduct a critical experiment that will allow us to decide between them or weigh the evidence supporting each position.

Schema, a psychological concept, represents an abstract generalization about behavior. The term is used at a more global level of thinking, so that routine behaviors may be thought to reflect the activation of a schema, but not all schemas are associated with a behavior—some are cognitive or perceptual, for example. A useful concept, the idea of a schema nevertheless is problematic because it has a less identifiable basis or referent than does a neural network (in fact, any schema is mediated by a neural network or set of networks). We can identify a neural network and study how it works (sort of), but there is a bit more arbitrariness in specifying what a schema is. A neural network has physical characteristics, whereas a schema is only a way of speaking about how people function. If you want to use a cognitive psychological level of analysis, you might speak of a behavioral schema mediating a behavior; from a neurophysiological perspective, you would think in terms of neural networks. Yet, the two ideas are closely related. The theory of neural networks may allow us to link theories about schemas to biology.

Finally, an *attractor* is a concept taken from the study of dynamics. In the context of neuropsychology, it is similar to a behavior in which one is inclined to engage (a habit) or a perception one is likely to have, in a given set of circumstances. A system's activity is drawn into an attractor in the same way that an individual is likely to behave habitually, or that the probability of activation of a neural network is great under certain circumstances. Again, the level of analysis differs, but whether one speaks in terms of behavior, habits, schemas, attractors, or neural networks, certain aspects of the essential phenomena are similar. To use these terms somewhat interchangeably may help illuminate certain aspects of their functioning, as long as we keep in mind the conceptual level (logical type) to which we are making reference.

If different levels of analysis are used appropriately in trying to understand human personality, the payoff is twofold. First, concordance among the various levels suggests the relative accuracy of the different theoretical models (and the corollary is that disagreement suggests that one or more of the models is flawed in the way it represents the phenomena). Second, different levels of analysis provide new insights across levels, raising new questions and permitting clearer perceptions of aspects of reality that may have been overlooked or forced into ill-fitting theoretical garb.

SCHEMAS AND THE AUTOMATIC AND NONCONSCIOUS ACTIVATION OF BEHAVIOR

Most human perceptual, cognitive, and behavioral activity is generated with little effort, habitually, and outside awareness. A neurologically intact individual engages in automatic behaviors (i.e., in appropriate situations) with little deliberate thought. In Shallice's theory of behavioral self-regulation (1988), both simple and complex behaviors may be thought of as being mediated by "schemata" (the term Shallice uses for lower-level, simple programs of behavior), or "scripts" or "memory organization packets" (Schank, 1982; Schank & Abelson, 1977). We will refer to these as *simple schemas* and *complex schemas,* respectively.

Schemas have a hierarchical organization. A simple schema consists of basic motor, perceptual, or cognitive processes, whereas a complex schema also involves a cognitive context for such simple schemas. For example, getting dressed is a complex schema composed of a number of simpler schemas, including putting on socks, tying shoestrings, and buttoning a shirt (each of which comprises modular subcomponents). Very basic habits, such as biting one's nails, the way one holds one's silverware, or a round-shouldered posture, also reflect the operation of simple schemas. More elaborate habits, such as social withdrawal in unfamiliar situations, or an arrogant manner of relating to other people, represent more complex schemas.

The hierarchical nesting of schemas facilitates their appropriate selection, although simple schemas (which might be useful in a number of tasks, many of which are potentially novel) are not neatly nested within complex schemas. For example, the complex schema of driving a concrete mixer truck involves many simple schemas, such as double-clutching when shifting gears, using both the main and auxiliary transmissions, and making sure the mixer drum continues turning so the concrete inside doesn't harden on its way to a construction site. Certain simple schemas involved in driving a concrete truck also are relevant to driving a car (signaling before turns), riding a bicycle (riding in the proper lane), and even walking (watching for oncoming vehicles before moving into an intersection). If you ordinarily drive a car with a standard manual transmission but you rent a car with an automatic transmission, you probably will find, at least occasionally, that the simple schema for depressing the clutch and shifting gears is activated even though it is unnecessary. You might even find yourself inadvertently applying the break with your left foot in a habitual process of looking for the clutch.

SELECTION AND ACTIVATION
OF ROUTINE SCHEMAS

Shallice (1988) has a fairly well-thought-out model for how behavioral schemas—both automatic/nonconscious and deliberate/conscious—are regulated. He refers to the system for the selection and activation of routine behavior as the *contention scheduling* system. He argues that the selection of a simple schema for activation is a function of several factors: (1) the overall state of the nervous system (e.g., just after awakening, drunkenness, hyperarousal, and so on); (2) the complex schema active at the time; (3) the possibility that competing schemas also are close to the threshold of activation; and (4) the level of neural input that the simple schema receives. According to Shallice, "selection of a schema occurs if its level of activation exceeds a given threshold; once selected, it remains active even if its level of activation falls, unless it attains its goal or is actively inhibited by a competitor or by any higher level controlling schema" (1988, p. 333). Thus, for example, if a woman is driving a car with her children in the backseat, the driving schema and its associated simple schemas are active and she drives more or less automatically, perhaps thinking about something entirely different. Should one of her children suddenly scream out as though injured, however, the driving schema may be disrupted. She then is more likely to respond automatically to the children (activating, e.g., the *response to an injured 3-year-old* complex schema), and the appropriate and automatic activation of driving schemas may be inhibited depending on the attentional resources demanded by the situation.

Norman and Shallice (1986) suggested that the basal ganglia are responsible for the selection of these routine schemas, and there are data indicating that these structures in fact are involved in mediating various kinds of automatic processes. For example, Seitz et al. (1990) studied the relative contributions of the prefrontal cortex and basal ganglia to the learning of motor tasks. They found that the prefrontal cortex was necessary in early stages of motor learning, when a task was novel and demanded conscious, deliberate effort. With practice, however, the prefrontal cortex demonstrated less activation. By the time performance of the task had become automatic (i.e., the task was no longer novel, no longer required thoughtful practice, and could be done with little thought or deliberate attention), there was more activity in the basal ganglia than in the prefrontal cortex.

Although the basal ganglia are important for habitual activity, the prefrontal cortex nevertheless appears to play a role in the activation of these automatic schemas, in that it is responsible for maintenance of the overall intention that guides behavior. That is, the prefrontal cortex regulates the complex schemas that guide the activation of simple schemas. For example, the complex *driving-a-car* schema involves a plan to drive the car to a specific place for a particular reason. Should the ability to use that controlling complex schema be impaired as a result of injury to the prefrontal cortex, the overall integrity of the behavior would be affected adversely.

DISRUPTION OF SCHEMAS

Action Slips and Parapraxes

In *The Psychopathology of Everyday Life*, Freud (1901/1966) discussed what he called *parapraxes*—phenomena involving apparently unintended actions. Among other things, these may involve slips of the tongue (e.g.,

"You have to learn to walk before you can crawl"), instances of forgetting (such as failing to recall an unpleasant meeting one wishes to avoid), or errors in carrying out actions. To most of these parapraxes, Freud attributed some kind of meaningful expression of unconscious forces. For example, he noted that during the days when he made frequent housecalls, "it often happened, when I stood before a door where I should have knocked or rung the bell, that I would pull the key of my own house from my pocket, only to replace it, quite abashed" (1901/1966, pp. 90–91). Freud interpreted this event as indicating that he was at a house where he felt "at home."

Perhaps some slips may be interpretable, at least in part, in a "psychodynamic" sense. In the case of Freud and his key, however, there is another equally plausible interpretation. The act of walking up to a door and taking out a key is one that occurs repeatedly and becomes quite automatic. How many times has the average adult done this in a lifetime, and how many times has the average adult tried to use a car key in the front door of his or her home or to use a house key at work? You arrive at home and reach for your keys without even thinking about the act. If Freud's mind were occupied by other thoughts, walking up to a door may have been all the stimulus required to trigger the simple schema of trying his key in the lock, instead of the more appropriate act—given the circumstances—of knocking on the door.

Whether or not you wish to accept Freud's explanation, there indeed must be an underlying neuropsychological mechanism that would permit such a slip. The slip was, after all, not completely inappropriate. Freud didn't walk up to the door, check the mailbox, and read the mail, nor did he go in and take off his shoes, rearrange the furniture, or call out, "Honey, I'm home."

Action slips, which are common in everyday life, may take a variety of forms (Norman, 1981). There are data suggesting that the average individual experiences several action slips, in one form or another, each day. Many involve actions rather than mistakes in speech. For example, during a power failure at home, I (J. G.) decided to make a phone call. I took a flashlight and went into my office to call. Holding the flashlight in my left hand, I held the phone in my right and pushed the buttons with my right thumb. Having finished entering the number, I then adjusted the position of the phone in my right hand and held the flashlight up to my left ear. Although I habitually dial the telephone with my right hand, I also habitually hold it in my left while I talk. Preoccupied with the power failure and the dropping temperature in the house, I made an action slip. I'm not certain, but I don't think any light was visible coming out of my right ear.

Action slips may occur as a result of different types of minor errors made by Shallice's contention scheduling system (1988). According to Norman (1981, p. 5), "there can be error in the selection of the intention or errors in the specification of the components. Even if the appropriate schemas are all activated, there can be errors of performance when a relevant schema is missed. There can also be errors resulting from the intrusion of unwanted activities from thoughts, from the occurrence of some event in the world that triggers an unintended response, or from a well-learned, familiar habit's taking control of action." Essentially, the system controlling automatic behavior fails to gain access to or to activate the appropriate schema for the circumstances. Given that the vast majority of human behavior is automatically and unconsciously directed, perhaps it's surprising that we make so few action slips.

Impaired Access, Defective Content, and Failures of Activation

A good deal of the neuropsychological evidence in support of the idea that schemas of this sort constitute the basis of much behavior comes from neurological disorders known as *apraxias* or *dyspraxias,* involving disturbances of purposeful activity: an apraxia is a disorder affecting the performance of some task; apraxias occur in the context of intact basic sensory, cognitive, and motor functioning, which means that these basic aspects of behavior are not responsible for the disorder. There are many types of apraxias. For example, *ideomotor apraxia* is an inability to perform simple purposeful gestures (Hécaen & Albert, 1978). When present, it may not be observed in spontaneous activity but can be elicited during neuropsychological assessment. The patient with ideomotor apraxia may be unable to do the following: (1) demonstrate symbolic expressive gestures (such as threatening someone by shaking a fist); (2) pretend to use objects that are not actually present (such as pretending one is pouring water from a pitcher into a glass); or (3) imitate meaningless gestures (such as holding the hand in an unfamiliar position). Such patients may be completely unable to perform the intended action or may perform a distorted, confused, or even bizarre approximation of the task. In some cases, an apraxic patient will use a body part as though it were the object (i.e., he or she may use the index finger as a "key" in a lock), and it is not unusual that a patient will attempt to facilitate performance of the task by talking himself or herself through it, using language to try to organize the behavior.

Ideational apraxia refers to an impaired capacity to perform somewhat more complex purposeful movements. The component acts of a schema may be performed adequately by themselves, but the overall sequence is disturbed. For example, if an examiner asks a patient with ideational apraxia to light a candle, "one is as likely . . . to see the patient strike the match against the wrong side of the box, or attempt to strike the wrong end of the match, or even attempt to strike the candle against the box, or present an unlit match to the candle. The patient is unable to conceive the desired action as a whole and organize the diverse partial acts that constitute the whole in their temporal and spatial relations" (Hécaen & Albert, 1978, p. 100).

The basic deficit in these kinds of apraxias appears to be a breakdown in the processes involved in activating various schemas; as McCarthy and Warrington (1990) noted, these schemas "are thought to be organized hierarchically, so that they can call up the components of complex actions. The component actions in an established motor programme can be run off relatively automatically, without 'thinking' about the action" (p. 119). The basic deficit could involve lack of access to knowledge (including procedural knowledge) about how to use objects, failure to gain access to a motor routine, or damage affecting the integrity of the schema itself (Heilman & Rothi, 1985).

NONCONSCIOUS BEHAVIORAL SCHEMAS AND THEIR DISORDERS: SUMMARY

To summarize, most nonconsciously activated behavior is likely to be organized hierarchically, simple schemas being nested within more complex schemas, which themselves are associated with more complex behavioral repertoires. Playing basketball, for example, involves a complex schema that contains subordinate schemas for dribbling, passing, shooting, playing defense, setting picks, and so on, each of which may be done automatically in a large number of ways. Activation of a complex schema (as a result of the activation of its underlying neural network) results in the activation of diverse component schemas that operate automatically. Complex schemas are characterized by the sort of modular architecture that we have encountered at other levels of organization within the brain, wherein individual modules or component processes can be activated within the context of diverse complex schemas. Apraxias demonstrate the existence of schemas that facilitate much nonconsciously activated behavior.

THE EXECUTIVE COGNITIVE FUNCTIONS AND DELIBERATE CONSCIOUS CONTROL

We now turn our attention to the second functional neural system associated with deliberate action. The *executive cognitive functions* of the brain involve relatively complex behavior. According to Luria (1966, 1980), these functions are the emergent properties of a system specialized for the planning, initiation, regulation, inhibition, and monitoring of behavior, and involving the prefrontal cortex and medial frontal cortex as important components (see also Fuster, 1997; Milner & Petrides, 1984; Stuss, 1992;

Stuss & Benson, 1986, 1987). Shallice (1988) referred to the functional system responsible for the executive abilities as the *supervisory attentional system*.

The executive functions are a somewhat heterogeneous group of higher cognitive abilities. Among other capacities, the executive functions include the following: (1) formulation of plans; (2) anticipation of the possible consequences of an intended action; (3) organization of one's approach to the solution of a problem; (4) taking an active approach to the solution of a problem, rather than passively responding with whatever comes to mind; (5) using an intention or plan to guide one's ongoing behavior; (6) critically monitoring the accuracy of one's performance, continually comparing the outcome with what was intended (often referred to as "insight"); (7) initiation of purposeful, goal-directed activity under appropriate circumstances; (8) responding adaptively to novel situations or stimuli; (9) inhibition of irrelevant or inappropriate behavior; (10) inhibition of distractibility; (11) keeping track of two or more activities simultaneously (control of working memory); (12) flexibly focusing and shifting attention; and (13) understanding another person's perspective. In short, the executive cognitive functions permit an individual to engage actively with life; to respond flexibly to unfamiliar situations; to inhibit irrelevant or routine behavior when it is advantageous to do so; and to learn from experience in real time.

THE NEUROANATOMY OF EXECUTIVE FUNCTIONING

By now it should be apparent that the model of the mind we are articulating emphasizes the dynamic relationships between many distributed areas of the brain in the emergence of complex behavior. Thus no complex neuropsychological activity can be localized within a specific structure. Nonetheless, the prefrontal cortex has been shown to be involved in the processes associated with executive functioning. Although the prefrontal cortex has a role in automatically activated behavioral processes as well, its activation, along with the activation of several other structures in the brain, appears critical in situations demanding the complex cognitive processing associated with deliberate behavior.

We first will look briefly at the anatomy of the prefrontal cortex, illustrating that its structure is well suited for supporting the complex integrative processes required for initiating and regulating complex behavior. The prefrontal cortex develops over a long period of time, not reaching full maturation until the individual is well into adulthood, reportedly sometimes as late as the end of the fourth decade. Its development is of crucial importance for the capacity to regulate behavior. We will discuss some disturbances of executive functioning among persons with neurological disorders. These so-called *dysexecutive syndromes,* while representing extreme cases, should nonetheless illustrate the modular basis of executive functioning.

Anatomy of the Prefrontal Cortex

The prefrontal area is considered to be an *association cortex,* meaning that it is involved in integrating functions mediated by other areas of cortex. As is the case with the visual cortex, the prefrontal cortex has been found to have vertically oriented cell columns, suggesting a modular structure for this region of the brain (Goldman-Rakic, 1984; Goldman & Nauta, 1977), and there are regions in which fibers from the opposite (contralateral) hemisphere alternate with neurons from the same (ipsilateral) hemisphere (Goldman-Rakic, 1984; Goldman-Rakic & Schwartz, 1982), thus possibly integrating interhemispheric functioning. Fuster (1989) maintains that the hierarchical, modular nature of the frontal lobes has as its highest level the participation of the prefrontal cortex in the production of behavior at a global, abstract level; he described the "supraordinate function" of the prefrontal cortex as "the formation of *temporal structures of behavior* with a unifying purpose or goal—in other words, the structuring of goal-directed behavior" (p. 158; emphasis in original).

The prefrontal cortex, which accounts for more than one-quarter of the human cortex, is defined by Fuster (1997) as the region of the cortex receiving neural input from the mediodorsal nucleus of the thalamus. In primates, projections from the mediodorsal thalamus have two major components (Fuster, 1997; Goldman-Rakic & Porrino, 1985). The *magnocellular* tract projects to the *orbital* (above the eyes) and *medial* (between the hemispheres) areas of the frontal lobes. The *parvocellular* fibers project to the superior and lateral surfaces of the prefrontal cortex, which are known as the *dorsolateral* prefrontal cortex (DLPC; see Figure 14.1). The prefrontal cortex also receives inputs from the hypothalamus, subthalamus, midbrain, and many regions of the cortex, so that it seems in part to serve as an anterior brain center for the convergence of information from different sensory modalities (Fuster, 1997). The prefrontal cortex is mutually interconnected with nearly every area from which it receives projections, and it projects as well to other areas such as the *putamen* and *caudate nucleus* of the basal ganglia, which appear *not* to send direct inputs to the prefrontal area (Fuster, 1997; they do, however, project indirectly to the prefrontal cortex via the globus pallidus and thalamus).

The distinction between the DLPC and the OMPC (orbitomedial prefrontal cortex) is important clinically and functionally (Luria, 1966, 1973, 1980), as both regions receive fibers from and project to different areas of the brain. Injury to one or the other area may produce rather differ-

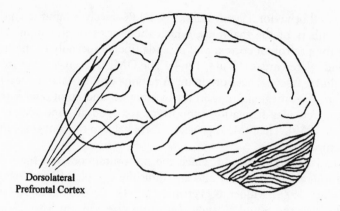

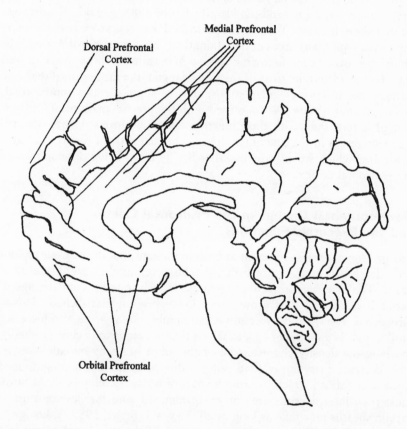

FIGURE 14.1. Lateral view of the left side of the brain (A) shows the approximate area of dorsolateral prefrontal cortex (DLPC), which includes the superior (dorsal) and lateral surfaces of the prefrontal area as well as the frontal pole. The sagittal (midline) view of the right side of the brain (B) shows the approximate areas of the medial, orbital, and dorsal prefrontal cortex.

ent cognitive and behavioral syndromes. The DLPC receives input from the parvocellular fibers of the thalamus, which themselves receive input primarily from the prefrontal cortex, and it sends fibers especially to the hippocampus and related areas (Nauta, 1964). The OMPC receives input from the magnocellular fibers. These originate in regions of the thalamus receiving input from the amygdala (important in emotion and emotional learning), midbrain reticular formation (important for arousal), and temporal cortex (Fuster, 1989). The OMPC projects fibers back to the amygdala and related structures.

The human frontal lobes, of which the prefrontal cortex is the most anterior portion, are functionally and anatomically complex (Fuster, 1989; Goldman-Rakic, 1984; Milner & Petrides, 1984). According to Roland (1984), aside from the cingulate and orbitofrontal regions, at least 17 different functional areas had been identified as of 1984, and others have been located since that time. Because the prefrontal cortex is so extensively interconnected with many areas of the brain, the behavior typical of frontal lobe syndromes may occur following lesions in certain of those areas as well (e.g., lesions of certain areas of the basal ganglia, the mediodorsal thalamic nucleus, the anterior cingulate gyrus, and the supplementary motor area). In this chapter we are less concerned with the precise anatomical localization of lesions than with their functional manifestations. Hence our primary interest is in the functional deficits characteristic of the dysexecutive syndrome, which we will discuss after briefly considering development of the prefrontal cortex.

Developmental Change in the Prefrontal Cortex and the Executive Functions

The prefrontal cortex is present at birth in humans, but the neurons are not fully developed and are not fully interconnected as they are in the adult brain. The dendrites branch and grow relatively rapidly until the age of about 2 years, and then grow more slowly beyond that (Schadé & Van Groenigen, 1961). In the meantime, the number of synapses also increases until about 24 months of age, at which time it begins to decline gradually, reaching the density characteristic of the adult brain by midadolescence. This decrease in synapses (and cells) is due to *apoptosis,* a programmed form of cell death which is a routine part of neural development. At birth, most prefrontal neurons are not yet myelinated, and the development of myelin sheaths may take as long as 20–30 years (Benes, 1989; Yakovlev & Lecours, 1967). Thus complete maturation of the prefrontal cortex is a process that occurs in tandem with experience across childhood, adolescence, and young adulthood.

Children's performance on tests of the executive functions improves in a nearly linear fashion across the school years (Levin et al., 1991; Weyandt

& Willis, 1994), although by the age of 12 years most children have not yet reached adult levels of performance (with some exceptions; e.g., see Welsh, Pennington, & Grossier, 1991). Those children with attention-deficit/hyperactivity disorder (ADHD) are more likely than normal children to perform poorly on certain tests of executive functioning (Barkley, 1997).

Luria (1961, 1966, 1979) devised an interesting approach to studying children's ability to use language to regulate their behavior, the results of which suggested that the prefrontal cortex becomes capable of mediating behavioral self-control between the ages of 4 and 7 years. In these studies, he gave children a rubber bulb and told them to squeeze it whenever a red light came on. Children between the ages of 24 and 30 months were unable to follow these simple instructions, even when the directions were given prior to performance of the task. When first given the instruction, they began squeezing the bulb immediately. When the red light came on, they tended to be distracted by it and stopped their squeezing. Each time they heard the word *squeeze* they responded not with a single squeeze, but with "a whole series of involuntary motor reactions which only gradually exhausted themselves. Even the direct negative instruction 'stop,' frequently led to excitation and to stronger, less controlled motor responses" (Luria, 1979, p. 107).

By the age of 3–4 years, most children could follow these simple instructions, yet showed some difficulty when told to squeeze at the presentation of the red light and to do nothing when the green light came on. The problem was not with memory; Luria found that they could remember the instructions adequately. They simply were unable to use those instructions as a guide for their behavior. Luria (1979) noted that behavior began to come under verbal control only after about the age of 4 years, and that by 6 years they could perform these tasks without errors.

At the other end of the lifespan, substantial evidence exists for both anatomical and functional decline in the frontal lobes and associated structures in the process of normal aging. This decline is not ubiquitous—some older people show little or no significant impairment in executive functioning—but it nevertheless appears that many otherwise normal elderly persons demonstrate varying degrees of disruption of those executive functions considered to be mediated by prefrontal cortex.

The anatomical data are interesting. In the course of normal aging there is a significant neuronal loss in many areas of the brain, including the prefrontal cortex (Adams & Victor, 1989; Terry, DeTeresa, & Hansen, 1987; Zatz, Jernigan, & Ahumada, 1982). Probably in association with this cell loss, there is a decrease in cerebral blood flow in the frontal regions of older persons (Gur et al., 1987; Pietrini, Horwitz, & Grady, 1992) and an increased likelihood of eliciting primitive reflexes (L. Jacobs & Grossman, 1980). Because of the intimate relationship between the prefrontal cortex and the mediodorsal thalamus, it also is important to note that the thalamus undergoes a significant loss of neurons during the aging process (Haug et al., 1983) and this also could affect those functions mediated by the prefrontal areas. Neuropsychological data suggest the existence of a decrement in executive cognitive functioning with advancing age (e.g., Whelihan & Lescher, 1985). Compared with younger individuals, elderly adults tend to perform poorly on tests of executive functioning. For example, Mittenberg et al. (1989) found that age was strongly correlated with three measures of executive ability. Libon and Goldberg (1990) compared adults aged 64–73 with older adults aged 75–95 and noted a decline in performance on tests of these functions. Daigneault, Braun, & Whitaker (1992) reported that subjects aged 45–65 performed more poorly than did younger subjects (aged 20–35) on four of six such measures and on three of six measures of perseveration; they concluded that aging affects prefrontal functioning and that "the prefrontal functions that seem to be most impaired are the regulation of behavior based on plans, abstract concepts, experimenter feedback, and one's own responses" (p. 110).

Other research (Grigsby, Kaye, & Robbins, 1992; Kaye & Grigsby, 1991; Kaye et al., 1990) has shown that many relatively healthy persons between the ages of 60 and 100 (or more) have significant difficulty with a number of tasks that assess behavioral control, a specific executive cognitive function (Luria, 1966, 1980). Older adults performed significantly more poorly than younger adults on the Behavioral Dyscontrol Scale (BDS), a measure consisting largely of tests of the control of motor activity. Their performance on the BDS was associated with the capacity for behavioral control and independent functioning (Kaye et al., 1990; Grigsby, Kaye, & Robbins, 1995; Grigsby et al., 2000; Suchy, Blint, & Osmon, 1997).

The contribution of the prefrontal cortex to adaptive functioning in novel and complex situations is well established (Fuster, 1989; Luria, 1980), and the problems with which older persons tend to have the most difficulty "typically involve speed, unfamiliar material, complexity of task, and active problem solving" (Lezak, 1983, p. 217). Thus subtle declines in frontal lobe functioning associated with normal aging may account for the frequently reported finding that, among older persons, performance on novel tasks is deficient relative to performance on routine tasks.

Consistent with evidence of prefrontal and thalamic cell loss are data indicating that working memory (i.e., the temporary storage of information which must be maintained and processed in the performance of concurrent cognitive tasks) becomes impaired with aging, a finding Baddeley (1986) attributes to an age-related decrease in information-processing capacity. The prefrontal area and mediodorsal thalamus are important components of a neural network that serves working memory (Friedman, Janas, & Goldman-Rakic, 1990).

THE DYSEXECUTIVE SYNDROME

The anatomical and functional complexity of the frontal lobes is associated with considerable variability in the nature of the syndromes observed following frontal lobe injury. Persons with prefrontal cortical lesions often demonstrate intact performance in a number of functional areas, and measures of IQ frequently are relatively unaffected (Stuss et al., 1983). Furthermore, such lesions may affect more than one functional system, so the pathological changes in cognitive and behavioral activity often are not consistent among patients. Because of the heterogeneity of disturbances following prefrontal injury, Baddeley (1986) argued against the use of the term *frontal* as a description of the kinds of symptoms observed following prefrontal injuries, and instead suggested the term *dysexecutive syndrome*. We next examine two specific executive functions: insight, and the capacity to regulate behavior.

Impairment of Insight

Prefrontal cortical lesions frequently affect the basic ability to observe oneself, to appraise one's own activity, and to compare it with what is intended or expected, whether those expectations are one's own or those of other people. This neuropsychological definition of "insight" emphasizes processes of a more fundamental nature than those typically associated with the term as it is used in psychiatric contexts. Among mental health professionals, the term *insight* usually has one of two meanings: (1) it may indicate than an individual is aware that an idea he or she has is crazy (as in a patient who has limited insight into his or her delusions); or (2) it frequently is used to mean that an individual understands his or her underlying motivations for engaging in a given behavior. Insight in the neuropsychological sense probably is a necessary but not sufficient condition for the possession of insight of the latter sort.

In the absence of insight, an individual is unable to monitor his or her behavior critically and accurately. Persons lacking in insight may engage in a variety of maladaptive behaviors, yet have no ability to observe their own activity, to assess whether it is appropriate, or to determine whether it reflects their initial intention. For example, one such patient, performing the Block Design subtest of the Wechsler Adult Intelligence Scale—Revised (WAIS-R), made several errors that would be obvious to most observers. In assembling designs that require the placement of nine blocks in a three-by-three square, he lined the blocks in two rows, one of five and one of four. He seemed satisfied with his performance, and when asked whether his reproduction exactly matched the stimulus figure, responded confidently that it did. In contrast, when the examiner took the blocks himself and deliberately assembled them incorrectly (much as the patient had just done), the patient readily recognized the discrepancy.

Failure to Initiate and Inhibit Certain Types of Behavior

Although the behavioral pathology characteristic of the dysexecutive syndrome has many determinants, it tends to fall into two broad categories: 1) failures to inhibit purposeless, irrelevant, or inappropriate behavior (disorders of inhibition); (2) failures to initiate and complete goal-directed activity (disorders of initiation). Both kinds of disorders are symptomatic of a behavioral dyscontrol syndrome. While one or the other type of behavior may dominate the clinical picture for a given individual, it is not unusual to see a combination of disinhibition and apathy.

Significant executive dysfunction commonly produces a marked dissociation between volition and action. Patients with a dysexecutive syndrome, although able to formulate and remember a specific intention to act in a certain way, may be incapable of *executing* the intended action appropriately. The ability to perform the act itself need not be impaired (i.e., the schemas are intact and the patient is not necessarily apraxic). Instead, the individual may demonstrate a complete failure to initiate the expected activity, or may lapse into stereotyped perseverative behavior, activating irrelevant behavioral schemas.

According to Luria (1966, 1980), the basic problem that such persons demonstrate is an inability to use an intention to guide behavior. The use of an intention in this way is a hierarchically organized process that occurs on different timescales. I may, for example, decide to brush my teeth. I go to the bathroom, get the brush and toothpaste, and do it. In that case, the intention guides my immediate behavior. It also may be the case that a somewhat more complex plan might regulate my activity for a few hours (e.g., I may decide to repair a damaged window frame), a few days (I may opt to write a chapter for this book), or a few years (I may foolishly decide to go back to graduate school and study for another doctorate). As one extends the time frame, one depends on higher-level schemas of increasing complexity, each somewhat more removed from the immediate details of ongoing behavior.

A person with a severe dysexecutive syndrome may be able to dress and undress himself, yet may not get dressed without being told to do so. He also may not complete the process of getting dressed unless he is prompted during the process. He may be unable to avoid undressing in public if the schema for undressing is activated—perhaps he finds that a button on his shirt has come undone, which serves as a cue to finish unbuttoning and removing the shirt. Depending on the quality of an individual's self-awareness regarding this kind of deficit, he or she may be oblivious to a manifestly flawed performance. If insight is better preserved, the individual may be surprised by such a lack of control and distressed by this awareness.

One behavior characteristic of the dysexecutive syndrome is *perseveration*, which we discussed in Chapter 8 on dynamic disorders. Generally, perseveration is considered to occur in any situation "in which elements of previous tasks or behavior(s) fuse with an ongoing task or behavior, or when a behavior or operation cannot be terminated" (E. Goldberg & Bilder, 1987, p. 161). There are several types of perseveration. In one kind, the patient shows a "pathological inertia" (Luria, 1980) in the performance of basic motor acts; once started on a routine motor task, the patient's movements are more likely to continue inappropriately than to terminate when the task is complete. For example, asked to draw a circle, the patient may continue the drawing movement until the circle is almost not recognizable as such. There is some evidence that this kind of pathology is characteristic of frontal lesions involving the basal ganglia (Luria, 1966, 1980).

A second kind of perseveration is more cognitive in nature. For example, a patient may be asked to draw a circle, and she does so correctly. Then she is asked to draw a triangle, which also is drawn adequately. This is followed by the command to draw a square, but the patient makes a triangle instead, perseverating on the previously drawn triangle. The next command, to draw another circle, is followed by yet another triangle. If she is asked about it, the patient is able to recall what she was told to draw, yet she does not recognize her error, nor does she respond correctly when she next is asked to draw another circle.

Goldberg and Bilder (1987) suggested that repetitive and overlearned behaviors (schemas, in other words) that can readily be performed automatically and nonconsciously are those most likely to lead to perseveration. Requiring rapid performance also is liable to exacerbate tendencies to perseverative behavior. This is because the neural network mediating the schema for an overlearned task is one that has a high probability of activation under certain circumstances. If a person with a dysexecutive syndrome attempts a relatively novel task, the performance of that task is more difficult than is performance of the overlearned task (it does not as yet have a well-developed schema to support it). If the prefrontal cortex cannot be activated properly to permit performance of the novel task, the likelihood of activation of the overlearned schema is quite high, and such behavior is liable to intrude on the performance of the novel task in a perseverative way. Perseveration may be most prevalent among persons with lesions of dorsolateral prefrontal cortex (Shallice, 1988).

Fuster (1980) discussed the way in which animals with DLPC lesions have difficulty with tests of learning that require them to shift their response to two different stimuli. For example, the animal may have learned initially to give behavior A in response to stimulus A*, and behavior B in response to stimulus B*. The experimenter then changes the task, and the animal now must respond to A^* with B, and to B^* with A. As Fuster noted (1980, p. 44), "the older the habit, the more familiar the discriminanda, the greater the difficulty that the frontal animal ordinarily shows in reversals." This is because the ease of activation of the formerly reinforced schema is greater than the ease of activation of the newly required schema. An intact DLPC is of considerable importance to the ability to inhibit habitual behavior (see Figure 14.1, above).

These findings are relevant to psychotherapy in that a patient may have learned a new way of behaving, but the older, more practiced, better established schema underlying the unwanted behavior may be more easily activated than the schema mediating the new behavior. Thus it is not at all unusual for a patient to return from a visit to her family only to report that "I forgot everything I thought I'd learned; I fell into all my old routines. I'm not getting anywhere." The old, familiar family situation plays an important role in determining her state, in which the easiest, most automatic, highly practiced, overlearned, habitual thing to do in response to her parents' behavior is to activate the old schemas. In order to engage in her more recently acquired behavioral repertoire, she would have to exert considerable effort, activating the prefrontal cortex in the process. Only after the newer behaviors had been practiced to the point that they themselves had become relatively automatic would she find it easier to deal with her parents differently without having to make a deliberate conscious effort.

Failure to Inhibit Inappropriate or Irrelevant Behavior

Impulsivity is common among persons with a dysexecutive syndrome, especially those whose lesions affect the OMPC (again, refer to Figure 14.1, above). In severe cases, the patient may demonstrate extreme distractibility, finding it difficult or impossible to inhibit responses to a wide range of internal and external stimuli. One example of this can be seen in the behavior of Calvin, a euphoric 25-year-old man who had sustained a severe bifrontal injury 3 years previously. Calvin was unable to stick to a topic in conversation because he consistently was distracted by his own thoughts or by sounds and sights in the room. He frequently would interrupt an ongoing conversation to comment on things he heard in the hallway or outdoors. At one point during an examination, he suddenly laughed, took a pencil and rubber band from the desk, and stood on a chair. Using the rubber band, he attached the pencil to a ceiling fire sprinkler, then returned to his own chair.

Lhermitte (1983) described a somewhat different kind of disinhibited behavior, which he called "utilization behavior." For example, a pencil and paper may be brought within reach of a patient, who then may impulsively take the pencil and begin to write or draw. If a pitcher of water and a glass are placed nearby, the patient may take the glass and pour water from the pitcher. These behaviors are elicited by the proximity of the salient objects, and the patient can't help but being carried along by the schemas thus activated. Lhermitte never observed behavior of this sort in neurologically intact individuals, nor was it seen in neurologically impaired patients with lesions outside the frontal cortex. Some of Lhermitte's patients explained that they thought they were supposed to use the objects. This "explanation" appeared inaccurate, however, in that Lhermitte could tell the patients not to use the objects, then distract their attention for less than a minute, following which they would grasp the glass, pencil, or whatever was being used as a stimulus item.

Failure to Initiate Purposeful Behavior

Disorders of initiation have been discussed as *apathy* by some investigators (e.g., R. S. Martin, 1991). These involve what appears at first to be a lack of motivation, characterized by diminished goal-directed behavior and cognition, and accompanied by a decrease in the usual emotional concomitants of goal-directed behavior (R. S. Martin, 1991). The lack of motivation is not attributable to intellectual impairment, emotional distress, or decreased level of consciousness. Sometimes apathy may be a *symptom* of depression, but it also exists in itself as a *syndrome*. Although apathetic persons not infrequently are diagnosed as depressed, emotional distress is generally either absent in this syndrome or is not of sufficient degree that it could produce the lack of motivation. Apathetic patients are unlikely to describe themselves as depressed, although they may be viewed that way by others. Depressed patients, on the other hand, typically describe themselves in such a way that one can identify them as being depressed.

Apathetic persons may fail to initiate or follow through with various simple self-care activities without being encouraged or told to do so. They may neglect to take care of such basic functions as eating, washing, brushing teeth, dressing, or getting out of bed. Some persons may neglect to use the toilet, with resulting incontinence. In severe cases, the syndrome is characterized by almost complete inactivity, unless some event or person prods the individual into action. It then becomes apparent that the deficit is not in the ability to perform the various tasks but in *initiating* any purposeful behavior.

LEARNING, DEVELOPMENT, AND THE ACQUISITION OF BEHAVIORAL CONTROL

The integrity of the prefrontal cortex, and hence of a considerable portion of the neurological substrate for behavioral control, is a necessary but not sufficient condition for the healthy regulation of behavior. Experience during early development also may be important for the acquisition of adequate behavioral controls. If one learns that the best way to get what one wants is to act out in some way, poorly controlled behavior may become habitual. For an individual who has not learned to control his impulses, if the neural substrate for control is intact there at least may be something to work with in therapy. In contrast, for a person with a head injury resulting from a pool cue striking the head in a bar fight, the therapeutic prognosis could be significantly different. An injury to the prefrontal cortex is not necessary for behavioral dyscontrol, however; even without acquired prefrontal lesions, ostensibly normal individuals vary somewhat with respect to the quality of their executive cognitive functioning. Moreover, both the modular architecture of the brain and normal population-based genetic variability make it likely that a certain percentage of persons with otherwise normal intellectual abilities will naturally have less than optimal executive abilities.

Luria (1980) found that both laboratory animals and humans with prefrontal lesions do not respond normally to operant conditioning. Presumably they are unable to comprehend the significance of the reinforcer and its relationship to their behavior. Individuals whose behavioral control is severely impaired as a result of a neurological disorder may be unable to regulate their own behavior, and thus require constant supervision from someone else, who essentially takes on the role of the patient's prefrontal cortex (as must be done with very young children whose prefrontal cortex is not yet mature). With lesser degrees of impairment, control may be impaired in conditions of fatigue or stress but be adequate under less difficult circumstances. It is a reasonable hypothesis that such individuals may be able to benefit from cognitive behavioral and behavioral methods.

THE DYSEXECUTIVE SYNDROME: CLINICAL CASES

Following are descriptions of the behavior of two individuals with different types of dysexecutive syndrome. These cases are intended to illustrate the kinds of behavior observed among persons with impaired executive functions. To a certain extent, knowledge of the disorders seen with prefrontal lesions is helpful for understanding how the prefrontal cortex and the executive functions operate within the context of normal personality functioning.

The details vary, but each individual had some kind of impairment in the ability to regulate behavior. Case 1 showed primarily disinhibited and inappropriate behavior, which got him into trouble in the community, earning him a reputation as "antisocial." Case 2 was apathetic for the most part. Brain-imaging studies or neurosurgical reports documented that both patients had significant pathology of the prefrontal cortex.

Case I

Bruno, a 29-year-old undergraduate student in physics, had sustained a serious injury to his prefrontal cortex. He experienced several weeks of unconsciousness, followed by what appeared to be a good return of cognitive functioning. When examined, he obtained a verbal IQ of about 130 and demonstrated few neuropsychological deficits apart from mildly impaired working memory, a slight decrease in the speed and capacity of information processing, and some difficulty in learning new motor tasks.

Bruno nevertheless showed a number of significant impairments, many of which were not demonstrable on formal assessment. He often was euphoric and stated that he never felt sad or depressed for more than a few minutes at a time. He joked frequently, remarking that his wife "screams at me in public a lot for joking too much," a trait which she told him was "getting on people's nerves." Bruno saw nothing wrong with what he did, thought it was his wife's problem, and wasn't concerned about whether it disturbed her. He acknowledged that sometimes it seemed that he might have "rubbed people the wrong way" but said it was "nothing that would make me evaluate my actions and exercise tact." He added, "It's a free society, and you can say what you want." His disinhibition thus was rationalized as though it were freely chosen behavior.

Bruno had been arrested twice following his accident. The first arrest followed a complaint by a woman that he had come running up behind her on the street at night, frightening her, and proceeding to tell a crude sexual joke. She shouted for help, and Bruno was restrained by three passersby until the police arrived. On another occasion, intending to buy a dog from an individual through a classified ad, Bruno took the bus to what he thought was the correct area of town, although he had forgotten to bring the exact address. He went onto a porch and, finding the front door open, walked in, calling the name of the individual who had advertised the dog in the paper. Hearing someone in the kitchen, he walked in that direction until he encountered an elderly woman, who was understandably startled by his presence. Bruno also was surprised; he apologized, said he must have the wrong address, and stated that he would leave and catch a bus. The woman called the police, and Bruno was apprehended at a nearby bus stop.

Bruno demonstrated several characteristics of a dysexecutive syndrome. He failed to plan ahead, as demonstrated by his not having brought the address with him. He failed to anticipate the possible consequences of his actions; he had chased after the woman on campus because he was lonely and wanted to talk with her, but he didn't consider how she might react to such an abrupt and intrusive introduction in a relatively isolated area of the campus at night. He also didn't anticipate that she might be offended by his sexual joking. He was impulsive and, despite previous similar unfortunate experiences, didn't seem to learn from what had happened before. He had no insight into how his behavior was an expression of impairment.

Case 2

Bart was a 16-year-old 10th grade student, with a verbal IQ of 87. Neurological data, including CT scans, indicated moderately severe bilateral atrophy of the prefrontal cortex. The etiology was unknown, as there was no history of any neurological insult. His social development had been very delayed, and his father described him as always having been "a strange bird." Bart showed a striking combination of disinhibition and inability to initiate purposeful behavior. He often sat silently for extended periods of time. His mother reported that she might go shopping for 3 hours and when she returned she would find him sitting in the same chair, almost as though he hadn't moved. When she asked him what he thought about while sitting there, he replied "nothing." In the company of very young children Bart became active, distractible, and disinhibited.

Even with direct probing, it was not possible to find out what was on Bart's mind. Either there was little cognitive activity or he was incapable of observing or describing it. He could not explain how he had attempted to solve problems of any kind, and in any event his attempts at solution were almost entirely passive. He seemed to answer questions with the first thing that came to his mind, with no critical analysis. He never joked spontaneously, and while he sometimes laughed at others' jokes, he was unable to explain what was funny. He never made complaints that might suggest he was sad or depressed, although his facial expression was ordinarily rather flat.

THE RELATIONSHIP BETWEEN MORAL JUDGMENT AND MORAL BEHAVIOR

The dissociation between what people do, what they *say* they do, and what they *think* they should do reflects the modular organization of brain functioning. The theory of dissociability of the various systems of the brain is consistent with Grinder's (1964) conclusion that moral behavior and moral reasoning develop along separate tracks. This is apparent in the findings of research on the relationship between moral judgment and behavior, which have demonstrated at best a tenuous link between the two (Rothman, 1980). An individual may possess the ability to engage in moral reasoning at what psychologists consider the highest levels (Kohlberg, 1976), but that ability does not necessarily predict what he or she will do in an actual situation. Emde et al. (1991) have given considerable attention to the important role of procedural learning in the early acquisition of moral behavior (which they refer to as the internalization of "do's" and "don'ts").

A number of studies, for example, have demonstrated moderate associations at best between the ability to make judgments about right and wrong and what one actually does. One paradigm often employed to study the link is one in which, for example, children are left alone in a room to perform some task and given an opportunity to cheat, unaware of the fact that they are being observed surreptitiously. Typically, such studies have found only a modest relationship between a subject's level of moral reasoning and whether the subject made an attempt to cheat (e.g., Schwartz et al., 1969).

A primary conclusion that can be drawn from this line of research is that moral reasoning influences behavior but does not predict it with any great degree of accuracy. It appears that a number of personal and situational factors determine whether a person will act in accordance with what he or she believes to be morally correct (Rothman, 1980), a finding consistent with our proposed model. Our interpretation of these results is that moral reasoning is learned by the semantic memory system whereas behavior is a function of both procedural learning (and hence the automatic schema-activating system) and, in certain circumstances, the executive functions. Most behavior is activated automatically and nonconsciously, and cheating or other forms of dishonesty may become habitual and rationalized. Under certain circumstances, activation of the prefrontal cortex may permit an individual to reflect actively on the situation, perhaps then to resist the pull toward some morally questionable behavior—or perhaps not.

Whether people behave morally, in large part, may be a function of habit. Some individuals may have acquired a set of readily activated procedural schemas for good behavior, in which case they may behave morally for the most part and may appear to act as though they were self-disciplined. In fact, it may be that they simply behave well automatically and nonconsciously. On the other hand, many people acquire habits that are widely considered to be wrong. For such individuals, to behave morally requires additional effort, including activation of the prefrontal cortex and executive functions in order to resist temptation (and even to be aware of the fact that they are in a situation to which there might be a more satisfactory response). With sufficient practice, ethical behavior might become relatively automatic. Yet, unless the neural network that mediates the procedurally learned schema for immorality is somehow disrupted or "unlearned," under many circumstances that schema may be automatically activated more readily than the schema for ethical conduct.

Acting against the grain of the automatic activation of behavioral schemas is extremely difficult, requiring considerable effort and discipline—a willingness and ability to arouse oneself out of automaticity and to behave differently than one is inclined to behave. For some individuals, behaviors characteristic of self-discipline itself may become easily activated schemas, producing the paradoxical result that true self-discipline might actually demand the difficult task of abandoning one's apparent self-discipline, since it has become such a deeply ingrained habit. In any event, abandoning this trait might be more difficult for the individual than to continue in his or her accustomed manner.

If a disorganized individual bought a book on getting organized, made a lot of effort to implement the suggestions in the book, and practiced those techniques consistently over time, he or she might be able to develop well-organized habits. But without considerable practice that change in behavior is unlikely to happen, because it won't become habitual. The CNS tends naturally to function so as to minimize energy expenditure at the level of neurons and neural networks, and the probability of backsliding into disorganization is much greater than the probability of staying organized. The same holds true for techniques that offer the promise of improving your memory. The techniques work only if you practice them so diligently that you don't even need to think about using them but rather employ them automatically.

The inference we draw from this line of research and thinking is that values—whether represented by laws, moral strictures, a code of ethics, religious prohibitions, some philosophy, or even a delusional system—serve at most only as a guide. Much of the time, they may function largely as a convenient source of material for rationalizing one's actions. It may be possible to teach the content of a value system, but unless an individual is motivated to make what sometimes must be an exceptional effort and uses a moral code as an intention to guide his or her behavior, values are just so much more content for the semantic memory system. Teaching values in school, itself not a bad idea, is an inadequate solution to the problem of bad behavior. For values to make a difference, an individual must deliberately and consciously use those ideas to guide his or her behavior. Over time, the behavior then may become less effortful and more automatic.

THE DETERMINANTS OF BEHAVIOR

Purposeful, Deliberate, Behavior as an Emergent Process

To whatever degree humans have the ability to behave purposefully and deliberately, such behavior emerges out of a medium created and circumscribed by a complex array of nonconscious processes and the vagaries of circumstance. A wide range of endogenous and environmental factors determines whether and to what extent an individual is able to engage in deliberate, relatively conscious activity at any particular time. Thus, as an emergent process, this kind of purposeful activity varies in its moment-to-moment expression in association with changes in any of the array of processes that contribute to its emergence.

Are Humans "Rational Actors"?

Does rationality guide behavior? The findings of neuroscience seem to offer strong support for the hypothesis that behavior regulated by the automatic schema activation system has little to do with rationality or logic. It is controlled by the interaction of habit and circumstance. It requires no deliberate thought; indeed, the automatic activation of this activity may be disrupted by the intrusion of deliberate conscious control. But habit is not a straitjacket, and the behaviors in which one engages are always a function of the complex interaction of brain and environment. The activation of any given simple schema depends on the type and level of input it receives. Thus, whether a given behavior occurs is a function of the complex schema active at the time, which in turn is determined by the state of the individual (mood, level of arousal, and so on) and the physical and social context. Moreover, an individual can override habit through deliberate, effortful activity, involving the activation of certain executive functions.

Therefore, we see that several functional systems act collaboratively to produce complex human behavior. These include the automatic schema activation system, the executive functions, the motivational and affective systems, reasoning, and various memory systems. Probably the least important determinant of behavior is rationality, while the most important are habits and the motivational/affective systems. An individual's affective status and his or her physiological motivational status, in conjunction with the level of arousal and activity level, are among the control parameters that determine his or her physiological and psychological state at any given time. This fundamental state tunes the nervous system (G. G. Globus, 1992) in such a way that the probabilities of activation of all schemas for all memory subsystems change, reflecting the influence of the predominant state. The sudden experience of rage, for example, decreases the likelihood of calm reflection and careful, reasoned, deliberate, and conscious action.

SUMMARY AND CONCLUSION

Most routine behavior is mediated by neural network-based schemas that can be automatically and unconsciously activated in different situations. The likelihood of activation of any of these attractors varies as a function of the individual's state and the condition of the environment. Some simple schemas are very precise and stereotyped, but most are characterized by a good deal of flexibility in the way they are played out.

Much of the behavior controlled by the automatic schema activation system can be initiated in such an effortless and unconscious way that the individual even may be unaware of performing certain tasks. This automaticity may lead to action slips, in which routine tasks are performed inappropriately, partially or completely outside the individual's awareness. It also accounts for the fact that one can do two things at once and barely be aware of one of them. Driving a car, for example, can be so automatic that one doesn't even remember consciously driving for some period of time ranging from seconds to minutes. Novelty, and situational demands for effort, may make automatic behavioral routines inappropriate in many circumstances, so there is a second system of the brain, mediated by prefrontal cortex and associated areas, that becomes active when habit will not suffice. Deliberate conscious action then may be activated, although it always occurs against the background of a considerable amount of automatic behavior of various kinds.

The functional system of insight permits one to monitor one's behavior, and to modify it in ways that might be more adaptive, in response to experience. The system involved in the regulation of behavior permits the individual to initiate purposeful, goal-directed activities that are essential to survival and to adaptation in a social environment. It also facilitates the inhibition of activity that may be inimical to the best interests of the person.

15

DEVELOPMENT, STABILITY, AND CHANGE OF CHARACTER

INTRODUCTION

The subject of this chapter is character, that aspect of personality consisting of the routine, typical things that people do repetitively. These tend to be habitual, and because they may be repeated many times over the course of the day and of one's life, they make people knowable and predictable. Character, like other aspects of personality, is an emergent property of the self-organizing activity of the brain and is an expression of procedural learning. When a person does something "out of character," it frequently is noted by that individual's associates and friends because it is unexpected. This chapter employs concepts discussed in the previous chapters on the modularity of memory (5), dynamics (6), and self-organization (6 & 7). Its purpose is to shed light on the development, stability, and change of character.

Psychoanalysts have devoted more attention to the problem of character than have the proponents of most other schools, so we will begin with a brief and highly selective discussion of what some of them had to say on the subject. At a descriptive level, their observations are similar to our own, although there are significant differences in how the mechanisms that form the basis for character are understood.

We will consider certain developmental factors that are relevant to the "acquisition" of character. Experience shapes and refines the expression of character. Although there are no clearly defined sensitive periods for character development, there is indirect evidence suggesting the relative importance of procedural learning in the earliest years of life for the subsequent unfolding of character. Procedural learning develops prior to declarative memory and therefore may be the vehicle through which these habitual behaviors are acquired.

Finally, we suggest that direct efforts to disrupt the procedural memory system may be required for character change to occur in psychotherapy. Talking about old events (i.e., episodic memories), or discussing ideas and information with a patient (the semantic memory system), may at best be indirect means of perturbing those behaviors in which people routinely engage. The modular organization of memory allows for the dissociation of procedural knowledge from declarative knowledge, so that learned processes can come to assume a certain automaticity. We contend that appreciation of the workings of procedural memory may increase the efficacy of therapeutic attempts to change character.

A BRIEF HISTORY OF THE CONCEPT OF CHARACTER

Since character is a concept derived primarily from psychoanalytic thinking, we will examine the views of those authors who concerned themselves most with the subject—Sigmund Freud, Otto Fenichel, Sándor Ferenczi, and Wilhelm Reich. We begin by considering Fenichel's definition and general description of character: the "habitual mode of bringing into harmony the tasks presented by internal demands and by the external world" (1945, p. 467). Fenichel emphasized "the habitual form of a given reaction, its relative constancy," and argued that character is "necessarily a function of the constant, organized, and integrating part of the personality which is the ego." Fenichel considered character to be largely, but not entirely, composed of defensive responses to conflicts between the ego, the instinctual drives, the external world, and the superego, and held that there are no "character attitudes" that "would be independent of instinctual conflicts" (p. 467). In other words, character is always a behavioral adaptation to conflict involving some kind of compromise.

Fenichel held the opinion that while some "expenditure of energy" is required to maintain the eccentricities of character, "it would be more exact to say that their formation corresponds to a single definite act of repression, so that the necessity for subsequent separate repressions, consuming more energy, and for separate anxiety experiences is avoided" (1945, p. 466). In other words, Fenichel thought that a characteristic behavior arose as a result of a one-time attempt to keep certain disturbing mental contents out of awareness.

How this one-time repression was maintained was not entirely clear in Fenichel's formulation, and he tended to speak metaphorically. As he saw it, conflict leads to various character traits which with time become "rigid and frozen." The conflict, which once was "urgent and alive," eventually becomes latent. Fenichel argued that, at least in general terms, "it is comparatively easy to see what has to be done; the requisite analytic task is to thaw the frozen energies of the inert attitude. It is, however, much more difficult to *fulfill* this task, to find the point where the defensive system is most insecure, where the neurotic defense is less rigid—the points and times, in other words, where the fight between instinct and defense has remained most alive" (1945, p. 538). Fenichel believed that by sniffing out and analyzing such conflicts, character might be changed.

In this context, Fenichel referred to Freud, who had suggested two ways to "remobilize old conflicts" and hence light a fire under the patient that might permit the resolution of character pathology: "Either we can bring about situations in which the conflict becomes actual or we can content ourselves with discussing it in analysis" (S. Freud, 1937, p. 333). Freud had assumed that the former course would either require the analyst to manipulate circumstances to contrive the reactivation of a conflict or require an intervention of fate to bring about events and situations similar to those that created the conflict in the first place. Like Fenichel after him, Freud was less than sanguine about the possibility that discussing the latent conflict could activate its expression in the analysis. Fenichel (1945, p. 538) described discussion of the conflict in analysis as "useless, since mere discussion will not help any more than reading Freud's works will cure a neurosis." Fenichel therefore rejected both of these options and argued that the therapeutic task instead was to provoke situations "in which the conflict becomes actual" not through any contrivance but through interpretation of the individual's character traits.

According to Fenichel (1945), the first task in treating character is for the therapist to make the patient "aware of the problematic nature of his behavior. After the patient has been wakened to amazement about what he does, he must become aware of the fact that he is compelled to act as he does, that he cannot act differently" (p. 537). Note that Fenichel was arguing here that the patient is somehow unaware of his character, that he has no control over his behavior, that it occurs more or less automatically. According to this prescription, the analyst must draw the patient's attention to the automatic, nonconscious behaviors that constitute character.

Fenichel maintained that both character and neurosis have their genesis in conflict. With neurosis, the conflict ostensibly remains somehow active, causing emotional distress. In the case of character, however, he thought the conflict was effectively forced out of awareness and made "rigid and frozen." Because of this freezing of character into rigid, automatic patterns of behavior, the repression of conflict is maintained, and it therefore is rare that an individual experiences conflict in association with his or her character. If character is to change, therapy must reignite the smoldering fires of conflict. To bring about character change, Fenichel proposed that the ossified conflict must be brought once again into awareness and analytically dissected.

Sándor Ferenczi (1925a/1980), although he shared many of Freud's and Fenichel's ideas, brought a somewhat different perspective to the understanding and treatment of character. In certain respects, the language he used is closer to our own formulation, despite the fact that he approached the phenomenon from a very different angle. Ferenczi proposed that character is composed of *habits*. Perhaps exaggerating the predictability of character, he said that it is "a kind of mechanization of a particular way of reaction, rather similar to an obsessional symptom. If you know the character of the individual, you can make him perform an action when you wish and as often as you wish, because he behaves like a machine" (1927/1955, pp. 66–67).

Ferenczi argued that the id is a kind of repository for habits (rather than a seething cauldron of sexual and aggressive impulses), a component of the mind in which "habit tendencies [are] piled up." In ordinary everyday functioning, these habits account for most behavior, although under certain circumstances, the ego has the capacity to override habit. Yet character is difficult to change, Ferenczi thought, because "each fresh adaptation demands expenditure of attention" by the ego. Since the energy dynamics of behavior favor the much less demanding habitual activity of character, "the ego is only stimulated when the necessity arises to deal with a new and disturbing stimulus, that is to say, when adaptation is essential." For Ferenczi, breaking a habit "implies that the conscious ego has taken over from the id a previously automatic method of discharge, in order to apply it in a new direction" (1925a/1980, p. 285).

Ferenczi contended that much behavior involves the automatic and unconscious activation of habits (character traits), and that in novel situations (or when one attempts to disrupt these habits in therapy) some psychological system (the ego) "must be stimulated" (1925a/1980, p. 285). We are wary of reading too much into Ferenczi's discussion in an attempt to find parallels with a neuroscience-based model. Nevertheless, there are interesting similarities between Ferenczi's conceptualization and the relationship between the automatic schema activation system and the deliberate conscious control mediated by the prefrontal cortex (discussed in Chapter 14). As we noted previously, habitual schemas are activated automatically under the influence of more complex schemas (intentions) through the mediation of the basal ganglia and prefrontal cortex. When it is necessary to override the routine activation of schemas, the prefrontal cortex becomes active and permits a more flexible, if effortful, response.

According to Ferenczi, "psycho-analysis can be regarded as a long-drawn-out fight against thought-habits" (1925a/1980, p. 285); for him, repetitively engaging in habitual behavior and thinking "is associated with an 'economy of mental expenditure,' compared with which seeking after new paths represents a fresh adaptation, [that is,] something relatively less pleasurable" (p. 285). Recall that in previous chapters we made a similar point when we discussed the dynamics of neural networks (Chapter 7) and the activation of automatic and deliberate behavioral schemas (Chapter 14). The pathways most likely to be activated in response to particular stimulation at any instant are those with the current highest probability of activation, and the probability of activation is in large part a function of repeated past experience, the environment, and one's current physiological state.

Ferenczi attributed the difficulty of changing character to "the fact that character traits, which are accepted by the ego, resemble symptoms concerning which the patient has no insight" (1925a/1980, p. 291). Not only does one have no concerns about one's character, but one essentially is unaware of the myriad behavioral processes that constitute his or her character (1920/1980). Ferenczi proposed that an "active technique" was required, an approach about which he was somewhat more enthusiastic in his earlier work (1919/1980, 1920/1980) than in later papers (1925b/1980). Because he considered psychoanalysis to be "really a fight against habits . . . directed towards substitution of real adaptations in place of those unsatisfactory habit-like methods of resolving conflict which we call symptoms" (1925a/1980, p. 286), Ferenczi thought it important to disrupt habits by "requiring what is inhibited, and inhibiting what is uninhibited" (1920/1980, p. 212). He encouraged his patients to do those things that they were most anxious to avoid (and which generally were not habitual, and so required deliberate conscious effort), and to avoid doing those things that were most pleasurable or most compelling (i.e., habits). Likewise, he applied his active approach to his patients' fantasy lives. He recommended that patients fantasize about the things they feared, and he attempted to prevent them from following more appealing fantasies (1923/1980).

As did Fenichel, Ferenczi pointed out the necessity of having initially to draw the patient's attention to habits, since ordinarily they occur outside of awareness. As a consequence, his active approach had the effect of disturbing "to no small degree the comfortable but torpid quiet of a stagnating analysis" (1920/1980, p. 212). Because active therapy works "against the grain," patients may find it aversive, and Ferenczi (1925b/1980) urged caution in the use of active methods, especially in the beginning of therapy, when the relationship between therapist and patient is tenuous.

The final psychoanalytic theorist we will discuss here is Wilhelm Reich (1949). Reich was very interested in the treatment of character pathology and in the differences between character and neurosis. He observed that one such difference is that, although neurotic symptoms frequently are experienced by the individual as alien or meaningless, character ordinarily is rationalized so that it is not experienced as pathological. Consequently, one of the more common explanations for one's characteristic behavior is simply "that's just the way I am."

Reich's ideas about character are derived in large part from his view of the phenomenon as a process rather than a thing. He was quite interested in "the *form* of expression" of an individual's habitual mode of being, noting that it "is far more important than the *ideational content*." In treating character, he often made use of "the form of expression *exclusively*" (1949, p. 45; emphasis in original). That is, rather than dealing with the content expressed by his patients, he focused on the manner in which the content was expressed. From Reich's perspective, character *is* the way in which the patient behaves, the attitude, tone of voice, facial expression, mannerisms, manner of carrying oneself, patterns of complex behavior, and so on.

A WORKING DEFINITION OF CHARACTER

Character, then, consists of habits, to a large extent procedurally learned, in which people engage constantly, repeatedly, automatically, and nonconsciously. Character consists of those habitual behaviors that give people their own distinctive styles of being in the world. The foundations of character are acquired early in life but undergo change over time in association with experience and neurocognitive development. Nonetheless, certain predispositions (e.g., arrogance or obsequiousness) tend to remain fairly stable despite changes in the precise details of how they may be manifested across development.

We maintain that most of what people do as a matter of routine is done automatically and unconsciously. It is an emergent property of the operation of the automatic schema activation system and expresses procedural learning. The idea that learning plays an important role in the formation of character is, of course, hardly novel. It has been appreciated for many years (e.g., Dollard & Miller, 1950; Pavlov, 1927; Thorndike, 1911), but the knowledge that there are multiple systems of learning and memory permits a more precise understanding of the processes by which personality development occurs. Learning theorists, for example, have concerned themselves primarily with classical and related types of conditioning, operant conditioning, and social learning. These are important, but the acquisition of character traits cannot be understood adequately without an appreciation of the contribution of procedural learning.

Character, like all psychological processes, is an emergent property of the brain's self-organizing activity. As such, expressions of character are actually the behavioral manifestations of the activation of neural networks with a high probability of activation. Thus, no matter how predictable a person's behavior, character is not a *thing*, but rather a set of processes that show variability in the probability of their expression from moment to moment. In addition, the activation and emergent manifestation of the behaviors associated with these processes can be described in dynamic, probabilistic terms. Thus no one *has* a character, and there is no such thing as character *structure*, although it often is difficult not to talk in those terms because people are so remarkably consistent in their thinking and behavior, and because there seems to be a nearly universal tendency to reify concepts. It thus may be more accurate to state that people *do* characteristic things (Grigsby & Hartlaub, 1994).

PROCEDURAL LEARNING AND CHARACTER

We propose that character results from the activation of neural networks that have been assembled as a consequence of procedural learning within the context of a specific temperament. Recall that procedural learning involves the acquisition of processes rather than information. These may be motor, cognitive, or perceptual skills, "defense mechanisms," the recognition of various types of patterns, or behavioral routines that have become automatic with repetition. Some are simple, whereas others may involve elaborate schemas that direct complex behavior.

Most procedurally learned schemas are activated automatically, probably by means of processes such as those described by Shallice (1988) and discussed earlier (in Chapter 14 on the regulation of behavior). The automatic, unconscious, repeated performance of routine behaviors is the essence of character. Activities that once may have been performed voluntarily become so ingrained over time that it is hard to imagine that they might be done differently. The individual tends to forget the circumstances under which a behavior was learned (if they ever were known), and the schema, mediated by a relatively specific neural network, acquires a functional autonomy independent of the original learning. The declarative memory system, which is structurally and functionally dissociable from the procedural learning system, is likely to be relatively unimportant in the maintenance of the character trait, although it may be involved in rationalization of the behavior if the behavior is consciously perceived. This dissociation between memory systems may account in part for Sigmund Freud's remark (1913/1958) concerning "the strange behaviour of patients, in being able to combine a conscious knowing with not knowing" (p. 142).

THE AUTOMATICITY OF CHARACTER

We previously discussed how, when speed and accuracy of performance are important, it is adaptive to behave automatically. Evolution has placed a premium on such organismic characteristics as rapid adaptation to change.

Animals that are able to survive while minimizing energy expenditure likewise are at a competitive advantage. Evolution thus must have favored those organisms possessing the capacity to engage in complex behavioral repertoires automatically, distributing different aspects of their activity among numerous hierarchically ordered systems and subsystems.

Reading, for example, would be very difficult if it always required the same effort that was necessary when one was learning to read. On the other hand, well-learned skills performed too thoughtfully or deliberately may not be executed properly. For example, a baseball player in a batting slump thinks a great deal about his swing and may receive advice from other people. This directs the player's attention to what ordinarily is an automatic process and tends to diminish the automatic quality of the activity, making it feel somewhat unnatural. This effortful focusing of conscious awareness on batting (or on any other automatically performed task) requires what Norman (1986) called deliberate conscious control, involving activation of the prefrontal cortex; this kind of processing, because it makes demands on one's limited working memory capacity, is "slow and serial, hence not very effective for some kinds of skills" (p. 544). As Norman pointed out, performance generally is better if it is automatic and nonconscious, rather than deliberate and conscious. In all likelihood, most skilled activities are best done with little thought. This is intuitively clear to athletes, artists, musicians, and others who become deeply absorbed in their work.

As one acquires various characterological processes (e.g., mannerisms, gestures, attitudes, ways of thinking about things, or complex behavioral schemas), these develop a high degree of automaticity. Yet, because procedural learning generally is a type of implicit learning, because it has no content, and because it is dissociated from the hippocampal declarative memory system, people generally are unconscious of the origins of most of their character. They don't know how they became the way they are or why they remain so, although they certainly may generate explanations that are plausible (Gazzaniga, 1985; Nisbett & Ross, 1980; Norman, 1986; T. D. Wilson, 1985).

Because important aspects of character can acquire automaticity and operate outside of awareness, "acting in character" becomes something over which the individual has little control in normal circumstances. This is apparent in the difficulty people commonly encounter in changing even inconsequential habits. To behave differently typically (although not always) requires awareness of one's habitual behavior, and considerable deliberate effort must be expended to behave contrary to one's usual tendencies, since the neural pathways most readily activated are those that subserve habitual activity. Deliberate effort to behave in ways that go against the grain is likely to involve activation of the prefrontal cortex, which is crucial "in the genesis of willed actions and required in situations where the routine selection of actions was unsatisfactory" (Shallice, 1988, p. 335).

A SENSITIVE PERIOD IN THE DEVELOPMENT OF CHARACTER

The first years of life may represent a sensitive period for the development of character. Tulving (1985) suggested that procedural learning ability develops prior to other forms of memory, and there are data to support a developmental dissociation between procedural and declarative memory systems, the former developing earlier (DiGiulio et al., 1994). DiGiulio and her collaborators administered tests of procedural and declarative learning to a sample of 88 children, half of whom were 8 years old and the other half of whom were 12 years old (22 of each sex at each age level); they found an interaction between age and type of test (procedural vs. declarative), and concluded that "procedural memory is functionally mature during a period of development where declarative memory continues to advance" (1994, p. 88).

There are few data concerning the existence of critical or sensitive periods in the acquisition of procedural knowledge, although certain commonly observed phenomena suggest that various kinds of skills are more readily acquired by younger children. For example, small children acquire motor skills more rapidly and thoroughly than do persons who try to learn the same skills in their 20's or 30's. The latter rarely reach the level of proficiency attained by those who learned at the age of 4 or 5 years. Improvement at such activities as video games, gymnastics, musical performance, and acquisition of second or third languages is similarly superior among younger individuals.

We postulate that the kind of procedural learning involved in the acquisition of character traits demonstrates a gradiential sensitive period; character is acquired by adulthood, after which time it ordinarily undergoes limited change. The processes involved in the development of character probably begin during the first year of life (well before the establishment of the hippocampal declarative memory system) and gradually diminish through adolescence. Adults, even very old ones, continue to be able to acquire new skills (Karni & Sagi, 1995), but speed of learning and the degree to which the skill can be perfected appear to decrease over time. Rarely, for example, does one hear of an accomplished musician who began studying music in adolescence; more commonly, study began before the age of 10, and often by 3 or 4 years.

Assuming the validity of this hypothesis, the automatic behaviors that constitute character would be acquired most strongly very early in life, with some modification over time as a result of experience and continued cognitive development. Character traits developed after adolescence could be expected to be less robust than those acquired early on, and probably would require a greater amount of repetition to become automatic. Even after becoming relatively automatic, the probability of their activation in a given situation might be less than the probability of activation of schemas learned early in life. If our supposition is accurate, it follows logically that character change is more difficult in adulthood than in childhood. A corollary is that effective character change probably would require disruption of existing schemas in addition to the acquisition of new ones.

TEMPERAMENT AND THE DEVELOPMENT OF CHARACTER

The process of character development, via the implicit processes of procedural learning, occurs in the context of certain basic phenotypic behavioral and cognitive orientations and capacities (Plomin et al., 1994). Fundamental, species-specific similarities in human neural organization account for much of the interindividual consistency in what we observe of both normal and pathological behavior, yet people differ widely from one another along certain basic dimensions of temperament and intelligence.

Phenotypic variations in neural organization and their associated temperamental traits may predispose an individual toward the development of a unique characterological orientation. Kagan et al. (1988), for example, argued that "most of the children we call inhibited belong to a qualitatively distinct category of infants who were born with a lower threshold for limbic–hypothalamic arousal to unexpected changes in the environment or novel events that cannot be assimilated easily" (p. 171). As Kagan and colleagues interpret their own data and the work of others, shyness results from a combination of this hypothesized physiological tendency in concert with "chronic environmental stress." Presumably, shy children are more likely to learn to respond to unpleasant situations in a relatively passive manner—by withdrawal, for example—than are active, engaging children, who may be liable to react to stress with increased motor activity. Kagan (1989) maintains that "the eventual display of inhibited behavior in the second year of life requires some form of environmental stress in order to actualize the temperamental disposition" (p. 673).

Although the role of temperament is fundamentally important in determining subsequent personality development, the evidence suggests that experience plays a crucial and continuing role in the developmental process. It seems probable that temperament is most likely to be decisive as a determinant of character when an individual's temperament is an "outlier" statistically speaking (i.e., when a child has an especially pronounced expression of one or more temperamental variables). The character formation of those with a more modal temperament might possibly be mediated to a greater degree by experience and learning; perhaps a less extreme temperament allows for greater plasticity of and variability in expressions of character.

Finally, as we discussed in Chapter 10 on temperament, there is persuasive evidence that temperamental style is critical in the formation of certain basic aspects of personality and in determining the child's fit with the environment (Stern, 1985; Thomas & Chess, 1977). Among hyperactive children, for example, it appears that those whose parents and social environment are best able to deal with their temperamental idiosyncrasies are likely to have the best outcomes as adults. When the fit between parent and child is less than optimal, there is a greater likelihood of subsequent psychopathology and behavioral difficulty (G. Weiss et al., 1985). Poor fit may thus predispose a person to character pathology.

PROCEDURAL LEARNING AND INTERPERSONAL TRANSACTIONS IN EARLY RELATIONSHIPS

While constitutional factors are unquestionably important, much of a person's character emerges from interactions with parents and other significant people. The requirements of adaptation demand that the mother and infant establish contact, and both contribute significantly to the interpersonal processes that are the vehicle for attachment. Procedural learning allows these transactions to become relatively automatic. The normal infant has the ability to adapt (within certain limits) to the psychosocial niche within which it finds itself, even though this niche may appear very idiosyncratic to an outside observer. Infants acquire an array of procedural memories (or habits) through their active participation in an ongoing series of complicated transactions with caregivers. Basic neurophysiological regulation is established within the context of these relationships, and subsequent behavioral self-regulation may rely heavily on these procedurally learned processes as well.

Basic patterns of behavior in interpersonal relationships are shaped by the interaction of the young child with its specific social environment, and these become habitual through modification of the nervous system. We suggest that important parts of the relational patterning observed in different "attachment styles" (Bowlby, 1969; Stern, 1985; J. Weiss & Sampson, 1986) are encoded as procedural memories that have a significant influence on how a person perceives and interacts with other people (again, within the context of temperament). These procedurally learned patterns are essential aspects of character.

Whereas some of a young child's transactions with the environment may require conscious attention, many of these processes are learned implicitly, becoming routinized and automatic, and hence allowing attention to be directed elsewhere. In interpersonal relationships, these procedural memories are reflected in a propensity to repeat certain habitual patterns of behavior automatically and nonconsciously. Procedural memories of a relational kind can be thought of as determining the nature of the relationships in which one participates.

Given the extraordinary complexity of the interpersonal world, it is essential that most of the time these processes operate automatically and without the need for conscious awareness. If one's procedurally learned relational behaviors have sufficient flexibility to allow for the possibility of recognizing new relational experience—in other words, if one is able to adjust and modify one's approach to one's circumstances when conditions warrant such an adaptation—things are likely to go well. When procedurally learned perceptual appraisals of the interpersonal world are applied rigidly in ways overdetermined by one's learning history, one can only find the relational configurations that one "knows" implicitly will be found in the interpersonal world. It becomes a thorny clinical problem to figure out how to facilitate a new adaptation in such situations.

CHARACTER AND THE PHENOMENOLOGY OF PROCEDURAL MEMORIES

Procedural knowledge can express itself in a number of ways: it may involve motor behavior, perceptual pattern recognition, cognitive appraisals or processes, or some combination of these. Thus, in practice, a person may intuitively recognize (rightly or wrongly) a given interpersonal situation to be of a certain kind and respond to it accordingly in a certain habitual way. By responding in a particular manner, he or she may increase the probability of evoking the reactions from others that he or she is prepared to encounter. All of this is done automatically, without premeditation or reflection, without motivation.

Automatized interpersonal routines of this sort do not require conscious or unconscious mental representations, images, motivations, or ideas to operate. Instead, while these relational procedural memories initially may have been acquired and refined within a specific relationship, once the behavioral–perceptual processes associated with the original relationship have become automatized via procedural learning, they are habits the activation of which is associated with a probability determined by the physiological state of the individual and the nature of the immediate environment. The original relational context can become, and usually is, dissociated from the habitual process itself. The procedure thus can be said to have become *decontextualized* (Ogden, 1994).

As noted previously, the brain functions in large part by recognizing and forming patterns (Kelso, 1995). Subtleties and inconsistencies may be missed in the recognition of patterns that appear to be familiar. This process of concretizing our perceptions of the world is mediated by procedural learning. That is, one's representation of experience is implicitly taken as *fact* and is assumed unquestioningly to be identical to whatever is being represented. We thereby "recognize" certain patterns, something at which the paranoid individual is exceptionally skilled. Thus, the deeply ashamed person may behave as though others are actual or potential critics who threaten to expose bad parts of the self. Transactions with others are conducted habitually on the spoken or unspoken presumption that the other is motivated to engender shame or to establish superiority. The factual basis of these procedurally learned appraisals of the other as critic remains largely unquestioned or even unacknowledged and is refractory to modification.

It is difficult to convey to individuals who are convinced of their unworthiness that others might see things differently. These people *know* that somewhere inside others must agree that they are despicable; others just won't admit it because they are too polite, too professional, or too timid to speak the truth. This sort of *knowing* is what we have in mind when we speak of perceptual procedural memories as operating as concretizations. It is a major therapeutic accomplishment when such persons can start to treat their concretely-acted-upon ideas as *ideas* of a very compelling kind, rather than as a pervasive, sometimes ineffable, and intuitively known truth. At the moment an individual becomes aware of this mismatch, a "gap" between the world and the person's perception of the world is created in consciousness.

DYNAMICS AND CHARACTER

Character also can be described in the language of probability and dynamics. Thus, people act according to character because they have a greater likelihood of activating a given array of nonconsciously initiated behaviors than of engaging in some "out-of-character" behavior. Characteristic behaviors can be thought of as attractors, and uncharacteristic behaviors may be thought of as repellors or attractors with very shallow basins of attraction. It is difficult for an individual to maintain a behavior associated with processes that are not attractors (like a marble balanced on a pinnacle between two troughs), because the neural networks associated with characteristic behavior have a greater likelihood of activation. Some people may be described as having especially wide or deep basins of attraction for given processes, so that in the first instance a wide range of situations can induce the associated expression of character. In the second instance, certain situations may induce an especially pronounced expression of character, with little likelihood of a different behavioral response.

It should be remembered that a behavioral schema that is an attractor at one time might not be an attractor, or even might be a repellor, at another. Manic behavior, for example, is very likely to be observed during a manic episode. However, when the individual is in a depressed or affectively neutral state, flight of ideas and wild grandiosity are highly unlikely and may represent a repellor. Physiological state plays a fundamental role in the determination of the probabilities that an individual will act in character or out of character. What is out of character may become characteristic of an individual, however, in association with some enduring change in physiological state (e.g., as a result of trauma and subsequent posttraumatic stress disorder).

MODULARITY AND CHARACTER

The mind's modular architecture reveals itself in certain characterological phenomena. For example, consciousness can be, and typically is, fully dissociable from processes associated with character. This nonconscious quality of character can be disrupted when people observe themselves on audio- or videotape. Seeing oneself as though from the outside in this way can direct awareness to qualities or characteristics in one's behavior of which one typically is oblivious.

Similarly, the "repression" that takes place in association with the acquisition of character in early childhood is primarily a function of the dissociability of procedural and declarative memory. Infantile amnesia, for example, is the term that refers to the fact that most people recall very few events prior to the age of 3–5 years. This phenomenon is probably a reflection of the relative immaturity of the episodic memory system in early childhood when compared with the neural substrates of emotional and procedural learning (Rudy & Morledge, 1994). Thus, cognitive, perceptual, and behavioral processes, including those associated with character, can be acquired at a time when memory for the events that led to the procedural knowledge may not be fully stable.

DISSOCIABILITY OF CHARACTER AND SELF

Character and self are dissociable functional systems. Each consists of different processes, and each has a different neural substrate. Character is composed especially of automatically and unconsciously activated procedurally learned behavioral schemas, whereas self consists of a hierarchy of schemas that primarily involve perceptual and emotional memory. Change may occur in one system and not in the other. Nevertheless, the two systems interact in a number of important ways.

For example, at any moment the currently active self-representation contributes to the physiological state of the individual, and this state affects the probability that any given characterological behavior will be activated. Thus there is a relatively strong association between self and character. Among other factors that influence state, and hence the expression of character, are level of arousal, activity level, the condition of the environment, health status, level of fatigue, and consumption of alcohol or other various drugs.

One important aspect of psychological well-being is the degree to which an individual's various personality systems are coherent and well integrated. Thus, the existence of very disparate and relatively independent self-representations may reflect a disturbance in the functional system of the self, but there also may be a similar lack of integration between different functional systems. For example, self and character ideally should be consistent with one another, so that one's behavior appears to be a genuine expression of their self-representation. In certain disorders, however, self and character may be very incongruous.

A classic example of this disjunction is the passive–aggressive individual. A passive–aggressive person behaves in a way that may be irritating and provocative and that appears to most observers to express hostility. Such an individual nevertheless routinely denies hostile intent, has an endless supply of sometimes plausible rationalizations for his or her behavior, and may put on a show of saccharine sweetness. Part of what makes it difficult to deal with such people is the contrast between their self-representations, professed intentions, and actual behavior. Because these dissociable sets of processes (character and self-representation) occur automatically and unconsciously, the individual has little awareness of the discrepancy that others see or the nature of the behavior. Reflecting on themselves, they are aware primarily of the self-representation, which essentially announces that "I am a nice person, without an angry bone in my body."

Successfully treating a passive–aggressive individual requires repeatedly drawing his or her attention to the habitual behavior and others' reaction to it, and to the discrepancy between his or her professed motives and rationalizations and the effect their behavior has on others. The behavior itself must become conscious, and the automaticity of the behavior must be disrupted, drawing into focus the discrepancy between these functional systems. Only then can the individual begin to take active control over the passive behavior, and the self-representation may begin to shift so that it comes to include the possibility that he or she might at times express aggression overtly.

VARIABILITY AND CHANGE IN CHARACTER

Despite the stability of character, it is important not to overemphasize the consistency in human behavior. Character undergoes variability over the short term as well as the long term. Character, like other learned processes, has a probabilistic neural basis. That is, learning has the effect of either increasing or decreasing the probability of certain behaviors. Thus over periods of days, weeks, and months, differing conditions in the internal or external environment may yield neurobehavioral outcomes that are "out of character" for a given individual. A person who is depressed, for example, has a greater probability of engaging automatically in behaviors associated with his or her depressed state than in behaviors associated with euphoria. As state shifts, so does behavior. Similarly, one's behavior—even automatically generated behavioral schemas—varies depending on who else is present. Thus, while there is an orderly pattern to an individual's character, the order is relatively complex, and no one's activity is as easy to predict as Ferenczi suggested when he described people as behaving "like a machine" (1927/1955, p. 67).

Further, because the brain remains a plastic, self-organized system throughout life, the capacity for long-term character change persists, so that uncharacteristic behaviors have the potential to become a stable part of a person's repertoire. This may, however, require considerable conscious, deliberate effort. Trauma, which involves conditions that are very favorable for synaptic modification (increased arousal along with perceptual and affective intensity leading to high-frequency firing of neurons in many pathways) frequently produces character change.

Psychiatric and psychological treatment also may affect character, although the effects usually are more gradual and not as dramatic as those associated with trauma. The use of various psychotropic medications may have a significant effect on how a person's character is manifested. The resulting changes, which frequently depend on continuation of medication, are similar to learning insofar as they "tune" the nervous system, altering the probability of activating various networks by changing the nature of synaptic responsivity. Psychotherapy and psychoanalysis involve environmental conditions that are significantly different from most social situations, and such a change in the context may facilitate a change in the probability of the utilization of certain neural circuits (i.e., it results in particular types of learning).

In any event, with few exceptions, character changes slowly and incrementally, as is the case with most procedural knowledge. This inertia is a function of the automatic, unconscious, highly overlearned quality of procedural knowledge, and the pace of change may be beneficial insofar as it maintains the stability of procedurally learned processes; more rapid learning might be disruptive to important schemas, and moreover, rapid change in schemas certainly would affect the operation of the automatic schema activation system.

KINDS OF CHARACTER PATHOLOGY

Our approach to understanding character suggests that there may be four distinct categories of character pathology. The first involves behavior that reflects disorders of temperament, such as in attention-deficit/hyperactivity disorder (ADHD). Here, certain aspects of temperament themselves are associated with problem behavior. The second involves behaviors that result from maladaptive learning, as might be the case in passive–aggressive personality disorder. The third category includes behaviors reflecting variations or disturbances in the functioning of either the automatic schema activation system or the prefrontal cortex. This type of pathology is most likely to be present when the primary difficulties are with the regulation of behavior. This might be the problem in disorders characterized by apathy, irrelevant and inappropriate behavior, and behavioral dyscontrol. Excessively inflexible, routine, automatic behavior (and even frank perseveration) may reflect difficulty with activation of the prefrontal cortex, as may significant distractibility. Finally, a fourth type of character pathology may reflect disturbed dynamics, as in certain quasi-periodic disturbances of mood (observed, e.g., in some individuals with borderline personality disorder).

REPRESSION AND THE DEVELOPMENT OF CHARACTER

Active effort need not be expended to maintain character; moreover, Fenichel's assertion to the contrary, neuropsychological data suggest that there probably is no "single definite act of repression" involved in most character formation (1945, p. 460). The genesis of character remains obscure not because of repression but because it is in the nature of procedural memories that they are unconscious, have no content, and are completely dissociable from declarative memory. The cause(s) of a repetitive behavior may be forgotten because there is no need (or ability) to remember the cause and because the acquisition of character, as with most procedural knowledge, tends to be an incremental process taking place over an extended period of time. Further, even a reconstruction of the presumed causes via the declarative memory system (i.e., interpretation) may at best be only a plausible explanation (Gazzaniga, 1985; Norman, 1986), a good guess. Although plausible, it is unlikely that such interpretations, in response to verbal descriptions of episodic and semantic memories, and presented verbally by the therapist (and hence encoded by the patient in verbal semantic memory), would affect significantly what has been procedurally learned and continues to be automatically activated.

Of functional importance for the individual who acquires procedural knowledge is that a novel behavior which was adaptive in a particular situation was learned and that it became automatic. Neither semantic nor episodic memory is necessary in this extremely efficient process, and it is not obvious that anything like the repression Freud hypothesized is operating here. Other forms of what is called repression—for example, following trauma—are likely themselves to reflect the procedurally learned restriction of access to awareness for certain information, and hence they themselves are manifestations of an automatic, unconsciously activated process.

In some cases it happens that a person will recall the circumstances surrounding the acquisition of a procedurally learned character process, when the automaticity of the process has been disrupted, and especially when its occurrence is prevented. Such associative memories may occur, but it seems likely that this "insight" is a consequence of (or simply concomitant with) a shift in character, and not the cause of that shift. Because the declarative and procedural learning systems frequently are associated in this way, it may be that an episodic memory, or an event somehow associated with an episodic memory, would lead to the activation of a procedurally learned schema.

THE THERAPEUTIC APPROACH TO CHARACTER

If character reflects procedural knowledge, one of the most direct and important methods of treating character pathology is to disrupt the automatic nature of the performance of certain processes. This was essentially Wilhelm Reich's method. Reich noted that "the character trait has to be continually pointed out so that the patient will attain the same attitude toward it as toward a symptom. Only rarely is this achieved easily" (1949, p. 67). If the therapist repeatedly points out character traits of which the patient ordinarily is unaware, their automatic performance is disturbed and learning (in other words, a change in the neural networks subserving the schema) may occur. The habitual behavior in a sense is "unlearned" as one tends to become increasingly aware of the behavior during its performance.

As an individual becomes more conscious of these behaviors, the behaviors become susceptible to influence by the system that regulates deliberate conscious control. Here is where Sándor Ferenczi's "active" therapy may be useful. If one wants to change one's character, it is not enough simply to become aware of an unconscious schema—one also must make an effort not to engage in it. Since some other behavior may need to substitute for the inhibited one, one must make an additional effort to behave in a way to which one is unaccustomed. In this manner, the individual gradually gains some capacity to exert control over these behaviors, as situations arise in which he or she actually feels able to make a choice about whether to engage in what previously had been automatic routines. The process is not easy, however, and the individual may be reluctant to go against the grain of character, since it is uncomfortable to do so and may require great effort. The probability of activation of those automatic schemas may remain high, but for once the individual may experience the possibility of *choosing* to behave in a particular way.

The resistance observed in response to an active treatment approach reflects the fact that to inhibit the habitual and to do something different requires deliberate effort. Without sufficient practice of a new activity and repeated disruption of previous learning, procedurally acquired character does not change. In contrast to a direct approach to the procedural learning system, a focus primarily on declarative memory might be expected to generate intellectual insight and maybe an understanding of one's past, while having a limited influence on character itself. Perhaps the objectives of a particular patient's treatment may be met by dealing primarily with the declarative memory system, but expectations for character change in such cases should be modest.

Character change is a difficult task not because the patient is deliberately resistant but because there seldom is much control over a neurally based, essentially automatic, unconscious process with a high probability of occurrence. As Gill (1982) noted, "the patient may be only peripherally aware of his suspiciousness, haughtiness, obsequiousness, or whatever" (p. 77). Disruption of the course of procedural memories such as we are describing here involves a gradual changing of the pattern of the neural networks that underlie a given behavior. By recruitment of the neuropsychological systems involved in deliberate conscious control during the performance of automatically activated character schemas, the nature of the behavioral performance may be affected, so that the behavior becomes less smooth, seamless, and automatic than usual (Norman, 1986). Reich's (1949) strategy therefore seems consistent with what we know of procedural memory.

While it is likely that character change may be brought about by a variety of means, one fairly direct route to changing a person's character may be through disrupting procedurally learned behavior by consistently directing the patient's attention to it, as Reich did. In some cases, however, it may be that specific aspects of certain personality disorders (e.g., splitting among persons with borderline personality disorder, or impulsivity among certain psychopaths) reflect neurological developmental variants or anomalies that in some instances may be quite subtle (e.g., D. Gardner, Lucas, & Cowdry, 1987). When this is the case, perhaps psychotherapy cannot bring about "normal" functioning. Therapy, however, may permit the individual to function adaptively within the constraints imposed by biology and irreversible developmental history (Gollin et al., 1988). As Fenichel observed, "what Freud once said about analysis in general is especially true of character analysis: Although it cannot alter the individual constitutionally and its effectiveness thus remains limited, it may change the patient into what he would have become had his life circumstances been more favorable" (1945, p. 540).

REPRESENTATIONS OF AND REACTIONS TO OTHERS' CHARACTER

People do characteristic things and, in observing them, we form abstract internal representations of those people. These representations are, in a sense, subtle caricatures of their personality styles. Through repetitive activation of these representations, we become bound by our perceptions of others' character just as they are bound by their own personality styles. Our perceptions of others' character is shaped by our experience with them. At the same time, in interacting with and getting to know other people, we develop our own habitual routines of behavior that are specific to each individual. There thus evolves an interpersonal set of routines that makes interaction more predictable and less spontaneous, a problem we discuss elsewhere (Grigsby & Stevens, 2000).

This combination of an internal representation of the other's character and of a tendency inevitably to become involved in a characterological *danse macabre* makes the treatment of character especially difficult. For example, an inflexible representation of the other may lead to mistaken attributions about behaviors that are "out of character" or even to a failure to recognize that the patient has engaged in a novel behavior that may be of considerable significance. Furthermore, the development of such a characterological duet, unconsciously and automatically choreographed, makes it very easy for the therapist to fail to understand his or her contribution to the patient's character as it is expressed in therapy.

SUMMARY AND CONCLUSION

Character encompasses those behaviors in which a person engages routinely, automatically, and unconsciously. Character makes a person knowable and predictable. It has as its foundation certain biological predispositions and capacities. A number of inherited and developmental–neural factors are important determinants of the form taken by character, including temperament, intellectual ability, and integrity of brain organization. These variables constrain and shape the development of character. Most of character reflects the activation of specific behavioral schemas by an automatic schema activation system, overruled sometimes by the prefrontal cortex. When routine characterological behaviors are inadequate or inappropriate to the situation, the neurologically normal individual experiences activation of the prefrontal cortex and of the executive functions, permitting deliberate conscious control to override what is habitual and automatic.

The apparent consistency of character is a manifestation of the differential probabilities of activation of various schemas in specific external and internal circumstances, which in turn are consequences of procedural learning. The first few years of life probably represent a sensitive period for the development of character. Tulving (1985) suggested that procedural memory develops prior to other forms of memory, and there are data to support a developmental dissociation between procedural and declarative memory systems, with the former developing earlier (DiGiulio et al., 1994). Nevertheless, it is likely that considerable modifiability remains throughout life because the brain retains its plastic capacity for procedural learning.

With few exceptions, character changes slowly. This resistance to change is a function of the automatic, unconscious, highly overlearned quality of procedural memory. While it is likely that character change may be brought about by a variety of means, we believe the most direct way to effect character change is by working with the procedural learning system rather than with declarative memories. In simplified form, this might involve two major activities. The first is to focus attention on the interpersonal therapy process, to observe, rather than interpret, what takes place, and repeatedly call attention to it. This in itself tends to disrupt the automaticity with which procedural learning ordinarily is expressed. The second therapeutic tactic is to engage in activities that directly disrupt what has been procedurally learned. This is what Ferenczi was addressing in his attempt to develop an "active therapy" (1920/1980, 1923/1980, 1925b/1980; K. A. Frank, 1992). It may be that specific aspects of certain personality disorders (such as splitting and impulsivity among persons with borderline personality disorder) reflect neurological developmental variants or anomalies. When this is the case, perhaps psychotherapy cannot bring about fully "normal" functioning. Therapy may, however, permit the individual to function adaptively within the constraints imposed by biology and irreversible developmental history.

Although there are few data concerning changes in the capacity for various kinds of procedural learning throughout childhood into adult life, it is a common observation that children frequently are more adept than adults at the acquisition of various motor skills, as well as in perceptual abilities and in the learning of foreign languages. Competing with their children on video games, for example, can easily frustrate even those adults who get a lot of practice. It is a reasonable hypothesis that a gradiential decrease in procedural learning capacity over time may account for some of the difficulties inherent in attempting to change character in adults.

This theory of character sets realistic limits on the extent to which one might expect character to change, since it is unlikely that basic temperament can be modified significantly. The theory further permits a rational examination of the role of different memory systems in the maintenance of personality traits, and leads us to question whether a therapeutic approach that relies primarily on the declarative memory system could have a significant impact on character. A therapeutic emphasis on the content that passes between therapist and patient (free association or interpretation, say), rather than on the process of the interaction, may be beneficial in some ways, but it seems likely that it would leave character unaffected.

There are a number of interesting implications of the fact that procedural memory antedates the development of declarative memory. First, evolution equips babies and toddlers with the capacity for procedural learning, permitting the development of behavioral repertoires for maintaining proximity to their parents. Infants learn how to transact with and feel their way through their immediate interpersonal environment by learning processes of interaction, without the use of verbally mediated declarative memory. With continued cognitive development, children gradually begin to acquire a different way of encoding experience based upon declarative (semantic and episodic) memory, and the representations of the world associated with this new way of encoding memory may or may not dovetail with the procedural knowledge of the earliest years of life. The time during which the procedural learning system is more dominant than the declarative memory system is likely to be critical for establishing the basic outlines of character. The subsequent acquisition of speech, and the capacity to affect the interpersonal world with language, may lead to a whole new mode of interpersonal relationship that may in fact be essentially split off from procedural knowledge.

16

BIOLOGY OF THE SELF

INTRODUCTION

In this chapter, we focus on the *self*: what would the self be if it were conceptualized as an emergent set of processes of a self-organizing modular distributed system? We will present neuropsychological research consistent with the hypothesis that the self, however it is construed, is likely to have a modular architecture. We will focus specifically on findings suggesting that any potential self-representation is mediated by a distributed neural network comprising an integrated set of perceptual, cognitive, and emotional subcomponents. Each network has a probability of activation determined by a number of different control parameters. Thus, physiological state, character, temperament, the social and nonhuman environment, and other factors affect the specific probabilities associated with activating any particular self-representation. As with other emergent properties, we assume that the process of self-representation interacts with and influences (to some degree) the biological and environmental conditions from which it emerges.

We believe it is conceptually useful and empirically justified to consider *self-representation* and *awareness of self* as dissociable phenomena. Thus there can exist self-representation without self-awareness. People with severe injury to the prefrontal cortex, for example, may have self-representations but have a severely limited ability to examine actively or reflect upon the self. We also suggest that self-representations are hierarchically organized. Some complex self-schemas are very abstract and relatively free from the ebb and flow of events. Others are entirely dependent on specific contextual variables or dynamic factors. Furthermore, people are capable of only a single unitary representation of self at any given moment in time.

Because the self is a process and not an entity, the psychological experience of self-continuity must be a sort of complex illusion that is re-created from moment to moment.

WHAT IS THE SELF?

The concept of the self is of fundamental importance for any attempt to explain human personality, but self is nevertheless difficult to define. In fact, trying to define the self can lead to peculiar intellectual contortions. Consider Søren Kierkegaard's definition of the self in *The Sickness unto Death* (1849/1954). He wrote that, "the self is a relation which relates itself to its own self, or it is that in the relation [which accounts for it] that the relation relates itself to its own self; the self is not the relation but [consists in the fact] that the relation relates itself to its own self" (p. 147). How clear it all becomes when expressed in this manner! Moreover, this definition raises several important questions. Most importantly, what hallucinogens were available to Kierkegaard and the philosophers of his day? Were they eating mushrooms or smoking opium? Should Kierkegaard have been forced to undergo random drug screening? Is it any wonder that he wrote *The Sickness unto Death* using a pseudonym ("Anti-Climacus")?

Schafer (1976) remarked on the difficulty inherent in discussions of the self. He noted that "self and identity are not things with boundaries, contents, locations, sizes, forces, and degrees of brittleness. And yet these terms have been used in theoretical discussion as if they refer to things with these properties" (p. 188). He further addressed the protean meanings associated with the term: "For example: I hit myself; I hate myself; I'm self-conscious; I'm self-sufficient; I feel like my old self; I'm selfish; my humiliation was self-inflicted; and I couldn't contain myself. Self does not mean exactly the same thing from one of these sentences to the next. It means my body, my personality, my actions, my competence, my continuity, my needs, my agency, and my subjective space. Self is thus a diffuse, multipurpose word" (pp. 189–190).

Concepts of the self tend to fall into one of two categories. Many theorists have considered the self to be a single, unitary mental structure that is stable and consistent over time (e.g., Allport, 1955). Others approach the problem from a different perspective, arguing that there are multiple selves, in some cases as a function of the environmental context (Allport, 1961; Lewis & Brooks-Gunn, 1979; Lichtenberg, 1975; Stern, 1985). The existence of multiple selves was the position of William James (1890), who maintained that there were separate selves for each of a person's many social roles. Mitchell (1993) suggested that self experience is emergent from the tension between the experience of a unitary self and the experience of multiple selves. Ogden (1994) argued that Freud saw the self as "decentered," emergent from the dialectic that existed between unconscious processes and a sense of self associated with consciousness. However self is conceived, it commonly is considered to be the participant-observer in experience, the "initiator of action" (Pine, 1985), and it usually is supposed to possess the quality of agency.

In the present model, we suggest that self is an emergent property of the brain's self-organizing modular architecture. (The modifier "self-" in the term *self-organizing* refers to a process discussed earlier, not to the concept of a self.) We maintain that there is no unitary self, nor in any strict sense could there be such a thing. At the same time, we do not contend that there are multiple selves. Instead, the "self" is actually composed of a large number of (often overlapping) internal representations of who one takes oneself to be. These representations vary as a function of physiological/emotional state and environmental conditions. Because of several factors, including the dynamics of neural networks and the limited capacity of conscious processing, people ordinarily can experience fully only one self-representation at a time. That is, one cannot fully experience oneself as simultaneously having two independent selves. Consequently, we experience a phenomenological sense of unitary selfhood.

ORGANIZATION OF THE SELF

We consider the self to be a complex, hierarchically organized functional system composed of many representations, each of which is a complex hierarchical system with many subcomponents of its own. In what follows, we have attempted to dissect out these subcomponents in order to reach a clearer understanding of the self. The reader should keep in mind that here we use the word *self* to refer to self-representations—models of what and who one is—and that we consider these representations separate from the *awareness* of those representations.

Self is an emergent property of a complex hierarchy of neural processes, a set of models of who one is, a complex network of representations, integrated into the model of the world created by the brain and qualitatively similar in important respects to that model. Each individual has many such representations, although only one self-schema can be fully active at any given time. As these self-representations develop through childhood, so does the capacity of the individual to organize and explain his or her experience.

MAJOR PURPOSES OF THE SELF

Having a self appears to serve several useful functions, among which the most important include the following: (1) providing one with information about one's physical presence in the world; (2) representing one's emotional and motivational state; (3) organizing and stabilizing one's interactions in the social sphere; and (4) explaining one's behavior and providing meaning to events. The first of these functions is addressed by the body schema, the most basic level of the hierarchical self. At a somewhat higher level, the self interprets various feelings, moods, and drive states (S. Schachter & Singer, 1962; Zajonc, 1980). At an even higher level, the self has an important social role (Mead, 1934/1974), an idea consistent with the findings of ethologists, primatologists, and others that species seeming to have clearly defined self-reflective awareness (humans, great apes, and possibly a few other species) have complex social environments and interactions (Gallup, 1970, 1982, 1994a, 1994b; Lethmate & Dücker, 1973; Miles, 1994; Parker, Mitchell, & Boccia, 1994; Patterson & Cohn, 1994; de Waal, 1996). In Chapter 11 on primate cognition, we reviewed research indicating that, among primates, the possession of reflective self-awareness appears to be associated with the capacity to participate in very complex social behavior. Finally, studies of corpus callosotomy ("split-brain") patients suggest the possibility that the self may provide reasons, after the fact, for nearly everything we do.

SELF-REPRESENTATIONS AND SELF-AWARENESS

Self-representation and self-awareness are dissociable processes mediated by different neural networks. Self-representations occupy a more basic place in the hierarchy of processes related to self than does reflective self-awareness. Like other perceptual data, self-representations are complex phenomena that may be associated with extensive cognitive elaboration. These perceptual representations of who a person is may gain access to consciousness by means of the same process through which visual or other perceptual stimuli enter awareness. At the risk of considerable oversimplification, self-awareness, which frequently is impaired by lesions of the prefrontal and parietal association areas, consists essentially of attention focused on currently active self-representations.

Lewis (1990, 1994) distinguished between these levels of the self hierarchy by referring to self-representations as "the machinery of the self," or "subjective self-awareness," and to self-awareness as "the idea of me," or "objective self-awareness" (see also Duval & Wicklund, 1972). Self-representations are psychologically essential for organisms to differentiate themselves from the environment and to be able to produce effects on the environment. This representational aspect of the self is common among animals. For example, a dog that has run into barbed wire once or twice quickly learns to jump between or over the wires, or to go around the fence. It has a means of representing its own body and its movements within the matrix of its representation of the world, and this permits adaptive behavior. On the other hand, dogs do not, or so it appears, have an "idea of me," an ability to reflect on themselves as individuals (Gallup, 1994a, 1994b; Parker et al., 1994).

Among humans, simple self-representations may be present from early infancy onward, while the capacity for self-recognition appears to be a developmental acquisition, possibly associated with a growth spurt in the prefrontal cortex, at about the age of 18 months (Lewis, 1990, 1994). Prior to that age, infants show no signs of recognizing themselves in a mirror (Lewis & Brooks-Gunn, 1979). According to Lewis (1994), "visual recognition of the self appears to occur no earlier than 15 months and, except for autistic children and children who do not possess a mental age of 15–18 months, it is achieved by all children by 24 months" (p. 23). Within the broad limits imposed by biology, self-schemas are learned from experience in the world, especially changes in the synaptic structure of the brain (Grigsby & Hartlaub, 1994; Grigsby et al., 1991).

These potentially activated self-representations are memories, and generally are automatically and unconsciously activated in the same way that other kinds of memories are activated. A self-representation is mediated by a distributed neural network that includes an integrated set of perceptual, cognitive, and emotional components. Such neural networks remain relatively constant over time, although they may vary considerably as a function of changes in either the internal or external environment. To a large extent, these networks represent an amalgam of declarative (especially perceptual) and emotional memories, and they may be strongly associated with episodic memories. In being mediated by these memory systems, self is distinct from character (which may be understood as a manifestation of procedural learning).

LIMITATIONS OF THE SELF AS A REPRESENTATION

Although the self is psychologically important, as a functional system it has a number of significant and fundamental limitations. First, the self "is an incomplete representation of the mind sufficient only to create the unique subjective experience of self-awareness" (Johnson-Laird, 1987, p. 256). An individual self-representation is a model, a convincing caricature with its roots in experience, especially experience early in life. It is who we learned that we are in relation to other people, and it is an accurate representation only insofar as it realistically reflects one's place in one's family and primary social group, and one's experience in bumping up against the world. The self also is limited in that it is privy to only a minuscule amount of the processing that takes place in the brain, so that the self cannot know most of what there might be to know about its own functioning; the self can only model this information in a shorthand manner.

Self-representations ordinarily do an adequate job of modeling one's identity, despite the fact that they are not entirely accurate. Psychologically, they are capable of conveying relevant information to an individual even if they are not representative of the biological phenomena. Besides being limited in the amount of information they can capture, self-representations are in other ways somewhat inaccurate as portrayals of oneself. First acquired in infancy in association with others' responses to and attributions about the developing child, self-representations are altered over time in conjunction with new experience and cognitive development. Yet, even among persons with an ideal temperament and developmental history, at best a self-representation can only be a plausible, reasonably accurate depiction of who one is. The distinction between a "true" and "false" self (Laing, 1960; Winnicott, 1960/1965), although it may be useful phenomenologically insofar as a true self better reflects one's experience, is in another sense misleading. There is no unitary self, and no self-representation is "real" or "true." All are partial, and only more or less accurate, depending on the situation.

THE HIERARCHICAL NATURE OF THE SELF

Self-representations are hierarchically organized, with more general, abstract schemas at higher levels of the hierarchy and more specific, context-dependent representations at lower levels (Cantor & Kihlstrom, 1987; Stuss & Benson, 1987). Other hierarchical models of self have been proposed (e.g., Kihlstrom & Klein, 1994; Schell et al., 1996, p. 171) but these tend to "focus on a particular type of self-knowledge—people's trait conceptions of themselves" (Schell, Klein, & Babey, 1996), and assume that (at least in lower levels of the hierarchy) self-representations are based on knowledge of one's own behavior.

An individual's typical behavior (i.e., his or her character) is dissociable from and relatively independent of the self. Self-representations do not reflect behavior quite so much as they reflect an idiosyncratic interpretation of oneself as a person, in large part in response to others' past reactions to oneself. Other people's reactions are most influential in shaping the self early in development, when their attitudes and behavior interact with temperament to establish a foundation for more abstract, pervasive self-schemas. Others' reactions typically diminish somewhat in importance as people mature, since the foundations of the self already have been acquired. Nevertheless, throughout life they remain a significant variable in determining the activation of both more general and context-specific self-schemas—a characteristic trait of both humans and apes.

The most basic representations in the hierarchy of self-schemas are concerned with the body. These form a kind of template for the development of later, more complex, socially learned representations. The body schema also plays an important role in the acquisition of the capacity to discriminate inner from outer, and self from other. Intermediate levels of the hierarchy consist of behavior- and situation-specific representations of varying degrees of complexity, whereas the highest levels consist of more abstract, general schemas. Regulation of the self system can operate in a top–down manner, in which more abstract schemas, such as those associated with a diffuse sense of well-being, or perhaps with feelings of emptiness and futility, determine context-specific self-representations (e.g., one may feel generally competent, worthwhile, and valued in dealing with one's coworkers). Even the lowest (somatic) levels of the hierarchy may be affected in this top–down manner, so that under the spell of a positive self-valuation, for example, an individual may be relatively unaffected by moderately severe pain.

The regulation of the self system also can operate in a bottom–up fashion, in which both situation-specific and more general levels of the hierarchy are influenced by the body schema. Chronic pain, illness, or the anxiety frequently experienced in the early stages of an acute illness thus may affect one's sense of self both in general terms (e.g., one feels as if one is defective or decaying), and in specific situations (as in the case of an individual who may feel that he or she is contaminating other people). Similarly, one's experience in daily situations may profoundly affect one's predominant self-schema. For example, Biff had been feeling euphoric after successful completion, earlier in the day, of a 3-year long engineering project. On his way to lunch he was cut off in traffic, and the driver of the other car spit chewing tobacco, hitting Biff's vehicle. Biff became furious and spent the next 2 days angrily brooding about "all the scumbags in the world who deserve to be killed" and feeling that he was himself "an angry asshole" and "potential serial killer." Twice in one day his global sense of self had been changed significantly by events.

THE SELF IS A MODULAR FUNCTIONAL SYSTEM

Phenomenologically, humans generally experience the self as a unitary thing. This reflects our limited capacity for conscious processing and the ability of the brain to bind perceptual experience from moment to moment so that we perceive the operation of multiple parallel processors as a seamless, synthetic whole. In fact, there are numerous representations of the self, mediated by numerous neural networks, many of which overlap to varying degrees. We maintain, consistent with others (e.g., Spezzano, 1993; Emde, 1980; Schore, 1996), that during development different self-schemas are organized around specific affective states, each including a corresponding model of the world. Because of the nature of perception, it seems probable that representations of the self and the world, although generated by different modular subsystems, ordinarily are fused—that they come as a complete package and are experienced "in" what might be described (for lack of a better term, knowing that there is no such "place," and given that the experience of self is an emergent property of the activity of many regions of the brain rather than the activity of a single structure) as a *representational space*.

Consequently, when one is depressed, one's perception of oneself and of the world has a particular quality that is relatively consistent from one depressive episode to another and is markedly different from what is experienced when one is experiencing other emotions. In the language of dynamics, the state of depression is an attractor. Its activation tends to be stable across timescales that range from hours to months. Depression organizes one's perceptual processes because cognitive representations of oneself as a bad, worthless, empty, meaningless person and of the world as a futile, withholding, frustrating, unsatisfying place are linked in a Hebbian manner, as a result of experience, with the specific affect of depression (Hebb, 1949). This linkage represents a form of mood-congruent memory. In other words, these self/world representations, or schemas, presumably are mediated via the activation of relatively stable, complex neural networks formed as a consequence of learning. These networks consist of complex arrays of modular subcomponents. The subsystems involved span various levels of the brain's processing hierarchy and include structures that mediate language, sensory imagery, body image, motivation and emotion, and the attribution of meaning to events, as well as simpler levels of integration (Grigsby et al., 1991).

SOCIAL LEARNING AND THE SELF

The development of self-representations is strongly influenced by socialization. It is within social structures and social transactions that one encounters the experience of self as *object* (Duval & Wicklund, 1972). Many authors have argued that what we experience as our self is, in important respects, a reflection of the appraisals of others. To some degree a child must have aspects of its self perceived by its parents and somehow be reflected from them for these aspects of self to gain representation. Infancy appears to be a sensitive period, during which the quality of the others' appraisal is decisive in terms developing basic ideas about one's self.

The affect of shame may have special status as an organizer of self-representations. Rudimentary notions of "good me" versus "bad me" may be established in conjunction with the experience of shame, and are associated with a dread of losing one's position within the larger social structure. Self-representing activity is likely to go to great lengths to exclude shameful experience from representation.

STABILITY AND CHANGE
OF SELF-REPRESENTATIONS

Although different self-schemas (neural networks) develop for different affective and emotional states, consistency in early interaction with one's parents (i.e., a stable history of learning who one is) and a relatively consistent emotional experience are likely in turn to promote a more or less consistent sense of self. Excessive variability and unpredictability, on the other hand, may encourage the organization of rather different self-representations that are *relatively* independent of one another. To a large extent, consistency may reflect the degree of similarity or overlap existing between the various self-networks. We hypothesize that vagaries of neurological integration (e.g., the quality and amount of reentrant signaling, or the depth of the basins of attraction of different self-schemas) set limits, for each individual, on the degree to which behavioral–cognitive consistency and organization may occur. It further seems a plausible hypothesis that variability in this putative biological predisposition toward consistency in sense of self is more or less normally distributed in the population.

It is likely that self-representations acquire stability (i.e., become readily accessible, relatively slow to change, and are activated regularly over the lifetime of the individual, given the proper circumstances) because they are essentially highly practiced, overlearned complex mnestic schemas. Since the processes associated with self-representation and self-awareness are bound by the principles of dynamics, the self-representation that one experiences at any given time is dependent upon events in both the internal and external environments. Furthermore, the activation of neural networks mediating various self-representations is a process over which the individual is likely to exercise no direct control and only limited indirect control. The process of shifting self-representations takes place nonconsciously for the most part, occurring automatically and habitually, and in accord with fundamental dynamic principles.

From what we know about the neuropsychology of memory, it is possible to formulate several hypotheses regarding certain aspects of self-representations. First, these schemas seem to involve primarily emotional (conditioned) memories in conjunction with perceptual (episodic) and some semantic memories. While self-representations may develop in parallel with the procedurally learned behaviors that constitute character, these systems are dissociable, and change in one should not necessarily bring about change in the other. Furthermore, the processes involved in changing self and character should differ. Procedural knowledge changes slowly and incrementally, whereas classical conditioning and the acquisition of episodic memories may occur quickly, and even precipitously in response to catastrophic events.

The capacity for rapid acquisition of perceptual and emotional memories is probably responsible for the fact that severe one-time trauma can induce striking changes in self-representations even among adults. It is not unusual, for example, for catastrophic trauma in adult life to leave an indi-, vidual with a profoundly reorganized sense of self and an associated pervasive sense of helplessness, hopelessness, and impotence. However, self-representations acquired in adulthood in general are liable to be less important determinants of psychological functioning than those acquired in early childhood (and perhaps revised or refined in association with subsequent brain maturation and experience), when there seems to be a critical period for development of the self.

Differences in developmental history may produce qualitative differences in the stability of certain aspects of self-schemas as a consequence of the timing and intensity of events. For example, the experience on one occasion of intense, possibly traumatic affect in response to some environmental impingement may bind together that affect with self and world representations to form a long-lasting self-schema with a high probability of activation. In a similar manner, other such events, inducing different affects, may produce a number of intense, relatively independent self-representations. This might be likely to occur, for example, in an unpredictable, inconsistent, and abusive caregiving relationship. Temperament and current state shape this process to some extent. Other self-schemas may develop in the context of more or less stable low levels of affective intensity regardless of the precise nature of the affect. One might anticipate differences in the degree to which one or the other type of memory would be resistant to change, as well as in the extent to which such schemas might come to dominate one's experience of self.

Assuming that each time a memory becomes conscious it undergoes some degree of change, or at least has the capacity to do so, the same is likely to hold true for the memories that represent the self. Any modifications that occur are likely to be a function of the state of the individual and the situation in which the self-schema is activated. The context of therapy therefore is important in part insofar as it facilitates some modification of the world representation and the affective aspect of a particular self-representation.

As a rule, however, self-representations are liable to change slowly. This is because existing representations have a history of being strongly reinforced, especially those that may have developed during a sensitive period in infancy and early childhood in association with intense affects. It also reflects the fact that the acquisition of a new self-representation as an adult generally is a slow process. First, the individual presumably would be long past the sensitive period for acquisition of such memories. Second, other conditions that contribute to such learning may not be present; for example, high levels of arousal, which potentiate the release of norepinephrine in the amygdala, facilitate the speed of acquisition and robustness of memory consolidation (Liang, Juler, & McGaugh, 1986; McGaugh, 1990). In the case of the memories that constitute the self, the experience of a strong affect also is likely to be an important factor. Thus it is likely that verbal, insight-oriented psychotherapies would induce change in self-representations only gradually. More emotionally intense therapeutic approaches, especially those involving high degrees of arousal, might facilitate more rapid learning of new self-representations.

The presence of high levels of arousal and emotional stimulation may account for the relatively rapid (although frequently somewhat transient) effects on a person's sense of self of such experiences as difficult wilderness encounters. Rock climbing, for example, may generate considerable anxiety as well as arousal, and if the situation is structured so the individual cannot fail, then he or she may learn that it is possible to master difficult, frightening situations and the experience of mastery may affect self-representations positively. It seems likely, however, in high-arousal therapeutic modalities, that the same conditions of arousal and emotional stimulation that might contribute to the ease of memory acquisition potentially permit both favorable *and* unfavorable outcomes; an intense, frightening situation handled badly by a therapist (as with the use of traumatic imagery in the treatment of posttraumatic stress disorder) may further traumatize a patient and perhaps teach him or her that therapy and therapists are not to be trusted.

REPRESENTATIONS OF THE SELF AND WORLD

As discussed previously, perception and imagery rely on the same neural substrate. Not only are there important qualitative similarities between imagery and perception, but examination of certain neuropathological syndromes indicates that self-representations and world representations are different facets of an identical process. The phenomenon of *unilateral spatial neglect,* for instance, raises important questions about the nature of perceptual buffers and the experience they mediate. In unilateral spatial neglect (as was discussed in Chapter 12), lesions of the right hemisphere may produce deficits in the perception of stimuli on the left side of space, in conjunction with a tendency to ignore what takes place on the left side. The severity of neglect varies, ranging from subtle and occasional inattention through a complete unawareness of the existence of things on the left.

It is common, for example, for many right hemisphere stroke patients to deny that the left side of their bodies is even a part of themselves. The left side is not perceived at all, or comes to be perceived as nonself when attention is directed to it. Any clinician experienced in working with stroke patients has seen a number of cases in which patients totally deny that the left side of their bodies even belongs to them. One patient who demonstrated unilateral *asomatognosia,* a denial or unawareness of hemiplegia (Hécaen & Albert, 1978), insisted that he was not paralyzed, when in fact he had a dense left-sided spastic hemiplegia affecting both distal and proximal musculature of both his leg and arm. When asked to raise his left arm, he did nothing. He was asked again and, somewhat irritated, he said he *had* raised it. Asked once more if he would repeat the motion, there still was no response. Other patients might raise the right arm instead of the left, insisting that nothing was amiss.

Since one's experience of the world and of oneself is all a matter of representations, we might consider that there is something wrong with the process of representing both the left side of the body and of the external environment among these stroke patients. When we examine the matter closely, we see that there are at least two main possibilities: either there is a loss of the ability to form a representation or a loss of the ability to direct attention to such a representation. In either case, the result is unilateral spatial neglect.

The research of Farah and her coauthors (Farah, 1989, 1990; Farah & Perronet, 1989; Farah et al., 1989) is consistent with other work showing that patients with significant unilateral neglect are unable to form mental images of the left side of objects (Bisiach & Luzzatti, 1978; Bisiach et al., 1981; Bisiach, Luzzatti, & Perani, 1979). For example, a 72-year-old patient with a right-sided stroke of the posterior temporal and inferior parietal areas was asked to imagine a piazza he had seen many times (the Piazza del Duomo, or cathedral square in Milan) and to describe what he "saw" in his imagination. The patient described only features that would be found in his right visual field if he were actually looking across the piazza in the required direction (Bisiach & Luzzatti, 1978). Subsequently the patient was asked to form an image of the same piazza from the opposite end; once again he described only features found in the right visual field, ignoring the details he had listed moments before. Similar findings were reported in the same paper for an 86-year-old woman with a right temporoparietal stroke. Bisiach et al. (1979) followed these case reports with a study of the ability to detect differences in pairs of visual patterns among 19 persons with right-hemisphere damage. Relative to control patients, the right-hemisphere injury subjects were more likely to make errors in judging similarity about differences on the left side of the pattern but not the right side.

In a third paper, Bisiach and his associates (1981) asked 50 persons with right-hemisphere lesions and 41 neurologically intact individuals to give a verbal description of the cathedral square in Milan, a place that was familiar to all of them. Their findings replicated those of the previous studies, suggesting that "the pattern of brain activity underlying these representations is to a degree isomorphic with the [perceptual] object being represented" (p. 549). It was unclear whether the left side of the visual buffer itself was defective—that is, whether it was impossible to form an image of the left side—or whether it was not possible to direct attention toward presumably latent but not consciously represented images on the left. Bisiach et al. (1981) favored the former interpretation, and research discussed in Chapter 12 provides some support for this explanation.

Not all sensory buffers are equally affected among persons with unilateral spatial neglect. The precise nature of the deficit is a function of the specific areas involved and the extent of the lesion(s). Nevertheless, it is quite common for right-hemisphere stroke patients to ignore both the left side of their bodies as well as all sensory input coming from the left side of space. Thus patients with dense neglect may be severely limited in their capacity to be aware of the left side of representational space, irrespective of whether they are perceiving the world, their bodies, or imagined pictures. For these patients, half of the body schema—a fundamental subcomponent of the sense of self—and half of the world disappear from their experience.

These data suggest that the distinction between representations of the self and of the world is at least somewhat arbitrary. Both self and world, as well as "internally" generated imagery, are represented in a similar neural/mental matrix. If we generalize from the research on visual imagery, in their fully synthesized, experienced form, the representations which appear in this matrix have a number of modular sensory subcomponents—visual, auditory, somesthetic, and others. There probably is no innate system that clearly differentiates inner from outer, self from nonself. While some capacity to make this discrimination may be constitutional (Lewis, 1994), to a certain extent the ability to make the judgments about self and nonself may be learned early in life, and probably in large part is a function of the sensory modality through which information is perceived. In other words, somesthetic, visceral, olfactory, gustatory, and affective stimuli, because they are up close and personal, are the perceptual data most likely to be important for the development of self-representations, while the distance senses of vision and hearing are of primary importance in representations of the world.

Certainly there is some degree of overlap between aspects of these different sensory representations. People are able to see most of the front of their bodies, for example, and can hear the rumbling in their gut after a big dinner of chicken enchiladas—and, in any event, the association of self-representations with specific models of the world reflects the integration of the many perceptual subsystems into a functional whole. Although composed of many modular constituents, it may be that, as represented in the mental medium, self-representations and world representations normally are interconnected. The temporal binding of stimuli would, in all likelihood, synthesize self-schemas, world representations, and affects into a seamless, apparently unified experience.

In order to have self-representations and be aware of them, there must be a neuronal system that allows for these psychological phenomena. Most animals, for example, probably have some kind of self-representations but do not seem to have self-awareness, although the apes and a few other species appear to be aware of themselves. In humans, there also may be relatively specific biological predispositions toward developing particular kinds of self within the constraints imposed by genetics. In autism, the self and self-awareness appear to be very deviant from what is observed among normal persons. But even among neurologically normal individuals it seems unlikely that the nature and organization of the neural matrix of the self, as well as the innate capacity for self-awareness, are invariant from one person to the next.

REPRESENTATION OF THE BODY: THE PHYSICAL ASPECT OF SELF

The first of an infant's self-representations to develop probably are associated with the body schema. In this section we examine in detail some disturbances of the body schema that have been observed as a consequence of neurological illness. The variety of disorders that may occur illustrate the complexity of the system underlying the most basic aspects of what Lewis refers to as the "machinery of the self" (1994). At the simplest level, this will demonstrate the dependence of these aspects of self-representation on an intact CNS. Additionally, careful analysis of the nature of these disturbances may cast light on the biological foundations of normal functioning that ordinarily are taken for granted.

The concept of a body schema can be traced back at least as far as Henry Head (see Head & Holmes, 1911; Head, 1920), who spoke of a "postural model" of the body, and Paul Schilder (1935), who first used the term *body schema (das Körperschema)* to mean "the picture of our own body which we form in our mind" (p. 11). The body schema is composed of both percepts and remembered representations of internal and external stimuli, and its current state is constantly changing. Although there may be a visual component to the body schema, it consists primarily of representations of the feeling of having and using a specific body. Schilder postulated that pain and the ability to control movement were major factors in the development of a body schema, although it seems likely that ordinary somatesthetic and visceral sensation also play important roles.

Like other functional systems, the body schema is hierarchical and modular in its architecture. While it includes a variety of somesthetic sensations of varying degrees of complexity (touch, pressure, pain, heat/cold, kinesthetic sense), it appears also to involve motor representations (Jeannerod, 1994). Felleman and Van Essen (1991) proposed a hierarchical structure for the sensorimotor system that involves 13 somatosensory and motor cortical areas, with 62 connecting pathways, spanning 10 or 11 hierarchical levels, and it seems likely that disorders of the body schema may be produced by lesions of any component of the somatesthetic hierarchy.

Loss (*anesthesia*), distortion (*paresthesia*), or unpleasantness of sensation (*dysesthesia*) may result from injury to either peripheral nerves or the primary somatosensory cortex, and any of these may affect the individual's perception of various parts of the body. Paresthesias, for example, sometimes can be quite bizarre sensations of heat, electrical current, or numbness and tingling. Not only do they draw attention to parts of the body of which a person ordinarily might be only dimly aware, but their unusual quality may affect the sense of self at a basic level.

At a higher level of integration are a number of disorders involving an inability to integrate or interpret intact primary somatesthetic sensation, or to create a representation of the body. These mostly are agnosias, such as the asomatognosia discussed earlier. The denial that one's left side is in fact one's own, and the assertion that it may belong to someone else, despite a preserved ability to examine one's body visually, certainly represents one of the more severe and dramatic distortions of the somatic foundation of selfhood. The primacy of belief in somatesthetic sensation over visual perception suggests the greater importance of the former in the construction of self-representations.

Another disorder of somatesthetic sensitivity, *allesthesia*, frequently accompanies unilateral asomatognosia (Bender, Schapiro, & Teuber, 1949; Hécaen & Albert, 1978). Allesthesia involves displacement of sensation from one location to another. What is most commonly observed is that a touch applied to the affected side of the body is experienced as a stimulus at the homologous point on the contralateral side. The palm of the left hand is touched by the examiner, for instance, and the patient reports the touch as being on the right palm. Lord Brain, a British neurologist, described a patient who seemed to have a variant of allesthesia in which motor representations were displaced (R. Brain, 1941). The patient noted that, upon movement of the left hand, "it seems as if I am using my right."

A somesthetic disturbance at a somewhat higher level of perception is *finger agnosia* (Kinsbourne & Warrington, 1962). This is a syndrome in which the individual has difficulty identifying individual fingers. As most commonly tested, the examiner touches one of the blindfolded patient's fingers, and it is difficult for the patient to determine which finger was touched. Persons with finger agnosia also may have difficulty naming or drawing fingers, and the deficit may affect their ability to perform these tasks either on themselves or on others. Finger agnosia is occasionally the only residual sign of an earlier *autotopagnosia,* a disorder first described by Pick (1908), involving a loss of the ability to identify and locate body parts. It may be either bilateral or unilateral (*hemiautotopagnosia*). Affected individuals, although able to examine their various body parts, are unable to name them. In some cases this may reflect an aphasic disturbance in which there appears to be a disconnection between centers required for naming and those required for recognition of anatomical details. One patient with this disorder, discussed by Yamadori and Albert (1973), was asked to point to his arm. He appeared very confused by the request, stood up and looked around, then returned to his seat, spelling the word "arm" to himself repeatedly. Unable to locate his arm, he finally apologized to the examiner for not knowing what it was. According to Hécaen and Albert (1978), some of these patients seem unable to form mental representations of the body and are unable to draw a human figure, or even crude cartoon stick figures.

One of the more exotic and bizarre sensory disturbances in the literature, most likely to be seen in demented patients, is *exosomesthesia,* a pathological extension of the body image described previously in Chapter 13 (Shapiro et al., 1952). It involves an impairment of the representation of both the environment and the self. Shapiro and associates reported the case of a patient who, when touched on the hand, said that the touch had been applied to objects in extrapersonal space rather than to his hand, despite the presence of conflicting visual information. The fact that these patients are unable to integrate the perceptual data obtained from different sensory systems, or even to persuade themselves of the accuracy of what they see, also suggests primacy of somatesthetic sensation over vision in its contribution to the body schema and to the foundations of the sense of self.

The perception of pain also may be perverted. For example, *asymbolia for pain* involves a diminished reaction to pain despite the fact that the individual remains able to discriminate basic sensations, such as the difference between the head and the point of a pin. Referring to earlier work he had done with E. Stengel on asymbolia for pain, Schilder (1935) described their first patient with this syndrome, a woman who "did not react to severe pinpricks, hitting with hard objects, or pinching" (p. 101). (He did not describe her response to having her nose rapped sharply several times in quick succession with a reflex hammer. One wonders how institutional review boards might have responded to Schilder and Stengel's research protocol.) The patient did not withdraw from painful stimuli, and although she "might sometimes say, 'it hurts,' " she "often readily offered the limb which had been hurt. She even hurt herself. The patient did not show any lack of attention concerning the pain, but on the contrary was very much interested in it" (Schilder, 1935, p. 102). On autopsy, this patient was found to have a lesion in the frontal lobe, and a second lesion extending from the temporal cortex into the posterior parietal area (the precise regions were not specified). Schilder speculated that asymbolia for pain involves an inability to associate the sensation of pain with the body schema. It also may be that the patient's frontal lesion left her indifferent to the pain (a finding also reported among persons who underwent prefrontal lobotomy as treatment for chronic pain; see Freeman & Watts, 1946; Poppen, 1946).

Hécaen and Albert (1978) discussed a number of phenomena that they referred to as paroxysmal illusions and hallucinations, unusual perceptions that occur especially as auras associated with seizures, or as components of migraine headaches. They may occur in some toxic states as well, or in conjunction with infectious illness of the CNS. Although these are quite interesting, we will discuss them only briefly.

The first is a sensation of "absence or loss of a body part," involving one side of the body or a portion thereof. According to Hécaen and Albert (1978), "the loss is usually preceded by paresthesias in the affected body part, followed abruptly by the impression that the body part is missing"; the individual "calls on his other senses to overcome this astonishing impression. He looks at or palpates the body part that seems to be missing" (p. 317), and it frequently requires this additional perceptual information to convince the patient that the part in question has not disappeared. This differs from the loss of the ability even to represent the body part insofar as the individual is at least aware of a sense of having lost part of his or her anatomy. Somewhat similar are "illusions of corporeal transformation," often seen in epilepsy or focal neurological lesions, in which weight, volume, density, thickness, or length seem to change. In *microsomatagnosia* it feels as though a body part has grown smaller, whereas in *macrosomatagnosia* the opposite sensation occurs.

Among the more bizarre of these illusions is the occurrence of paroxysmal phantom limbs. These are rare, and appear to have been reported only in association with seizure disorders. Hécaen and Albert (1978, p. 318) describe these as proceeding through a phase of paresthesias, following which "the patient has the impression of having a supernumerary limb, usually in an abnormal position." In some cases, the affected person will describe a sensation of having an extra hand, or perhaps several extra hands, and there are reports of a few patients having had concurrent visual hallucinations of the extra extremities.

Finally, there are combined visual and somatesthetic illusions, including *micropsia, macropsia,* and *autoscopic* phenomena. In micropsia and macropsia (previously mentioned in Chapter 13), which are frequently experienced in association with feelings of depersonalization and derealization, there is an Alice in Wonderland quality: in the former, one feels as though one has either grown enormously in size while everything else has shrunk; in the latter, one feels that one has grown quite small and is dwarfed by the surroundings. Autoscopic phenomena (Lhermitte, 1951) involve an illusory or hallucinated observation of oneself outside one's body, an extreme form of the sensation of being outside oneself, watching oneself, that frequently is a major component of depersonalization. According to Lhermitte, one believes that one's image is outside oneself and that there is a "spiritual and material" connection with the phantom. Lukianowicz (1958) attributed many of these experiences to migraine auras. Autoscopic phenomena have been described a number of times in fictional literature, including Fyodor Dostoevsky's short novel *The Double* (1846/1945). Given the fact that Dostoevsky himself had epilepsy, it is possible that he may sometimes have experienced autoscopy himself.

These intriguing disorders of the body schema illustrate the very complex, hierarchically organized systems involved in this fundamental somatic aspect of self-representation. In normal functioning, the brain must create a sensorimotor representation of the body that is coextensive with the entire body and that permits rapid, intuitive identification and location of all body parts. The body schema must move exactly as we move, and it reacts by changing in response to a variety of sensory stimuli.

DEFECTIVE SELF-AWARENESS AND DISTURBANCES OF THE BODY SCHEMA

Insight into one's performance and abilities may be affected in any of at least four different ways (E. Goldberg & Barr, 1991; Stuss, 1991). First, a person may be unable even to represent (or attend to the representation of) some part of the body and hence be unable to represent or perceive his or her impairment. This is liable to result from parietal lobe injuries, which disrupt the neural basis of the body schema. It also may become impossible to form stable representations that can mediate the performance of various cognitive, motor, or perceptual tasks. For example, in the case of motor tasks, Jeannerod (1994) argued that *motor imagery* is essential to their performance. These images represent the action, providing the individual with the feeling of executing it. According to Jeannerod, "representing the self in movement . . . requires a representation of the body as the generator of acting forces" and, as is the case with the sensory buffers, he asserts that "these 'representation' neurons are the same as those activated during preparation for actual acts" (1994, p. 189).

The motor representations of which Jeannerod writes are interesting for several reasons. For one, evidence exists to suggest that in the acquisition of motor skills, a combination of mental practice, using imagery, and actual physical practice, produces outcomes that are superior to either mental or physical practice alone. Apparently, as with visual imagery, the same neural substrate is used in each case. In addition, it is interesting that even observing certain movements made by other individuals may lead to the activation of these motor representations. For example, experimental work demonstrates that, in monkeys, certain neurons in the premotor cortex of the frontal lobes are active prior to and during the performance of various actions (Rizzolatti et al., 1988). Moreover, the same populations of neurons are active while the monkeys merely observe a human performing the identical action (Di Pellegrino et al., 1992). According to Rizzolatti (1994), when a second monkey, placed near the monkey from which the investigators recorded neuronal activity, was allowed to reach for food, "the recorded neurons fired every time the second monkey grasped the food, in strict temporal relation with this movement" (p. 220).

A second way in which insight may be impaired is when a person is aware of his or her deficits but maintains an indifferent attitude toward them, apparently failing to understand their severity or significance. Luria (1969) described this as a "disturbance of the critical attitude." This kind of deficit is liable to result from injuries to prefrontal cortex. Fulton and Bailey (1929) described the attitude of such anosognosic persons toward their deficits as one of "fatuous equanimity." Even when the person's attention is directed bluntly toward the defect, the problem is denied—often with a rather indifferent or even insouciant attitude, although sometimes irritably. If the patient is asked to perform a task requiring the deficient function, deficits in the performance are overlooked, as was the case with the asomatognosic patient reported by Olsen and Ruby (1941), described below. The response of persons with a less severe version of anosognosia may be exemplified by indifference rather than denial. Hécaen and Albert (1978), for example, described a patient who, when asked to lift his paralyzed left hand insisted repeatedly on raising his right hand. When he was told that he was raising the wrong hand, his indifferent response was that "I can't on the left; especially with my arm" (p. 304). Following this statement he was again asked to raise his left arm, and he nonchalantly raised the right one.

A third avenue to impaired insight may exist when you are unable actively to compare your performance or capacities with your ordinary reference standard in order to monitor actively the accuracy and appropriateness of your behavior. Luria (1966) suggested that in such cases the unawareness results from a failure to compare one's performance with what one intends to do or is instructed to do. This also is likely to reflect lesions of the prefrontal cortex (Luria, 1980), and may be associated with the indifference, or even euphoria, commonly seen in conjunction with certain lesions of the prefrontal areas.

Finally, awareness of one's deficits may be limited by a degradation of systems that ordinarily provide one with feedback about one's behavior (E. Goldberg & Barr, 1991). This may be the case among persons with aphasic disorders that primarily affect language comprehension (as among persons with Wernicke's aphasia). These usually are associated with lesions of the posterior temporal cortex.

The anosognosic syndrome may assume extreme proportions. Olsen and Ruby's patient (1941), for example, not only denied that she was hemiplegic on the left side, but she insisted that the left arm and leg belonged either to the physician or to some other individual who was sleeping in her bed. The physician demonstrated to her that her left arm was indeed attached to her own shoulder, to which she responded, "My eyes and my feelings are not in agreement; and I must believe what I feel. I sense by looking that they are as if they are mine, but I feel that they are not; and I cannot believe my eyes." This disorder represents a severe disturbance of very fundamental aspects of the body schema. It seems that if an individual has lost the ability to represent part of his or her body, it may be impossible even to imagine that those body parts might possibly belong to oneself.

Anosognosia also may exist in conjunction with other neuropsychological disorders. For example, Olsen and Ruby's patient had a disturbance of the body schema (*asomatognosia*). In her case, there may have been a distortion, or complete destruction, of the perceptual schema that permitted her to be aware of the left side of her body. If the patient described by Olsen and Ruby (1941) had damage to a modular component of a distributed system that permits awareness of a complete body schema, with the result that part of that schema was defective, she may have had no ability even to sense that the left side of her body should feel like part of her. Either the neural basis of the schema itself or the access of that schema to consciousness was affected.

The modular architecture of the system is evident also in the intra-individual variability observed among persons with defective insight. Moreover, clinical experience suggests that some individuals may have deficient insight concerning specific kinds of performances (e.g., memory or cognitive tasks), while insight regarding other kinds of task (such as motor functioning, which may be easier for the individual to observe) is relatively intact.

These deficits in self-awareness are physiological in origin and should not be confused with psychological obstacles to the formulation of certain kinds of knowledge about oneself. In some cases, even very fundamental aspects of self-representation (such as basic physical integrity) are distorted. In other cases, the deficiencies are much more ephemeral and elusive. What is apparent in all of them, however, is a defective ability to form or to be aware of representations that ordinarily are crucial to the experience of normal selfhood.

CORPUS CALLOSOTOMY AND THE MODULARITY OF SELF

The idea that we have multiple selves is an old one, but some of the most compelling evidence for the idea that the self is other than unitary may have derived from the findings of commissurotomy studies (Gazzaniga, 1985; Gazzaniga et al., 1977), which suggest the possibility that people may have parallel multiple selves. Puccetti (1981) even made a case for what he called "mental duality," arguing that "the function of the corpus callosum is to duplicate conscious experience on both sides of the brain" (p. 99), but his proposal has met with considerable controversy (e.g., see Bogen, 1981; Brown, 1981; Churchland, 1981; Eccles, 1981; Geschwind, 1981; Joynt, 1981; LeDoux & Gazzaniga, 1981).

Among the early investigators of the effects of callosotomy were K. U. Smith and Akelaitis (1942), who concerned themselves primarily with the effects of callosotomy on motor skills and on handedness. Perhaps most interesting in their discussion of a series of 18 patients was the occasional occurrence of antagonistic behavior between the two hands: one patient, for example, would be seen doing such things as "attempting to put on an article of clothing with the right hand and pulling it off with the left"; another patient "displayed persistent movement antagonisms . . . such as picking up a deck of cards, putting it down and picking it up" (p. 529). Most of these reactions were transient but nevertheless demonstrated a loss of unified control over motor behavior.

More recently, Gazzaniga, Bogen, and Sperry (1962) reported their findings from the examination of a 48-year-old, right-handed man ("W. J.") who had been having generalized seizures for 15 years following a brain injury sustained during World War II. W. J. could perform spontaneous simple skilled movements with his left hand (such as eating, drinking, and putting on glasses), but if he was asked to perform them by the examiner, the left hand often did nothing, or failed to make an adequate response. In short, he appeared to be apraxic with the left hand in response to a verbal instruction, but not apraxic in spontaneous behavior.[1] In contrast, the performance of the right hand was entirely normal. Gazzaniga and colleagues noted that "frequently, when his left hand had been fumbling ineffectively at some task, he would become exasperated and reach across with the right hand to grab the left and place it in the proper position" (1962, p. 1767). The patient's wife also reported antagonistic behavior such as that described by Smith and Akelaitis (1942). For example, he would pick up the newspaper with his right hand, set it down with the left, then pick it up again with the right hand. Problems of this sort also occurred in dressing and undressing, among other activities, "at times on a scale sufficient to be distinctly bothersome."

Even more bizarre antagonisms, reminiscent of Peter Sellers's character Dr. Strangelove (in the 1964 Stanley Kubrick film of that name), were reported by Kurt Goldstein (1908). His patient's left hand would, on occasion, grab the patient by the throat and attempt to choke her. It was necessary to restrain the rebellious hand in these circumstances. The left hand

---

[1]Technically, W. J. was not apraxic although unable to perform the requested tasks with his left hand. The problem was that his right hemisphere, having no capacity for language, could not understand and then carry out the instructions.

engaged in other troublesome behavior as well, such as pulling the sheets and blankets off the bed. Interestingly, as another indication of the independence of the two hands in persons with a severed corpus callosum, it has been reported that the left and right hands of callosotomy patients may be able to perform two different tasks simultaneously without interhemispheric interference, something generally impossible for persons with an intact set of cerebral commissures.

At this juncture, two implications of these phenomena in particular are noteworthy. First, split-brain patients demonstrate a lack of unified control of the two hands together. The left hand, in certain circumstances, appears to be marching to the sound of a different drummer—an unsettling situation if it happens to be doing something one doesn't want it to do. In addition, without access to the verbal left hemisphere, the left hand (the movements of which are controlled by the right brain) is unable to perform activities in response to verbal command without cuing from the right hand. Schemas for motor behavior can be activated automatically and unconsciously in the course of spontaneous activity, but the cannot be initiated appropriately when it is necessary to use a verbal intention to regulate the behavior.

The right cerebral hemisphere receives visual information from the left visual field, while the left hemisphere gets its input from the right visual field. This peculiar situation, described previously in Chapter 12 on consciousness, permits the independent examination of one or the other hemisphere in persons who have undergone callosotomy. With such a protocol, the patient is instructed to look at a point in the center of a screen and, using a tachistoscope, the examiner briefly presents visual stimuli to one hemisphere, the other, or both. Among right-handed subjects, the brief duration of the presentation ensures that what was shown in the left hemifield projects only to the mute right brain and what was shown in the right hemifield projects only to the verbal left brain (Gazzaniga & LeDoux, 1978).

For example, the examiner might simultaneously project an image of a dinosaur to the left brain (right visual field) and an image of a mouse to the right brain (left visual field). The subject is then asked what pictures were shown and responds that she saw a dinosaur. "Anything else?" asks the examiner, and the response is "No." If, however, the subject is presented with pictures of several different objects, including a mouse, the left hand points confidently to the mouse. The left hemisphere did not report the mouse because it did not see it and because it had no access to the stimuli seen by the right hemisphere. The right hemisphere, however, knows that it saw the mouse. Because it has control of the left hand, it uses that hand to point to a picture of what it saw. This experimental protocol sets the stage for some very interesting studies, one of which we will discuss next.

Multiple Selves in a Single Brain?

Studies of callosotomy patients appear to demonstrate—if not the presence of separate, independent selves—at least the modularity of the functional system that mediates selfhood. In his review of the research, Sperry (1982) discussed the relative independence of the hemispheres and concluded that each hemisphere appears capable of using "its own percepts, mental images, associations, and ideas" (p. 1224). Moreover, a patient's right hemisphere is able "to recognize his or her face among an array of portrait photos, and in doing so, generates appropriate emotional reactions and displays a good sense of humor requiring subtle social evaluations" (p. 1225). Overall, the findings "suggest the presence of a normal and well-developed sense of self and personal relations along with a surprising knowledgeability in general" (p. 1225), as well as an ability to anticipate the future.

One of Gazzaniga's split-brain patients, a 15-year-old boy identified as "P. S." (discussed previously in Chapter 12), had a right hemisphere that was "mute" but was able to read, and with the left hand could spell out words using Scrabble letters. Gazzaniga presented questions verbally to P. S. but left out key phrases. The missing phrases were projected to P. S.'s right hemisphere using the tachistoscope. For example, he was asked "Who?" The words presented by the tachistoscope in this case were "are you?" In response, the left hand selected the appropriate letters and correctly spelled out the name "Paul." In like manner, the right hemisphere was asked the name of Paul's girlfriend, his favorite hobby, and his favorite person, and it responded accurately to all of these. The right hemisphere could report correctly that the following day would be Sunday, and it described its mood as "good." Interestingly, when asked what job it would like to have, the right hemisphere responded "automobile race," in contrast to the verbal hemisphere's stated preference for becoming a draftsman (Gazzaniga & LeDoux, 1978, p. 143). The authors noted the following details:

> The right hemisphere in P. S. possesses qualities that are deserving of conscious status. His right hemisphere has a sense of self, for it knows the name it collectively shares with the left. It has feelings, for it can describe its mood. It has a sense of who it likes and what it likes, for it can name its favorite people and its favorite hobby. The right hemisphere in P. S. also has a sense of the future, for it knows what day tomorrow is. Furthermore, it has goals and aspirations for the future, for it can name its occupational choice. (Gazzaniga & LeDoux, 1978, pp. 143–144)

Puccetti (1981), on the basis of such data as these, argued that the split-brain studies suggest there are two "selves." His position generated considerable comment. As Joynt (1981) wrote regarding Puccetti's paper, "consciousness is like the Trinity: if it is explained so that you understand it, it hasn't been explained correctly." He criticized Puccetti's (1981) attempt to posit "mental duality" on the basis of the callosotomy studies and to "draw a fence around" the two hemispheres, when in fact "there are many fences and they are forever shifting" (Joynt, 1981, p. 108). Just as the apparently unitary self of everyday experience is unmasked by commissurotomy, so may the right and left hemisphere "selves" be made up of various subcomponents.

In certain callosotomy patients (and here Gazzaniga and LeDoux [1978] suggest that it may be only those cases in which the right hemisphere possesses some capacity for language), and under carefully designed conditions, different facets of the self system stand exposed. Such evidence of split awareness is not apparent among persons with an intact corpus callosum. Presumably this is in part because the dominant (usually left) hemisphere exerts an inhibitory influence over the nondominant hemisphere when the two are joined by the cerebral commissures. Because the brain is a self-organizing system, with the synthesizing emergent properties peculiar to such systems, most of the time people feel they have a stable, consistent, and unitary sense of self.

Given our definition of self as one's current emergent self-representation, it seems clear that there are potentially a great many "selves." Our tentative inference, perhaps in accord with Joynt's (1981) is that "the self" is capable of fractionation so that different combinations of brain subsystems may yield different patterns of emergent self-like properties. Whether one wishes to consider these to be separate "selves" or not, it seems plain that the functional system we call the self is composed of a large number of self-representations, organized at different levels of complexity, and that the specific representation in awareness at any given time is a function of internal and external context. Each self-representation (which is mediated by a neural network) is in essence a subcomponent of the functional system of the self, and each of these neural networks is composed in turn of a number of modular units (including affect, perception, and cognition), each of which also is a modular system.

THE SENSE OF CONSISTENCY OF SELF

The brain's remarkable capacity for synthesis allows for a unitary experience of self in spite of the fact that it is constructed of countless modular components. Most people, most of the time, perceive themselves as consistent and whole. Even persons with cyclothymic or bipolar disorders who show regular oscillations in mood usually describe their selves in a way that is consistent with their mood. A manic person, while manic, may feel unlimited power and grandiosity, and may expect always to remain that way.

When depressed, however, he might as easily feel worthless, experiencing the world as a cruel and unsatisfying place. In the face of all one's possible self-representations, the sense of relative consistency that most people experience over time probably is a function of several factors.

We previously discussed the idea that the self, like other emergent psychological processes, can be characterized by its tendency to maintain itself in the vicinity of critical states. The reader will recall that this mode of functioning leaves the system perched near the edge of bifurcation. As a result of minor variations in internal control parameters or environmental conditions, new organizations of self-representation may emerge. We also have seen that states near criticality, despite their likelihood of bifurcation, are nonetheless characterized by a certain stability. This dynamic stability is responsible for a sense of continuity of the self.

Limitations on the content and temporal duration of conscious processing also may serve to inhibit the experience of having more than one self. Consciousness will entertain only a small amount of information at any given time, and—without rehearsal—most of what passes through awareness is forgotten in as little as 20 seconds. Given the complexity of the neural arrays subserving self-representations, it is likely that under normal circumstances an individual would be incapable of intensely experiencing more than one complex self–world representation at a time. When one representation passes out of awareness to be replaced by another, the continuity of consciousness generally is unbroken, providing a sense of continuity to experience despite the shift in sense of self. Under ordinary circumstances, within the context of any given self-representation, an individual usually feels consistent and feels that this experience reflects the person he or she actually is.

Another likely factor in this process is the fact that competitive, mutually inhibitory processes are common in the nervous system. These serve the purpose of permitting the activation of specific behaviors or representations while inhibiting the activation of others that may be irrelevant or inappropriate. These processes occur at the level of interactions between individual cells (as is the case with mutual lateral inhibition in the visual cortex) and at the level of large populations of cells. When activated, some cells, and some populations of cells, exert inhibitory influences on other cells or cell groups. One inference we can draw from the work with callosotomy patients, for example, and from the tendency they show toward relative independence of the two hemispheres, is that the dominant hemisphere in normal individuals serves to regulate expression of the nondominant hemisphere, providing a single final common pathway (instead of two final common pathways) for all types of activity.

For many individuals, the current self-representation at times may reflect a sort of emergent compromise between different self-representations (recall our previous discussion of phase space—a self-representation at any given time potentially could be mapped in some multidimensional self phase-space). We assume that self-representations and world representations are mnestically associated with specific affects in a more or less coherent neural network and that the activation of an affect thus induces activation of a self-schema. The emotional aspect of affects, presumably mediated by structures such as the amygdala, and interacting with motivational state (e.g., lateral hypothalamic activity and the sensation of hunger), level of arousal, and activity level, varies across time even within the context of a single predominant mood such as depression. Hence, location of mood in "state space" may be rather variable, although it tends to fall into certain attractors. Consequently, an individual may experience varying degrees of retarded depression, agitated depression, or something in between, and may have feelings of self-loathing, or emptiness and futility. The precise combination of these at any given time may determine the exact nature of the self-schema that is activated, by recruiting different but overlapping ensembles of neurons. It also is likely that there is considerable overlap from one self-schema to another with respect to the neurons, and patterns of neurons, that are involved.

Finally, studies of certain commissurotomy patients (Gazzaniga, 1985; Gazzaniga & LeDoux, 1978; Gazzaniga et al., 1977) have suggested that the primary possession of language by the left hemisphere may provide a sense of unity to experience. Certainly, the facility with which the verbal hemisphere can explain behavior initiated by either hemisphere suggests that the possession of language could generate a sense of more or less coherent meaningfulness.

PSYCHOPATHOLOGY AND THE MODULAR SELF

It seems probable that the modular, hierarchical nature of the self gives rise to many of the disturbances of the self system observed in schizophrenia, posttraumatic stress, dissociation, and disorders such as the borderline personality. The extreme "splitting" of the self observed in severely borderline patients, for example, is possible because the self is not unitary but is fundamentally composed of a number of distinct self-representations. In fact we suggest that individuals who possess an extreme form of borderline personality organization may have a constitutional predisposition (perhaps involving a reduced efficiency of neural integration) as a substrate for the relative independence of very contradictory self-representations and world representations. The idea that borderline patients may have a subtle neurological deficit is not new, as findings of an increased incidence of soft neurological signs among persons with personality disorders previously have been reported (Cowdry, Pickar, & Davies, 1985; D. Gardner et al., 1987; Quitkin, Rifkin, & Klein, 1976; Shaffer et al., 1985).

It appears likely that certain kinds of psychopathology may result from "synthetic" failures. Without minimizing the importance of experience in the development of these character disorders, we argue that borderline personality disorder (or any other type of psychopathology characterized by splitting, dissociation, or fragmentation) likely involves a disruption of certain aspects of the brain's capacity for integration of the various self-representations. This hypothesis also suggests an explanation for the fact that, given qualitatively similar adverse early environments, some individuals will develop a borderline personality disorder whereas others will show much better organization in their psychological functioning.

Psychopathology of the self also may reflect a disturbance of the balance, near criticality, between the brain's tendency to operate in a routine, stable, automatic manner, on the one hand, and its propensity to enter bifurcations, on the other. Thus, some individuals may be unable to respond to diverse social contexts with adaptive shifts in role behavior, instead behaving in a somewhat stereotyped, relatively rigid manner across situations. It seems that a good deal of character pathology can be understood as reflecting an inability to recognize and respond appropriately to the demands of different social situations. Conversely, some pathology may be secondary to a self system that is too prone to bifurcation. Some traumatized individuals, or persons who are easily dysregulated for various reasons, may be prone to such maladaptive bifurcations of self-representations.

Navigating psychological development requires a periodic reorganization and modification of self-representations, a process requiring considerable psychological flexibility. Adolescents, for example, seem deliberately to seek different models of self, in the service of allowing the emergence of new representations that facilitate separation and individuation. They may actively repudiate self-representations consistent with earlier developmental periods. An inability to redefine oneself in accord with developmental demands while maintaining some sense of continuity could possibly lead to developmental psychopathology.

Finally, some failures to represent experience or aspects of the self adequately might limit behavior potential and could be implicated in psychopathology. Fonagy has proposed that one type of failure of representation results from a deficiency in the capacity for what he calls "mentalizing" of experience (e.g., see Fonagy, 1991; Target & Fonagy, 1996).

SUMMARY AND CONCLUSION

From our perspective, the functional system of the self is composed of a large number of hierarchically organized self-representations, each subserved by different but generally overlapping neural networks. The hierarchy includes schemas at different levels of complexity, from high-level abstract representations that regulate the activation of intermediate- and lower-level representations, down to basic aspects of the body schema. Activation of schemas may operate in either a top–down or bottom–up manner.

Each of these schemas includes a representation of the self as well as of the world, seamlessly bound together with a specific affect. Self and world are experienced simultaneously in the same "representational space," and many of the distinctions between the two (especially subtle ones), which are arbitrary from the brain's perspective, are learned early in development. The self consists of an amalgam of emotional and perceptual memories, and may include semantic memory as well. As such, its acquisition and change involve different processes, are facilitated by different means, and occur on a different timescale than does acquisition and change of character.

Such disorders as borderline personality and dissociative states may reflect disturbances in which the neuropsychological integration of the self system is deficient. Neurological disorders may produce a fundamental disruption of the cognitive foundations of the functional system of self, whereas in neurologically intact individuals, self-pathology may be more likely to involve more traditional disorders, such as pathological narcissism or psychopathy, and to reflect the influence of temperament and learning.

17

GENERAL PRINCIPLES OF CHANGE

INTRODUCTION

A major aim of this book has been to elucidate the biological underpinnings of stability and change in personality. We therefore have dealt with this issue in bits and pieces scattered throughout the preceding pages, but in this final chapter we hope to distill certain fundamental principles of change with which any viable personality theory must be in agreement. In attempting to present in a more organized fashion a number of ideas pertaining to personality change, we offer tentative answers to several important questions. How and in what ways do people change? What kinds of behavior change are really possible? What are the limits on the kind of changes that can occur? At a neural level, how does change occur, and can these processes be controlled? What factors promote or retard change?

Philosophers, physicians, behavioral scientists, and laypeople have addressed these questions, with varying degrees of success in developing implicit or explicit theories about the mechanisms of change. The history of psychology is replete with efforts to develop systematic strategies to change behavior. Insight, catharsis, abreaction, social learning, operant conditioning, classical conditioning, self-actualization, self-acceptance, hypnotic suggestion, corrective emotional experience, ego integration, habituation, relaxation, meditation, medication, implosion, *in vivo* flooding, punishment, education, making the unconscious conscious, and systematic desensitization are among the many means proposed for inducing change. Some of these mechanisms are better researched, supported, and understood than others. For example, there is, no scientific documentation of the efficacy of past lives therapy, but a considerable amount of supportive evidence exists for upholding the value of treating phobias by means of systematic desensitization. Similarly, classical conditioning is much easier to explain, identify, and demonstrate than is self-actualization.

PERSONALITY TENDS TO BE RELATIVELY STABLE OVER TIME

Personality tends to remain consistent across a lifetime. In a summary of the literature on the stability of personality, McCrae and Costa (1994) concluded that one of the most definitive findings of psychological research is that "an adult's personality profile as a whole will change little over time" (p. 173). Trauma, serious injury or illness, mystical experience, or other significant events may produce a lasting effect on a person's attitudes and behavior, but even in such cases certain aspects of personality functioning remain constant.

Attending a high school reunion provides considerable evidence that some things never change. Former classmates no longer have the same adolescent concerns but nevertheless are recognizable in many ways—attitudes, gestures, manner of speech all may be strikingly similar. It even may be the case that they find themselves drawn to old patterns of interaction—an expression of interpersonal procedural learning processes, such as were just discussed in Chapter 16. The same kind of phenomena characterize family reunions. Procedural learning possesses a sort of inertial quality. All things being equal, we tend to behave, think, perceive, and feel in habitual ways across time. Those neural networks are activated that have the greatest probability of activation at any moment, and they tend to be attractors that demonstrate considerable stability over time. As a result, there are indications of stability nearly everywhere we look. Yet, sometimes people seem to change.

SOME KINDS OF PERSONALITY CHANGE OCCUR CONTINUALLY

Despite the fact that it appears stable over time, personality is characterized by constant change. The manifestations of personality have a probabilistic basis; variability in the environment and in the state of the individual alter the probabilities that he or she will engage in certain behaviors and experience specific representations of self and world. Infradian, circadian, and ultradian rhythms influence state, as do myriad perceptual, neuroendocrine, and other factors. Personality thus is a constantly fluctuating emergent property of the activity of self-organizing neural systems (e.g., Globus,

1992; Grigsby et al., 1991). But just as individual grains of sand dropped onto a sandpile produce many small avalanches but relatively few large ones, much of the change that occurs in personality from moment to moment goes unnoticed whereas major shifts in different aspects of personality functioning are infrequent.

Personality is a self-organizing system, an emergent property of the activity of the CNS. Self-organizing systems, by their very nature, fluctuate continually in response to alterations in local conditions. A system's global fluctuations themselves lead to change in local conditions, in turn inducing changes in the global state of the system. This circular feedback process never stops. The manifestations of personality have a probabilistic basis, and those probabilities are determined by the state of the individual and of the environment. Consequently, personality undergoes constant, unpredictable change (D. D. Smith, 1991, 1992, 1993).

While some of these changes are long lasting, associated with synaptic plasticity in response to experience, many changes in neural (and hence psychological) activity are transient, involving responses to stimuli from either the external or the internal environment. The brain "is in constant structural and functional flux" (Black, 1991, p. 3). This activity is mediated by continual changes in ionic conductance, by variability in environmental conditions, by "chemical modulation of transmitter synthesis, release, transport, and reuptake" (G. G. Globus, 1992, p. 301), by glial cell buffering of ionic concentration, and be many other factors. In this way "there is continual tuning going on [and] not even theoretical probabilities are fixed but change moment to moment" (G. G. Globus, 1992, p. 303).

The various systems of personality at any given time are the emergent properties of transiently stable neural attractors. That is, they are stable only as long as the individual's physiological state and other internal and external control parameters regulate the ebb and flow of activity in different neural networks. The system fluctuates constantly, and while most of these dynamic fluctuations are quite subtle, some are more marked. Depending on the conditions at any given time, these fluctuations may lead to bifurcations—alterations in the functioning of the system—which in turn may become stable attractors themselves.

On the psychological level, many such changes are observable. These tend to be as ephemeral as the brief neurochemical processes that mediate them. For example, in the course of a conversation, one may change one's mind several times in deciding how to deal with a certain situation. Momentarily, one may feel persuaded of the correctness of a particular course of action, but this conviction may ebb and flow as one considers different arguments. Examples of similar kinds of change are legion: inspired by a pep talk, one may feel a surge of confidence and energy that lasts all of 15 minutes; suddenly irritated by a friend's subtly insulting comment, one might forget about it in a matter of seconds, or respond recklessly in a way that threatens the relationship; failing to perceive approval on the faces of his audience, a speaker may change his subject, or begin to feel anxious and become disorganized in his presentation.

More enduring changes in functioning involve alterations of synaptic efficacy, changing the probability that activity in one array of neurons will lead to a response in another. In psychological terms, synaptic plasticity alters the likelihood that an individual will have certain experiences or will engage in certain behaviors, in specific situations. Keeping these basic principles in mind is essential if we are to understand different processes of personality change.

CHANGE IN A HIERARCHICAL SYSTEM

The brain's self-organizing activity is a function of its modular, hierarchical architecture. Therefore, change may occur within or across different modular components and subcomponents of the brain and within or across different levels of the brain's hierarchical systems. For example, much of the change that occurs in response to visual experience within a certain critical period during infancy appears to involve the connections between neurons in "lower" levels of the primary visual cortex. In contrast, the changes occurring in the brain of a fellow in neuroradiology who is becoming adept at reading magnetic resonance angiograms involve higher levels of the visual hierarchy.

The same holds true for other functional systems, such as the regulation of behavior. For example, a young child's acquisition of the capacity to control his or her behavior is facilitated by the development of prefrontal cortex and related systems that mediate executive cognitive abilities. Although it may be influenced by experience, this kind of development differs from the establishment of neural networks in response to parental reactions to the child's behavior. It differs as well from the kind of change that must take place when one decides to undertake a prolonged course of action. A decision to go to graduate school requires the use of a very abstract intention to direct many aspects of one's behavior over the course of several years.

THE DYNAMICS OF CHANGE

As a self-organizing system, the brain tends to dwell in or near critical states. As such, much of the brain's operation involves the activation of transiently stable attractors (neural networks). Overall, its activity is marked by a constantly shifting pattern of activation of networks, the activity of which is a function of the state and the environment at each instant. Changes in certain internal or external conditions may lead to bifurcations, involving significant changes in the way the brain functions. Such bifurcations themselves may become stable attractors. Thus, a traumatic experience might cause an abrupt shift in overall brain functioning, accompanied by sympathetic hyperarousal and a freezing response. The learning that takes place in association with such an experience (classical conditioning, episodic memory with vivid traumatic imagery, and procedural learning) may result in a traumatic state and posttraumatic behavioral adaptation that are relatively stable over time and readily activated by a wide range of stimuli.

Psychotherapy also can be conceptualized in terms of dynamics. For example, by maintaining the proper tension in a therapeutic relationship (perhaps by preventing the interaction from becoming too automatic and routine, avoiding the inertia induced by procedural learning), the therapist may be able to maintain the relationship in a close-to-critical state that can facilitate change. Insufficient tension threatens stagnation through the acquisition of largely automatic and nonconscious behavioral schemas that are enacted jointly by the therapist and patient. Excessive tension, on the other hand, may be destabilizing, preventing the development of an effective working relationship and possibly leading to negative therapeutic outcomes.

NEURAL PLASTICITY AND SENSITIVE PERIODS

We owe our capacity to adjust to new circumstances, and to learn and change as a result of experience, to synaptic plasticity. Yet the nervous system does not remain equally malleable across the lifespan. Indeed, it is influenced by a variety of developmental factors. For example, we have seen that there are sensitive periods for the development of certain functions during which the brain may be at its most plastic.

It appears likely that there is a kind of sensitive period during early childhood for the acquisition of character traits and models of self and world (for a discussion of related issues, see Schore, 1996). This is manifested in the fact that basic character dispositions, as well as fundamental properties of self-representations and world representations, evolve rapidly in the first years, at which time they appear to be extremely sensitive to environmental influences. In adulthood, self-representations change much more slowly than they do in the first few years of life, so that more intense or more sustained experience is necessary to effect major changes in the sense of self. Severe trauma—either sudden and cataclysmic or chronic and involving somewhat less intense arousal—can induce relatively sudden and enduring changes in self even among mature adults, permanently altering their experience of selfhood and of life in general.

The same type of thing has been noted by researchers who study the development of gender identity, who have observed that the foundations of stereotypical feminine and masculine personality styles are well established by the end of the second or third year of life (Coates, 1992; Coates, Friedman, & Wolfe, 1991; Money & Ehrhardt, 1972). After that age, gender identity generally is so firmly grounded that anomalous identities commonly are refractory to change through therapy or any other means. Consequently, by the time one reaches adolescence, one's gender identity (even if ambiguous) is well established and is likely to remain fairly constant.[1]

If a child lacks appropriate experience during a true sensitive period (e.g., during the first 6 months of life for attachment, or during the first 5 or 6 years for language), the nervous system undergoes significant changes that are likely to be irreversible. The sequelae of such a developmental history cannot be undone. Thus, failure to attach to a loving caregiver in infancy, or severe disruption of such an attachment at that time, is likely to produce lifelong indelible effects which are manifested both physiologically and psychologically (Field, 1996). Complete absence of a caregiver may render a child forever unable to form close attachments. Among monkeys, "total social isolation for a substantial period of time (e.g., 6 months) in a newborn infant effectively inhibits development of social responses" (Bramblett, 1994, p. 27).

On the other hand, if an existing primary attachment is disturbed in some way (possibly due to parental death, or disrupted by pathological parents), the child presumably will be able to form attachments, but these are likely to be idiosyncratic and maladaptive, as was seen in Harry F. Harlow's studies of maternal deprivation among infant monkeys (Harlow, 1958; Harlow & Harlow, 1973). Disturbed patterns of relationship that are acquired during sensitive periods become templates for subsequent relationships. For example, Pratt and Sackett (1967) studied juvenile monkeys raised in different social settings for a period of 9 months: some had experienced total isolation, some had been partially isolated, and some had been raised among peers. Monkeys tended to prefer associating with other monkeys who shared similar experience (although those raised in total isolation preferred to spend time by themselves), and thus apparently have a similar capacity for attachment.

CHANGES IN NEURAL PLASTICITY ACROSS THE LIFESPAN

It seems that a general decline in neural plasticity across the lifespan may be an especially important constraint on a person's capacity for significant

---

[1] It is unclear to what extent this aspect of identity reflects more basic biological influences, although early learning is likely to play an important role as well.

personality change. Character traits are acquired more rapidly by children than by adults, presumably as a function of greater plasticity during childhood. Although adults remain able to develop habits and may be able to change their character to some extent, the ease with which they do so is probably not as great as it is for children. Perhaps the kind of procedural learning involved in character acquisition is distributed along a temporal gradient, becoming less robust and being acquired with less facility as one ages.

To illustrate the facility with which children acquire the foundations of character structure, consider how quickly they learn to emulate the behavior of parents and siblings—especially when they are very young—and of friends and peers in older childhood and adolescence. Children pick up habits with no apparent effort. Adolescents are notorious for acquiring habitual verbal expressions and behaviors from their peers. The same general phenomenon is observed among young children, who may imitate their parents and siblings. Yet, in contrast to the rapidity of procedural learning among children, by adulthood nontrivial habits are acquired only with persistent practice.

TEMPERAMENT IMPOSES CERTAIN LIMITS ON CHANGE

Temperament is a fundamental template for the organization of personality. Operating on this template, procedural learning shapes character. We are persuaded that temperament, perhaps especially extremes of the sort discussed by Kagan and his associates (see Kagan, 1989; Kagan & Snidman, 1991; Kagan et al., 1992, 1998), sets limits on the possible extent and nature of personal change. In other words, temperament is more likely to guide the development of personality style than to be changed by experience. Under favorable circumstances, a good fit between child and environment permits the acquisition of behavioral routines, via procedural learning, that are adaptive not only in the family but within the wider social context as well.[2]

When the fit is less than optimal, basic temperament is unlikely to change significantly but temperamental predispositions probably shape the development of characteristic maladaptive behavioral responses. Thus an active and outgoing child probably is unlikely to become avoidant and bookish in response to environmental stress, whereas an inhibited child

---

[2]Some adaptations may facilitate getting along in the family but may be counterproductive in other relationships. For example, a learned tendency to withdraw from others, acquired in response to intrusive psychotic parents, may be helpful in the family but not with peers or teachers.

might. In some cases, traumatic, chronically abusive, or otherwise intense kinds of experiences—especially early in life—may be powerful enough to alter certain basic temperamental dispositions. Trauma, for example, may produce conditioned hyperarousal of the sympathetic nervous system (Blanchard, Kolb, & Prins, 1991; Butler et al., 1990; McFall, Veith, & Murburg, 1992; Perry, 1994; Perry & Pate, 1994; Perry et al., 1995), and it is a reasonable hypothesis that the effects of a trauma will vary as a function of an individual's temperament.

Different aspects of temperament may be more or less malleable as a result of experience. Activity level seems relatively resistant to modification except by pharmacological means, and sometimes transiently as a result of environmental manipulation (such as restriction of stimulation for some hyperactive kids). The autonomic nervous system, on the other hand, may be relatively conditionable. We consider it likely that many individuals with personality disorders, perhaps especially borderline and psychopathic personality disorders, would demonstrate variations in certain aspects of brain organization predisposing them to develop specific kinds of psychopathology (Cowdry, Pickar, & Davies, 1985; D. Gardner et al., 1987; Hare, 1978). Among individuals for whom this is the case, the prognosis for change through psychotherapeutic or behavioral intervention is likely to be poorer than when psychopathology is primarily the result of learning. Among autistic persons, who presumably have significant neurobiological abnormalities, there is little likelihood that therapy or medication will enable the individual to approach "normal" functioning.

CHANGES IN PHYSIOLOGICAL STATE

Physiological state can be conceptualized as a complex, multidimensional control parameter influencing behavior by affecting the probabilities associated with the activation of specific neural networks. States themselves, as emergent properties of the brain's self-organizing dynamics, are constantly undergoing change as a result of shifts in internal and external circumstances. Furthermore, physiological state plays an important role in the acquisition of new learning.

An individual's state at any instant is a major determinant of his or her behavior, attitudes, perceptions, and memories. As state changes, so does behavior, and thus state is associated with both adaptive and maladaptive behavior. There are two broad categories of disturbances of state: in some pathological conditions such as depression, the "content" of a particular state is pathological; in other conditions, the problem lies in the regulation of state. Disorders of this sort may be either periodic (e.g., cyclic variability in mood) or aperiodic (emotional lability).

   In disorders of state, associated behavioral pathology (such as suicidal thoughts or behavior) is secondary to the state itself, and the most efficacious approach to treatment may be to treat the state directly. The most rapid and reliable way to change a state is probably through pharmacological means. For example, a CNS stimulant such as methylphenidate (Ritalin) might quickly render a distractible, hyperactive child more compliant and attentive (as we noted in Chapter 10). Antidepressants, over a period of a few weeks, may significantly affect one's predominant mood. Diazepam (Valium) relaxes skeletal muscle and generally alleviates anxiety. Consumption of alcohol, a CNS depressant, may lead to disinhibited behavior.

   These changes are effected by a kind of neurochemical *tuning* of the brain. Although it is true that a specific drug may bind preferentially with one or another receptor protein or may specifically affect a single neurotransmitter (perhaps by inhibiting reuptake of serotonin in certain synapses), there is more to depression than simply a serotonergic disorder. It is highly unlikely that transient, although perhaps chronically maintained, chemical changes at a class of synapses will affect only those synapses; instead, the use of various drugs changes the dynamics of widely distributed neural networks. The induction of a changed state—an emergent property of these altered dynamics—thus has the potential to affect nearly all psychological activity. Therapeutically useful psychotropic drugs are those that tune the nervous system in ways that, for the most part, improve mood or behavior while having minimal adverse effects. They may directly influence only a single receptor protein, but functional changes at the targeted neurons are likely to shift dynamic patterns of activity throughout the entire brain. Similarly, the side effects of various medications may represent unintended or undesirable consequences of this tuning (as is the case, e.g., with the "extrapyramidal" symptoms associated with neuroleptics).

   Not all pharmacological influences are temporary. For example, there is evidence that some of the methoxylated amphetamines (such drugs as 3,4-methylenedioxyamphetamine, MDA, and 3,4-methylenedioxymethamphetamine, MDMA; Grinspoon & Bakalar, 1979) may produce permanent changes in the number of serotonin receptors in the brain. The same holds true for certain other drugs. One recent study (Jentsch et al., 1997) reported that after 2 weeks of twice daily treatment with the dissociative anesthetic phencyclidine (PCP), vervet monkeys demonstrated both lasting impairment of executive cognitive functions and persistent reduction of dopamine utilization in the prefrontal cortex. It is unclear how long such effects might be manifested, but the changes reported by these investigators persisted well past the time when they could have been attributed to direct action of PCP. Such drugs have the potential to produce enduring effects on one's state.

   Physiological state also may be affected, albeit indirectly, by the external environment and by one's own behavior. As we demonstrated in our discussion of dynamics in Chapters 6–10 and 13, changes in the nature or intensity of sensory stimulation may affect state. For example, the behavior of some hyperactive children improves when there are few distracting stimuli, whereas for others improvement may be observed when they are exposed to increased levels of stimulation. To a certain extent, an individual may be able to control his or her state by regulating the environment. An individual who is easily overstimulated may habitually avoid crowds and prefer to be alone. Another kind of self-regulation may be observed among those depressed people who deepen the mood (probably unwittingly) by listening to depressing music; in contrast, others deal with their depression by seeking out excitement, pleasurable sensation, or interaction with other people.

Finally, an individual may affect his or her state by means of cognitive or perceptual strategies. Cognitive therapists who suggest that their patients adopt a more positive attitude toward unpleasant experiences are adopting an approach espoused many centuries ago by the Stoic philosophers Marcus Aurelius (A.D. 121–180), Epictetus, (ca. A.D. 55–135), and Seneca (ca. 4 B.C.–A.D. 65).[3] Such methods have an indirect influence on state and require the individual to expend some effort in going against the grain. If I am angry about what someone has said to me, it may be necessary for me to engage in a low-probability behavior (i.e., one not easily activated in my current state) to get over it. In other words, I might have to make a deliberate effort and avoid the path of least resistance if I intend to have an influence on my state. Even so, because the state I seek cannot be accessed directly and immediately, my efforts may be futile. It is very difficult, for example, suddenly to make oneself angry, or happy, or sad, without some strategy such as imagining an event one has experienced which produced that specific feeling.

Self-hypnosis, biofeedback, and relaxation techniques may be used to alter one's state. In each case, however, it is important that such methods—whatever one chooses to do—be practiced repeatedly until they become overlearned and automatic. In other words, they must be procedurally learned. If they cannot be used automatically and nonconsciously, irrespective of the state in which one finds oneself, they may be ineffective.

---

[3]In his *Meditations* (VIII.47), Marcus Aurelius advised, "if thou art pained by any external thing, it is not this that disturbs thee, but thy own judgment about it. And it is in thy power to wipe out this judgment now. But if anything in thy own disposition gives thee pain, who hinders thee from correcting thy opinion?" (Marcus Aurelius, 1991). Epictetus, in *The Enchiridion* (1948, p. 19), maintained that "men are disturbed not by things, but by the views which they take of things." Seneca held up the example of Zeno of Citium (ca. 335–263 B.C., the founder of Stoicism, who was told that all he owned had been lost in a shipwreck. Zeno responded that "Fortune bids me philosophize with a lighter pack" (Seneca, 1958, p. 100).

SOME TRANSIENT CHANGES
ARE STATE DEPENDENT

It is common for people to have experiences that they believe are life trans-
forming, only to have the effects fade in a matter of hours, days, weeks, or
months. Falling in love, so-called near death experiences, and many situations involving intense affect and arousal (religious revivals, say) may have
such effects. These experiences are associated with specific states, and state
naturally changes over time. Unless one is able to re-create the internal and
external circumstances associated with the original experience, it is unlikely
to recur. Even if one could re-create those circumstances, the fact that one is
making a deliberate attempt to do so may have a significant effect on the
state, rendering it difficult or impossible to achieve what one experienced
previously without effort.

In the case of dangerous activities undertaken for the sake of an adrenergic rush, nothing can ever be quite the same as the first time, when the
situation was novel and it was unclear what to expect. Moreover, one has
learned something from the first experience. Thus it may become necessary
to continually introduce new complications into the activity that will make
it novel again.

LEVEL OF AROUSAL AND CHANGE

Arousal (an important contributor to state), mediated by adrenergic processes and their effects on the amygdala, appears to potentiate the effects of
learning (McGaugh, 1990; McGaugh et al., 1993). High levels of arousal
are present in many traumatic situations and may account for the vivid,
seemingly indelible, intrusive imagery associated with recollections of such
events. Many attempts have been made to use this traumatic imagery therapeutically, with varying degrees of success.

Breuer and Freud (1895/1957), Ferenczi (1923/1980), and Jung (1928/
1959) were among the first to suggest that the systematic use of visual fantasy images with certain patients might be productive. Other authors subsequently have proposed specific uses of imagery (e.g., A. Lazarus, 1981;
Leuner, 1969; Schultz & Luthe, 1959; J. L. Singer, 1974; Stampfl & Levis,
1967; Wolpe, 1958). Fairbank and Keane (1982) and Keane and Kaloupek
(1982) reported the successful use of imaginal flooding in therapy with
combat veterans with posttraumatic stress disorder (PTSD). How such approaches work is not entirely clear. According to Wolpe (1958), the therapeutic value of reviewing anxiety-arousing imagery lies in the concomitant
use of relaxation ("reciprocal inhibition") to lessen the arousal and anxiety.
Other authors have suggested that the use of *guided* imagery provides the
patient with a sense of control over the images.

One approach to the use of imagery in treating PTSD—involving no relaxation, guidance, hypnosis, eye movements, or other such techniques—was described by Grigsby (1987). The patient discussed in that paper, a combat veteran, was simply asked to close his eyes and imagine himself in a specific situation he had described previously, making the image as vivid as possible by attending to auditory, visual, and olfactory stimuli, as well as to the emotions associated with the imagery. This quickly led to a high level of arousal (presumably classically conditioned at the time of the incident), moderately intense affect (although considerably less than with many abreactive therapies), hyperventilation, and involuntary movements resembling myoclonic jerks. These phenomena continued for a little over an hour, punctuated by occasional discussions of what the patient was experiencing. Over a series of 8 or 10 sessions, this approach led to substantial resolution of the patient's PTSD, eliminating the intrusive imagery and significantly alleviating long-standing feelings of guilt (J. P. Grigsby, 1987). Although it is unclear precisely to what we might attribute the efficacy of this and related techniques that rely on visual imagery, we discuss it here because we believe one important element of the successful use of this method may be the arousal it produces.

Just as high levels of arousal produce relatively enduring memories of trauma, it seems a reasonable hypothesis that they might lead to modification of those memories when carefully used in psychotherapy. When the patient is highly aroused, new learning is enhanced. He or she may be able to experience the traumatic memories without suffering harm, in the safe context of a therapeutic relationship. By doing so, the meaning associated with the memories undergoes an important shift; the feelings of helplessness and hopelessness induced by the trauma may be experienced as manageable. It seems plausible that the arousal associated with the recollection of traumatic images—in this approach or in others—thus may leave the patient feeling better able to deal with the associated memories and feelings. The traumatic state itself may become less compelling, and self-representations and world representations learned in association with the trauma may be similarly lose their intensity.

The fact that arousal is associated with robust learning also may account for occasional negative therapeutic reactions when imagery or abreactive approaches are used. When the therapist handles the situation properly, patients may learn that they can master the trauma, that they in fact are no longer as powerless, helpless, and hopeless as they were during the actual event. When the therapist handles the situation poorly, on the other hand, the recall may retraumatize the patient, with high levels of arousal serving further to reinforce the feeling that everything is as bad as it seemed.

High levels of arousal in situations experienced as potentially dangerous may be responsible for some of the therapeutic effect and changes in self-concept frequently attributed to wilderness experience courses and certain other activities (e.g., self-defense courses that attempt realistic simulations of assault as part of the training). When properly conducted, these courses may enable an individual to perform certain risky tasks, such as rock climbing, in a situation in which the chance of failure is minimized. The perception of risk produces arousal, and mastery of the situation in the context of a supportive group environment may have a beneficial effect on certain representations of self and the world.

LEARNING, INHIBITION OF LEARNING, AND CHANGE

Behaviorists and learning theorists realized long ago that to understand development and change in personality, it was necessary to understand the role of learning. All learning presumably involves the modification of synaptic structure, with consequent change in the probabilities of activation of different neural networks. If we accept the proposition that learning is the emergent psychological property associated with experience-dependent changes in neural networks, then it becomes clear that it is important to understand the neural basis of various learning phenomena; the ability to study learning on both the biological and psychological levels of analysis significantly enhances our ability to do this.

All personality change is mediated by complex neurobiological processes. All lasting personality change involves permanent modifications of synapses so the probabilities of activation of different networks change accordingly. Some kinds of structural change result in more permanent modifications—or stronger connections—than do other types of change.

For example, consider *habituation* and *sensitization*, two very basic learning processes. In habituation, one's response to a repeated, innocuous stimulus decreases over time. If you live near an airport, for example, you may have become so used to the sound of airplanes flying overhead that you seldom notice them. An especially loud airplane, however, may produce *dishabituation*, so that once again you become aware of the noise.

Sensitization in some respects is the opposite of habituation. Sensitization involves an *increase* in responsivity to a range of stimuli following the presentation of an intense or unpleasant stimulus. Dishabituation may be a type of sensitization. Thus, you may have habituated to the sound of airplanes flying over your house. Then one day a plane crashes into your neighborhood just a few blocks away. This may produce dishabituation, and also may leave you very aware not only of all the airplanes overhead but of the motorcycles and other loud vehicles passing by your home as well.

Although habituation and sensitization are relatively simple processes, the molecular and cellular processes involved in both are relatively complex and are best understood in fairly simple organisms (Dudai, 1989). Spencer, Thompson, and Neilson (1966) conducted research suggesting that habituation involves an inhibition of synaptic responsivity. Kandel and his associates (Kandel, 1991b; Kandel et al., 1983) found that, at least in the sea hare, *Aplysia californica*, sensitization involves a potentiation of synaptic transmission. In humans, sensitization may be important in the development of an increased startle response as a chronic outcome of certain traumatic experiences.

Habituation can be reversed, but what about more complex kinds of learning? Let's consider classical conditioning (Kim & Thompson, 1997; Pavlov, 1927; Rescorla & Wagner, 1972; Thompson, 1988), in which a stimulus that initially elicits no response is paired, in temporal proximity, with a stimulus that does elicit a response. This second stimulus is called the *unconditioned stimulus (US)*, since it spontaneously causes the animal to behave in a particular way (as, when the smell of food causes a dog to salivate). This spontaneous reaction is called the *unconditioned response (UR)*. The first stimulus, which must precede the unconditioned stimulus, is referred to as the *conditioned stimulus (CS)*, since with time the animal becomes conditioned to respond to the US.

Ivan P. Pavlov's well-known experiments with dogs involved pairing a neutral signal—the ringing of a bell, or a light turning on—with the presentation of food, which typically causes dogs to salivate. Initially the neutral signal produced no reaction in Pavlov's animals, but it was repeatedly presented immediately prior to feeding and eventually became an indicator that meat was about to arrive. Over time, presentation of the CS itself, without the meat, caused the animal to salivate. Although a classically conditioned response may be long lasting, it also may undergo *extinction* if the CS is never again accompanied by the US. Thus, assume that we teach a dog that a buzzer means food is on the way and the dog learns the connection. Then, if we stop following up the buzzer with food, the dog eventually will stop salivating when it hears the buzzer.

However, the original connections serving the CS–US link in a classically conditioned response seem not to disappear as a result of extinction. This is suggested by the fact that following extinction, the original classically conditioned response may be reacquired very quickly and even spontaneously (Jacobs & Nadel, 1985; Rescorla & Heth, 1975). In other words, complete *unlearning* of a conditioned stimulus–response relationship seems not to occur. Instead, the animal undergoes new learning that overrides the older learning, (i.e., there is a change in probabilities).

Certain classically conditioned CS–US links may be acquired rapidly, often after only one learning trial. Kolb (1984) and Kolb and Mutalipassi (1982) argued that classical conditioning plays a major role in the development of posttraumatic phenomena among combat veterans. In particular, they postulated a "persistent conditioned emotional response to external stimuli reminiscent of battle sounds" (Kolb, 1984, p. 241). Kolb suggested that many traumatized combat veterans are prone to respond to such stimuli "with immediate and excessive physiological arousal in cardiovascular and neuromuscular systems" (p. 241).

Research findings regarding the return of classically conditioned learning following extinction raise an important question: once learned, is anything ever really *unlearned*? The answer is not yet clear, but the evidence suggests that, although the slate can never be wiped entirely clean, memories (and the neural networks that mediate them) may be *changed* over time, especially as awareness is directed toward them when they are active. This is because most types of memories evolve over time. Although some individuals maintain that memories are veridical representations of events, it is difficult to see how psychotherapy could produce any kind of significant change in personality if memories, upon which much of personality is based, were immutable.

Thus, new learning presumably often supplants other learning, but depending on the individual's state and the environmental circumstances, the probability of activation of older learned behaviors may be greater than the likelihood of activation of newly learned ones. This can account for the patient who goes home to visit her family and finds herself falling into the same old patterns of behavior that she thought she had shed. The problem is that being in that old, familiar context induced an old, familiar state. The presence of that state made engaging in the behaviors learned specifically to deal with her family much more likely to occur than were more mature behaviors, acquired at a later date.

IMPLICATIONS OF INFANTILE AMNESIA FOR PSYCHOTHERAPY

With the exception of isolated memories, most people recall little of the first 3–5 years of their lives owing to the immaturity during those years of the declarative memory system. This developmental phenomenon is likely to be the source of so-called infantile amnesia (Rudy & Morledge, 1994). Procedural learning and classical conditioning, however, both are operational during this time, and learning via these systems is liable to be implicit, or nonconscious. Thus the child is in a position that ensures the acquisition of many habits and responses, without recall for the events that may have induced such learning. While it is possible that emotional and perceptual memories (phenomenologically, these probably involve primarily the experience of some state) could be recalled from that early time, and while early procedurally learned processes also are likely to be preserved in some form (with these memories modified, of course, as a result of subsequent experience), the recollection of any significant number of episodic memories is very unlikely.

The unavailability of episodic memories from early childhood suggests that therapeutic approaches which attempt to recover or work with such memories may be incapable of producing reliable recall. The attempt to deal with early childhood memories, especially using verbal discussion and interpretation, therefore may be efficacious primarily insofar as it provides patients with a cognitive framework for understanding certain emotional and process phenomena, the meaning of which otherwise is obscure. The therapeutic interpretations made in such a therapy may be correct or incorrect, but if they are plausible to the patient, they may well be acceptable and even therapeutically useful in certain ways. It seems unlikely, however, that they will facilitate recollections from the first few years of life. Unfortunately, most therapists have neither the time, the inclination, nor the ability to seek independent verification of their interpretations, so that such interpretations represent a "best guess" by therapists who are disposed to see certain kinds of patterns in their patients and to draw inferences accordingly.

The availability of nondeclarative memories from early childhood, on the other hand, suggests that therapeutic approaches to working with these types of memories may have some efficacy. Methods of this sort are not uncommon. Ferenczi (1920/1980, 1923/1980, 1925b/1980) and Reich (1949), for example, developed interesting psychoanalytic approaches to the therapy of character pathology, and Levine (see Levine & Frederick, 1997) has devised a technique that relies on awareness of somatesthetic and motor imagery, and procedural learning. There are many other approaches that may in fact have a reasonable neuroscientific rationale (and perhaps many more that do not), but that discussion is outside the scope of this chapter.

CHARACTER CHANGE

As we discussed previously, if character reflects procedural knowledge, one of the most direct and important methods of treating character pathology is to disrupt the automatic nature of the performance of those processes. Often the first step in perturbing the operation of procedurally learned processes is to bring the nonconscious behavior into the patient's awareness. This has the effect of disrupting what ordinarily is an automatic process, and repeated disruptions of this sort further interfere with its automaticity. By increasing an individual's awareness of such behaviors, the procedural memories are modified somewhat over time, especially as they become increasingly likely to be associated with awareness. At first, the effort of the therapist is required in order to make the patient conscious of the manifestations of character. If the therapist succeeds in capturing the patient's interest in these phenomena, the patient's own motivation may play a significant role in working independently on character issues (although an outside observer—the therapist—may be required to point out nonconscious behaviors of which the patient has not yet become aware).

Such procedurally learned behaviors will continue to occur largely outside the patient's control, but the process of repeatedly focusing attention on them may make it possible for the prefrontal systems involved in deliberate conscious control to come into play more readily. When this happens, the patient acquires some capacity to choose to behave differently, to do something other than what comes naturally. The choice may be difficult, however, since it is much easier to engage in familiar, practiced, relatively automatic behavior than to make effortful, deliberate attempts to do things differently. With repeated practice, however (in other words, with repetition of a new, more adaptive behavior in lieu of what is automatic and habitual), the probability of the new behavior is increased, and it may itself become relatively automatic over time. If it does not become somewhat automatic, character hasn't really changed, since it is impossible for a person to go through life making conscious, deliberate choices all day long.

Because character is hierarchically ordered, the most significant changes are those that affect character schemas at a relatively high level, rather than motor habits or simple behaviors. Nonetheless, work must take place on all levels of the hierarchy, and probably it is necessary to deal with many lower-level phenomena before an individual is amenable to modification of higher levels of the hierarchy. This kind of therapeutic work is difficult and demanding, requiring considerable discipline, caution, and self-understanding on the part of the therapist, and a trusting therapy relationship. It is likely that the patient will frequently feel criticized for things he or she can't help doing. Moreover, as the patient begins to gain some sense of control over formerly automatic behavior, there may be a kind of inertia associated with the fact that it is much easier to let one's character do what it is used to doing than to struggle against the current. It thus also requires considerable self-discipline on the part of the patient.

Finally, it is important to recall that character change reflects alterations of the probabilities associated with the activation of different neural networks. Old characterological tendencies will maintain a relatively high probability of activation even as they may be displaced gradually to some extent by the establishment of networks associated with new behavior. To paraphrase General Douglas MacArthur, old habits never die, although they might fade away. Hence, these "old" habitual behaviors, even though less likely to be activated, nevertheless may be readily called up nonconsciously under certain circumstances. They are unlikely ever to disappear entirely from an individual's behavioral repertoire. If no learned behavior is actually ever unlearned, from a dynamic perspective, old behaviors are instead supplanted to some degree by the activity of newly acquired networks which have come to assume a greater probability of activation.

INSIGHT

"Insight" is likely to have a limited ability to produce change in character, except indirectly. Given the dissociability of declarative, procedural, and emotional memory systems, and the rationalizing propensity of the brain, merely *knowing that you habitually do something a certain way* is not the same thing as actually *starting to do something a different way*. While it often is argued that insight itself produces change, in general it has a less than sterling track record. We believe this is because gaining insight is only a first step toward any kind of significant change.

Consider our discussion of character change, for example. The first insight the patient must achieve is awareness of the fact that he or she is acting in a certain way. In itself, this awareness does nothing to change the patient's behavior but only permits the individual to work toward gaining some control. The same holds true for the therapy of perceptual concretizations—no real change can occur until one becomes aware that one views the world in a particular idiosyncratic way and that this unquestioned assumption plays an important role in determining one's relationships with the world. Insight, for the most part, is a precursor to processes that effect change.

In some cases it happens that a person will recall the circumstances surrounding the acquisition of a procedurally learned character process when the automaticity of the process has been disrupted and especially when its occurrence is prevented. Such associative memories may occur, but it seems likely that this awareness is a consequence of—or simply associated with—a shift in character, not the cause of that shift. Because the declarative and procedural learning systems frequently are associated in this way, it may be that an episodic memory, or an event somehow associated with an episodic memory, can lead to the activation of a procedurally learned schema. Similar phenomena have been observed frequently in implosive therapy (Stampfl & Levis, 1967), but it appears that in those cases the insight results from the emotional experience.

SUMMARY AND CONCLUSION

We have attempted to explore a few of the many factors influencing stability and change in personality. We began by reminding the reader that the model we have outlined considers the brain—and its mind—to be in a constant state of flux and that neural and psychological processes at all levels of analysis thus can be expected to show some degree of change from moment to moment. Interestingly, these continual fluctuations take place in the context of a relatively stable personality organization.

The brain changes as a result of experience. While many questions concerning this neural plasticity remain to be answered, enough is known to propose a model of the processes involved in personality change. Personality, like the brain, has a modular architecture. We therefore infer that different aspects of personality are acquired through the action of different memory systems, probably during sensitive periods for such learning. Assuming the correctness of our inference, effective treatment of these different aspects of personality presumably requires that we approach each through the medium of the appropriate memory system. Hence, for example, character may best be addressed through the use of methods that directly affect procedural knowledge, whereas other phenomena may be dealt with adequately via the episodic memory system.

The recall of memories of any type has a probabilistic basis. The likelihood of activation of the neural network mediating a specific memory at any instant is a function of the individual's state and of the environment. This has a number of important corollaries. One is that certain apparent changes in behavior or attitude may be transient, linked as they are to a state that itself is only transient. A second is that the induction of changes in state—directly, by means of drugs, or indirectly by other means (such as exercise, or regulating the intensity of stimulation)—can be expected to yield changes in behavior. A third is that, while in one state, an individual may have considerable difficulty engaging in a behavior associated with another state. If it is desirable for the behavior to be activated in both states, one must—repeatedly, and rather effortfully and deliberately—engage in the behavior when one is in the state in which the behavior is relatively unlikely to occur.

Behavior change is an emergent property of change in the synaptic structure of the brain. The changes characteristic of learning appear to be robust, so that once learned, it may be that most things cannot be completely unlearned. Subsequent learning from experience thus involves the reorganization of neural networks and a resetting of the probabilities of their activation. This process is facilitated by the fact that different aspects of memories change over time as a function of state, the environment, and the specific way in which one experiences the memory on any given occasion. Such changes may be temporary, reflecting only brief neurochemical influences, but they also may be long lasting. The latter type of change may be especially likely under conditions of high levels of arousal.

This model also imposes constraints on the nature and extent of change that are possible. Extremes of temperament, for example, presumably reflecting strongly heritable constitutional characteristics, are likely to be modified significantly only by such extraordinarily powerful influences as traumatic events. In like manner, memories acquired during critical periods of development may be relatively indelible, especially compared with memories acquired after such periods have passed. Finally, attempting to change one memory system through techniques that are appropriate to another may yield disappointing results. We believe the neuroscientific analysis of personality will permit a rational approach to determining what needs to be changed, what *can* be changed, and how to go about it.

FINAL THOUGHTS

In Chapter 1, we argued that "personality reflects the emergent properties of a dynamic, hierarchically ordered, modular, distributed, self-organizing functional system, the primary objective of which is the successful adaptation of the individual to his or her physical and social environment." We noted that the remainder of the book would be spent unpacking, examining, and explaining this single sentence, and attempting to demonstrate the utility of a neuroscientific understanding of the phenomena of personality. Those readers who understood what we meant at the outset presumably were able to skip ahead to this conclusion. For those who found these ideas somewhat less than intuitively obvious, we hope this volume has accomplished its objective.

We have attempted to work on the task of understanding the fundamental links between biology and human personality. Although we believe that the current state of neuroscience provides us with solid theoretical and experimental grounds upon which to address important questions about personality, the effort raises many more questions than it answers. Any such conceptual approach, like the phenomena it studies, will be dynamic and changing. Our focus has been on the biological and dynamic foundations of personality theory, rather than the detailed ramifications of brain–behavior relationships: the former have a more solid empirical basis; the latter have yet to be worked out in detail. It is a fairly safe bet, for example, that the brain is modular and that personality must reflect that organization as well. In contrast, we don't yet have a good understanding of the neurotransmitter systems and neural centers involved in a child's emotional reaction to maternal deprivation.

We have been concerned primarily with presentation of the model, not with a detailed discussion of how it might be applied clinically. The clinical issues are not unimportant, but we have given them relatively less attention because we thought their detailed consideration was beyond the scope of this book. Nevertheless, the model appears to us to have significant implications for the clinical diagnosis, assessment, and treatment of psychological disorders, as well as for the understanding of normal functioning. Even the outline we have sketched seems to point in obvious directions for psychotherapy. The concept of character as the manifestation of procedural learning, for example, clarifies a long-standing and thorny problem for clinicians, and suggests a rational approach to the problem.

Considerable work will be necessary to draw out the meaning of this model for the clinical setting, and to analyze the relationships between this material and traditional theories of personality. In presenting our ideas here, we are not arguing for a complete overthrow of previous understandings of personality. On the contrary—many aspects of existing theories are well worked out and represent valuable contributions to our understanding of human psychology. Instead, we believe that neuroscience provides a frame of reference within which these more psychological theories may be situated, permitting a careful and critical analysis of their individual merits. Perhaps most importantly, we believe that this model facilitates our ability to ask—and answer—substantive research questions about personality.

REFERENCES

Abeles M: (1991) *Corticonics: Neural circuits of the cerebral cortex.* Cambridge, UK: Cambridge University Press.

Abraham RH, Shaw CD: (1992) *Dynamics: The geometry of behavior.* Redwood City, CA: Addison-Wesley.

Ackner B: (1954) Depersonalization: I. Aetiology and phenomenology. *Journal of Mental Science,* 100, 838–853.

Adams RD, Victor M: (1989) *Principles of neurology.* 4th ed. New York: McGraw-Hill.

Adams RD, Victor M, Ropper AH: (1997) *Principles of neurology.* 6th ed. New York: McGraw-Hill.

Alexander GE, Crutcher MD: (1990) Functional architecture of basal ganglia circuits: Neural substrates of parallel processing. *Trends in Neurosciences,* 13, 266–271.

Alexander MP, Albert ML: (1983) The anatomical basis of visual agnosia. In A Kertesz (ed.), *Localization in neuropsychology.* New York: Academic Press.

Allen LS, Gorski RA: (1991) Sexual dimorphism of the anterior commissure and massa intermedia of the human brain. *Journal of Comparative Neurology,* 312, 97–104.

Allport GW: (1955) *Becoming.* New Haven, CT: Yale University Press.

Allport GW: (1961) *Pattern and growth in personality.* New York: Holt, Rinehart & Winston.

Alvarez P, Squire LR: (1994) Memory consolidation and the medial temporal lobe: A simple network model. *Proceedings of the National Academy of Sciences USA,* 91, 7041–7045.

American Psychiatric Association: (1994) *Diagnostic and statistical manual of mental disorders.* 4th ed. Washington, DC: Author.

Anderson JR: (1984) Monkeys with mirrors: Some questions for primate psychology. *International Journal of Primatology,* 5, 81–98.

Appollonio IM, Grafman J, Schwartz V, Massaquoi S, Hallett M: (1993) Memory in patients with cerebellar degeneration. *Neurology,* 43, 1536–1544.

Arbib MA, Érdi P, Szentágothai J: (1998) *Neural organization: Structure, function, and dynamics.* Cambridge, MA: MIT Press.

Arlow J, Brenner C: (1964) *Psychoanalytic concepts and the structural theory.* New York: International Universities Press.

Arnold MB: (1960) *Emotion and personality.* New York: Columbia University Press.

Artola A, Singer W: (1993) Long-term depression of excitatory synaptic transmission and its relationship to long-term potentiation. *Trends in Neurosciences,* **16,** 480–487.

August GJ, Stewart MA, Holmes CS: (1983) A four-year follow-up of hyperactive boys with and without conduct disorder. *British Journal of Psychiatry,* **143,** 192–198.

Baars BJ: (1988) *A cognitive theory of consciousness.* Cambridge, UK: Cambridge University Press.

Baars BJ: (1997) *In the theater of consciousness: The workspace of the mind.* New York: Oxford University Press.

Baars BJ, Newman J: (1994) A neurobiological interpretation of Global Workspace Theory. In A Revonuso & M Camppinen (eds.), *Consciousness in philosophy and cognitive neuroscience.* Hillsdale, NJ: Erlbaum.

Babinski J: (1914) Contribution à l'étude des trouble mentaux dans l'hémiplégie cérébrale (anosognosie). *Revue de Neurologie,* **27,** 845–847.

Babloyantz A: (1990) Chaotic dynamics in brain activity. In E. Basar (ed.), *Chaos in brain function.* Berlin: Springer-Verlag.

Babloyantz A, Destexhe A: (1986) Low-dimensional chaos in an instance of epilepsy. *Proceedings of the National Academy of Sciences USA,* **83,** 3513–3517.

Bachevalier J, Mishkin M: (1984) An early and a late developing system for learning and retention in infant monkeys. *Behavioral Neuroscience,* **96,** 770–778.

Baddeley AD: (1986) *Working memory.* Oxford, UK: Oxford University Press.

Baddeley A: (1990) *Human memory: Theory and practice.* Hove, Sussex, UK: Erlbaum.

Baddeley A: (1992) Working memory. *Science,* **255,** 556–9.

Baddeley AD, Wilson B: (1986) Amnesia, autobiographical memory and confabulation. In D Rubin (ed.), *Autobiographical memory.* New York: Cambridge University Press.

Bailey JM, Pillard RC: (1991) A genetic study of male sexual orientation. *Archives of General Psychiatry,* **48,** 1089–1096.

Bailey JM, Pillard RC, Neale MC, Agyei Y: (1993) Heritable factors influence sexual orientation in women. *Archives of General Psychiatry,* **50,** 217–223.

Bak P: (1996) *How nature works.* New York: Springer-Verlag.

Banks G, Short P, Martinez AJ, Latchaw R, Ratcliff G, Boller F: (1989) The alien hand syndrome: Clinical and postmortem findings. *Archives of Neurology,* **46,** 456–459.

Barkley RA: (1997) *ADHD and the nature of self-control.* New York: Guilford Press.

Bauer RM: (1984) Autonomic recognition of names and faces in prosopagnosia: A neuropsychological application of the guilty knowledge test. *Neuropsychologia,* **22,** 457–469.

Bear MF, Abraham WC: (1996) Long-term depression in hippocampus. *Annual Review of Neuroscience,* **19,** 437–462.

Beckstead RM, Morse JR, Norgren R: (1980) The nucleus of the solitary tract in the monkey: Projections to the thalamus and brainstem nuclei. *Journal of Comparative Neurology,* **190,** 259–283.

Bellak L, Hurvich M, Gediman HK: (1973) *Ego functions in schizophrenics, neurotics, and normals: A systematic study of conceptual, diagnostic, and therapeutic aspects.* New York: Wiley.

Bender MB, Schapiro MF, Teuber H-L: (1949) Allesthesia and disturbance of the body schema. *Archives of Neurology and Psychiatry,* **62,** 222–231.

Benes FM: (1989) Myelination of cortical–hippocampal relays during late adolescence: Anatomical correlates to the onset of schizophrenia. *Schizophrenia Bulletin,* **15,** 585–594.

Benson DF, Gardner H, Meadows JC: (1976) Reduplicative paramnesia. *Neurology,* **26,** 147–153.

Beres D: (1956) Ego deviation and the concept of schizophrenia. *Psychoanalytic Study of the Child,* **11,** 164–235.

Berns GS, Cohen JD, Mintun MA: (1997) Brain regions responsive to novelty in the absence of awareness. *Science,* **276,** 1272–1275.

Bernstein N: (1967) The co-ordination and regulation of movements. Oxford, UK: Pergamon Press.

Berton P: (1988) *The Arctic Grail: The quest for the North West Passage and the North Pole, 1818–1909.* Toronto: McClelland & Stewart.

Bion WR: (1959) *Experiences in groups.* New York: Basic Books.

Bisiach E, Capitani E, Luzzatti C, Perani D: (1981) Brain and conscious representation of outside reality. *Neuropsychologia,* **19,** 543–551.

Bisiach E, Luzzatti C: (1978) Unilateral neglect of representational space. *Cortex,* **14,** 129–133.

Bisiach E, Luzzatti C, Perani D: (1979) Unilateral neglect, representational schema, and consciousness. *Brain,* **102,** 609–618.

Bisiach E, Rusconi ML, Vallar G: (1991) Remission of somatoparaphrenic delusion through vestibular stimulation. *Neuropsychologia,* **29,** 1029–1031.

Black IB: (1991) *Information in the brain: A molecular perspective.* Cambridge, MA: MIT Press.

Blake MJF: (1967) Time of day effects of performance in a range of tasks. *Psychonomic Science,* **9,** 349–350.

Blakemore C, Cooper GF: (1970) Development of the brain depends on the visual environment. *Nature,* **228,** 477–478.

Blanchard E, Kolb L, Prins A: (1991) Psychophysiological responses in the diagnosis of posttraumatic stress disorder in Vietnam veterans. *Journal of Nervous and Mental Disease,* **179,** 99–103.

Blaney PH: (1986) Affect and memory: A review. *Psychological Bulletin,* **99,** 229–246.

Bliss TV, Lømo T: (1973) Long-lasting potentiation of synaptic transmission in the dentate area of the anaesthetized rabbit following stimulation of the perforant path. *Journal of Physiology (London),* **232,** 331–356.

Blumenthal AL: (1977) *The process of cognition.* Englewood Cliffs, NJ: Prentice-Hall.

Blumer D: (1975) Temporal lobe epilepsy and its psychiatric significance. In DF Benson & D Blumer (eds.), *Psychiatric aspects of neurologic disease*. Orlando, FL: Grune & Stratton.

Bodamer J: (1947) Die Prosop-agnosie. *Archiv für Psychiatrie und Nervenkrankheiten*, **179**, 6–53.

Boesch C: (1991) Teaching among wild chimpanzees. *Animal Behavior*, **41**, 530–532.

Bogen JE: (1981) Mental numerosity: Is one head better than two. *Behavioral and Brain Sciences*, **4**, 100–101.

Bogen JE: (1995) On the neurophysiology of consciousness: I. An overview. *Consciousness and Cognition*, **4**, 15–24.

Bogen JE, Fisher ED, Vogel PJ: (1965) Cerebral commissurotomy: a second case report. *Journal of the American Medical Association*, **194**, 1328–1329.

Bonner JT: (1980) *The evolution of culture in animals*. Princeton, NJ: Princeton University Press.

Bornstein RF, Pittman TS (eds.): (1992) *Perception without awareness*. New York: Guilford Press.

Bouchard TJ Jr: (1994) Genes, environment, and personality. *Science*, **264**, 1700–1701.

Bouchard TJ Jr, Lykken DT, McGue M, Segal NL, Tellegen A: (1990) Sources of human psychological differences: The Minnesota Study of Twins Reared Apart. *Science*, **250**, 223–228.

Bouchard TJ Jr, McGue M: (1981) Familial studies of intelligence: A review. *Science*, **163**, 139–149.

Bouyer JJ, Montaron MF, Vahnee JM, Albert MP, Rougeul A: (1987) Anatomical localization of cortical beta rhythms in cat. *Neuroscience*, **22**, 863–869.

Bower GH, Miller NE: (1958) Rewarding and punishing effects from stimulating the same place in the rat's brain. *Journal of Comparative and Physiological Psychology*, **51**, 69–72.

Bower GH, Monteiro KP, Gilligan SG: (1978) Emotional mood as a context for learning and recall. *Journal of Verbal Learning and Verbal Behavior*, **17**, 573–578.

Bowlby J: (1969) *Attachment and loss, Vol. 1, Attachment*. London: Hogarth Press.

Brain R: (1941) Visual disorientation with special reference to the lesions of the right cerebral hemisphere. *Brain*, **64**, 244–272.

Bramblett CA: (1994) *Patterns of primate behavior*. 2nd ed. Prospect Heights, IL: Waveland Press.

Breedlove SM: (1992) Sexual dimorphism in the vertebrate nervous system. *Journal of Neuroscience*, **12**, 4133–4142.

Brehm JW, Cohen AR: (1962) *Explorations in cognitive dissonance*. New York: Wiley.

Breuer J, Freud S: (1895/1957) *Studies on hysteria*. New York: Basic Books.

Brinciotti M, Trasatti G, Pelliccia A, Matricardi M: (1992) Pattern-sensitive epilepsy: Genetic aspects in two families. *Epilepsia*, **33**, 88–92.

Brock MA: (1991) Chronobiology and aging. *Journal of the American Geriatrics Society*, **39**, 74–91.

Brown JW: (1981) Structural levels and mental duality. *Behavioral and Brain Sciences*, **4**, 102–103.

Bruner JS: (1957) On perceptual readiness. *Psychological Review,* 64, 123–152.

Bruner J: (1992) Another look at New Look 1. *American Psychologist,* 47, 780–783.

Buchsbaum MS, Wu J, DeLisi LE, Holcomb H, Kessler R, Johnson J, King AC, Hazlett E, Langston K, Post RM: (1986) Frontal cortex and basal ganglia metabolic rates assessed by positron emission tomography with [18F]2-deoxyglucose in affective illness. *Journal of Affective Disorders,* 10, 137–152.

Bunnell BN: (1966) Amygdaloid lesions and social dominance in the hooded rat. *Psychonomic Science,* 6, 93–94.

Buss AH, Plomin R: (1975) *A temperament theory of personality development.* New York: Wiley.

Buss AH, Plomin R: (1984) *Temperament: Early developing personality traits.* Hillsdale, NJ: Erlbaum.

Buss DM, Haselton MG, Shackelford TK, Bleske AL, Wakefield JC: (1998) Adaptations, exaptations, and spandrels. *American Psychologist,* 53, 533–548.

Butler R, Braff D, Rausch J, Jenkins M, Sprock J, Geyer, M: (1990) Physiological evidence of exaggerated startle response in a subgroup of Vietnam veterans with combat-related PTSD. *American Journal of Psychiatry,* 147, 1308–1312.

Buzsáki G, Grastyan E, Kellenyi L, Czopf J: (1979) Dynamic phase-shifts between theta generators in the rat hippocampus. *Acta Physiologica Academiae Scientarum Hungaricae,* 53, 41–45.

Buzsáki G, Horváth Z, Urioste R, Hetke J, Wise K: (1992) High-frequency network oscillation in the hippocampus. *Science,* 256, 1025–1027.

Bygott JD: (1979) Agonistic behaviour, dominance, and social structure in wild chimpanzees of the Gombe National Park. In DA Hamburg & ER McCown (eds.), *The great apes.* Menlo Park, CA: Benjamin/Cummings.

Byrne RW, Whiten A: (1985) Tactical deception of familiar individuals in baboons *(Papio ursinus). Animal Behavior,* 33, 669–673,

Campion J, Latto R: (1985) Apperceptive agnosia due to carbon monoxide poisoning: An interpretation based on critical band masking from disseminated lesions. *Behavioural Brain Research,* 15, 227–240.

Cantor N, Kihlstrom JK: (1987) *Personality and social intelligence.* Englewood Cliffs, NJ: Prentice-Hall.

Cappa S, Sterzi R, Vallar G, Bisiach E: (1987) Remission of hemineglect and anosognosia during vestibular stimulation. *Neuropsychologia,* 25, 775–782.

Carter DA, Phillips AG: (1975) Intracranial self-stimulation at sites in the dorsal medulla oblongata. *Brain Research,* 94, 155–160.

Cassella JV, Davis M: (1986) Neural structures mediating acoustic and tactile startle reflexes and the acoustically-elicited pinna response in rats. *Society for Neuroscience Abstracts,* 12, 1273.

Castellucci VF, Carew TJ, Kandel ER: (1978) Cellular analysis of long-term habituation of the gill-withdrawal reflex of *Aplysia californica. Science,* 202, 1306–1308.

Castillo RJ: (1990) Depersonalization and meditation. *Psychiatry,* 53, 158–168.

Cattell J: (1966) Depersonalization phenomena. In S Arieti (ed.), *American handbook of psychiatry,* Vol. 3. New York: Basic Books.

Chatrian GE, Lettich E, Miller LH, Green JR: (1970) Pattern-sensitive epilepsy: Genetic aspects in two families. *Epilepsia,* 33, 88–92.

Chevalier G, Deniau JM: (1990) Disinhibition as a basic process in the expression of striatal functions. *Trends in Neurosciences,* **13**, 241–244.

Chi CC, Flynn JP: (1971) Neural pathways associated with hypothalamically elicited attack behavior in cats. *Science,* **171**, 703–706.

Chipuer HM, Rovine M, Plomin R: (1990) LISREL modelling: Genetic and environmental influences on IQ revisited. *Intelligence,* **14**, 11–29.

Chomsky N: (1988) *Language and problems of knowledge.* Cambridge, MA: MIT Press.

Chugani HT, Phelps ME, Mazziotta JC: (1987) Positron emission tomography study of human brain functional development. *Annals of Neurology,* **22**, 487–497.

Churchland PS: (1981) How many angels . . . ? *Behavioral and Brain Sciences,* **4**, 103–104.

Coates S: (1992) The etiology of boyhood gender identity disorder: An integrative model. In JW Barron, MN Eagle, & DL Wolitzky (eds.), *Interface of psychoanalysis and psychology.* Washington, DC: American Psychological Association.

Coates S, Friedman RC, Wolfe S: (1991) The etiology of boyhood gender identity disorder: A model for integrating temperament, development, and psychodynamics. *Psychoanalytic Dialogues,* **1**, 481–523.

Cohen NH: (1984) Preserved learning capacity in amnesia: Evidence for multiple memory systems. In LR Squire & N Butters (eds.), *Neuropsychology of memory.* New York: Guilford Press.

Cohen NJ, Squire LR: (1980) Preserved learning and retention of pattern-analyzing skill in amnesia: Dissociation of knowing how and knowing that. *Science,* **210**, 207–209.

Cohen RM, Gross M, Nordahl TE, Semple WE, Rosenthal N: (1992) Preliminary data on the metabolic brain pattern of patients with winter seasonal affective disorder. *Archives of General Psychiatry,* **49**, 545–552.

Collier J: (1988) The dynamics of biological order. In BH Weber, DJ Depew, & JD Smith (eds.), *Entropy, information, and evolution: New perspectives on physical and biological evolution.* Cambridge, MA: MIT Press.

Conover KL, Shizgal P: (1994) Competition and summation between rewarding effects of sucrose and lateral hypothalamic stimulation in the rat. *Behavioral Neuroscience,* **108**, 537–548.

Cooper AF, Porter R: (1976) Visual acuity and ocular pathology in the paranoid and affective psychoses of later life. *Journal of Psychosomatic Research,* **20**, 107–114.

Cowdry RW, Pickar D, Davies R: (1985) Symptoms and EEG findings in the borderline syndrome. *International Journal of Psychiatry in Medicine,* **15**, 201–210.

Cowey A, Stoerig P: (1991) The neurobiology of blindsight. *Trends in Neurosciences,* **14**, 140.

Crammer L: (1959) Periodic psychoses. *British Medical Journal,* **i**, 545–549.

Crick F: (1984) The function of the thalamic reticular complex: The searchlight hypothesis. *Proceedings of the National Academy of Sciences USA,* **81**, 4586–4590.

Crick F, Koch C: (1990) Towards a neurobiological theory of consciousness. *Seminars in Neuroscience,* **2**, 263–275.

Cruikshank SJ, Weinberger NM: (1996) Evidence for the Hebbian hypothesis in experience-dependent physiological plasticity of neocortex: A critical review. *Brain Research Reviews, 22*, 191–228.

Curry FK, Gregory HH: (1969) The performance of stutterers on dichotic listening tasks thought to reflect cerebral dominance. *Journal of Speech and Hearing Research, 12*, 73–82.

Cyander M, Berman N, Hein A: (1973) Cats reared in stroboscopic illumination: Effects on receptive fields. *Proceedings of the National Academy of Sciences USA, 70*, 1353–1354.

Czeisler CA, Kronauer RE, Allan JS, Duffy JF, Jewett ME, Brown EN, Ronda JM: (1989) Bright light induction of strong (type 0) resetting of the human circadian pacemaker. *Science, 244*, 1328–1333.

Daigneault S, Braun CMJ, Whitaker HA: (1992) Early effects of normal aging on perseverative and nonperseverative prefrontal measures. *Developmental Neuropsychology, 8*, 99–114.

Daly DD: (1975) Ictal clinical manifestations of complex partial seizures. In JK Penry & DD Daly (eds.), *Complex partial seizures and their treatment.* New York: Raven Press.

Daly DD, Mulder DW: (1957) Gelastic epilepsy. *Neurology, 7*, 189–192.

Damasio AR: (1990) Category-related recognition defects as a clue to the neural substrates of knowledge. *Trends in Neurosciences, 13*, 95–98.

Damasio AR, Damasio H: (1994) Cortical systems underlying knowledge retrieval: Evidence from human lesion studies. In TA Poggio & AD Glaser (eds.), *Exploring brain functions: Models in neuroscience.* New York: Wiley.

Damasio A, Damasio H, Tranel D: (1989) Impairments of visual recognition as clues to the processes of categorization and memory. In G Edelman, E Gall, & M Cowan (eds.), *Signal sense: Local and global order in perceptual maps* (Neuroscience Institute Monograph). New York: Wiley.

Damasio A, Damasio H, Van Hoesen GW: (1982) Prosopagnosia: Anatomic basis and behavioral mechanisms. *Neurology, 32*, 331–341.

Damasio AR, Van Hoesen GW: (1983) Emotional disturbances associated with focal lesions of the limbic frontal lobe. In K Heilman & P Satz (eds.), *The neuropsychology of human emotion.* New York: Guilford Press.

Damasio H, Damasio AR: (1989) *Lesion analysis in neuropsychology.* New York: Oxford University Press.

Dansky LV, Andermann E, Andermann F: (1980) Marriage and fertility in epileptic patients. *Epilepsia, 21*, 261–271.

Darwin C: (1859/1958) *The origin of species.* New York: Penguin.

Davidson RJ: (1992) Emotion and affective style: Hemispheric substrates. *Psychological Science, 3*, 39–43.

Davis KD, Tasker RR, Kiss ZHT, Hutchison WD, Dostrovsky JO: (1995) Visceral pain evoked by thalamic microstimulation in humans. *NeuroReport, 6*, 369–374.

Davis M: (1992a) Analysis of aversive memories using the fear-potentiated startle paradigm. In LR Squire & N Butters (eds.), *Neuropsychology of memory.* 2nd ed. New York: Guilford Press.

Davis M: (1992b) The role of the amygdala in fear-potentiated startle: Implications for animal models of anxiety. *Trends in Phramacological Science, 13*, 35–41.

Dawkins R, Krebs JR: (1978) Animal signals: Information or manipulation. In JR

Krebs & NB Davies (eds.), *Behavioural ecology: An evolutionary approach.* London: Blackwell.

DeArmond SJ, Fusco MM, Dewe, MM: (1989) *Structure of the human brain: A photographic atlas.* 3rd ed. New York: Oxford University Press.

Deecke L, Grözinger B, Kornhuber HH: (1976) Voluntary finger movement in man: Cerebral potentials and theory. *Biological Cybernetics, 23,* 99–119.

Delgado JMR, Hamlin H, Chapman WP: (1952) Techniques of intracranial electrode implacement and stimulation and its possible therapeutic value in psychotic patients. *Confinia Neurologica, 12,* 315–319.

Delgado JMR, Roberts WW, Miller NE: (1954) Learning motivated by electrical stimulation of the brain. *American Journal of Physiology, 179,* 587–593.

Dennett DC: (1991) *Consciousness explained.* Boston: Little, Brown.

Dennett DC, Kinsbourne M: (1992) Time and the observer: The where and when of consciousness in the brain. *Behavioral and Brain Sciences, 15,* 183–247.

De Renzi E, Perani D, Cartesimo GA, Silveri MC, Fazio F: (1994) Prosopagnosia can be associated with damage confined to the right hemisphere: An MRI and PET study and a review of the literature. *Neuropsychologia, 32,* 893–902.

Devinsky O, Feldmann E, Burrowes K, Bromfield E: (1989) Autoscopic phenomena with seizures. *Archives of Neurology, 46,* 1080–1088.

Devlin B, Daniels M, Roeder K: (1997) The heritability of IQ. *Nature, 388,* 468–471.

de Waal F: (1982) *Chimpanzee politics.* Baltimore: Johns Hopkins University Press.

de Waal F: (1996) *Good natured: The origins of right and wrong in humans and other animals.* Cambridge, MA: Harvard University Press.

Dewhurst K, Beard AW: (1970) Sudden religious conversions in temporal lobe epilepsy. *British Journal of Psychiatry, 117,* 497–507.

Diamond A: (1991) Frontal lobe involvement in cognitive changes during the first year of life. In KR Gibson & AC Petersen (eds.), *Brain maturation and cognitive development.* New York: Aldine/de Gruyter.

Dicks D, Myers RE, Kling A: (1979) Uncus and amygdala lesions: Effects on social behavior in the free-ranging rhesus monkey. *Science, 165,* 69–71.

DiGiulio DV, Seidenberg M, O'Leary DS, Raz N: (1994) Procedural and declarative memory: A developmental study. *Brain and Cognition, 25,* 79–91.

Di Pellegrino G, Fadiga L, Fogassi L, Gallese V, Rizzolatti G: (1992) Understanding motor events: A neurophysiological study. *Experimental Brain Research, 91,* 176–180.

Dixon JC: (1963) Depersonalization phenomena in a sample population of college students. *British Journal of Psychiatry, 109,* 371–375.

Dobzhansky T, Eldrige N: (1982) *Genetics and the origin of the species.* SJ Gould (ed.). New York: Columbia University Press. (Work originally published 1937.)

Dollard J, Miller NE: (1950) *Personality and psychotherapy: An analysis in terms of learning, thinking, and culture.* New York: McGraw-Hill.

Dostoevsky F: (1846/1945) The double. In *The short novels of Dostoevsky.* Translated by C Garnett. New York: Dial Press. (Russian title: *Dvoinik.*)

Douglas RJ, Martin KAC: (1991) A functional microcircuit for cat visual cortex. *Journal of Physiology, 440,* 735–739.

Drevets WC, Raichle ME: (1995) Positron emission tomographic imaging studies of human emotional disorders. In MS Gazzaniga (ed.), *The cognitive neurosciences.* Cambridge, MA: MIT Press.

Drevets WC, Videen TO, Price JL, Preskorn SH, Carmichael ST, Raichle ME: (1992) A functional anatomical study of unipolar depression. *Journal of Neuroscience,* **12,** 3628–3641.

Dudai Y: (1989) *The neurobiology of memory: Concepts, findings, trends.* Oxford, UK: Oxford University Press.

Dunnett SB, Lane DM, Winn P: (1985) Ibotenic acid lesions of the lateral hypothalamus: Comparison with 6-hydroxydopamine-induced sensorimotor deficits. *Neuroscience,* **14,** 509–518.

Duval S, Wicklund RA: (1972) *A theory of objective self awareness.* New York: Academic Press.

Eastwood MR, Corbin S, Reed M: (1981) Hearing impairment and paraphrenia. *Journal of Otolaryngology,* **10,** 306–308.

Ebbinghaus H: (1885/1964) *Memory: A contribution to experimental psychology.* New York: Dover.

Eccles JC: (1981) Mental dualism and commissurotomy. *Behavioral and Brain Sciences,* **4,** 105.

Eccles JC: (1984) The cerebral neocortex: A theory of its operation. In EG Jones & A Peters (eds.), *Cerebral cortex: Functional properties of cortical cells,* Vol. 2. New York: Plenum Press.

Eclancher F, Karli P: (1971) Comportement d'agression interspécifique et comportement alimentaire du rat: Effets de lésions des noyaux ventromédians de l'hypothalamus. *Brain Research,* **26,** 71–79.

Edelman GM: (1979) Group selection and phasic reentrant signaling: A theory of higher brain function. In FO Schmitt & FG Worden (eds.), *The neurosciences: Fourth study program.* Cambridge, MA: MIT Press.

Edelman GM: (1987) *Neural Darwinism: Theory of neuronal group selection.* New York: Basic Books.

Egger MD, Flynn JP: (1962) Amygdaloid suppression of hypothalamically elicited attack behavior. *Science,* **136,** 43–44.

Eich E: (1995) Searching for mood dependent memory. *Psychological Science,* **6,** 67–75.

Ekman P, Levenson RW, Friesen WV: (1983) Autonomic nervous system activity distinguishes among emotions. *Science,* **221,** 1208–1210.

Emde RN: (1980) Toward a psychoanalytic theory of affect. In SI Greenspan & GH Pollock (eds.), *The course of life: Psychoanalytic contributions towards understanding personality development.* Rockville, MD: National Institute of Mental Health.

Emde RN, Biringen Z, Clyman RB, Oppenheim D: (1991) The moral self of infancy: Affective core and procedural knowledge. *Developmental Review,* **11,** 251–270.

Engel J Jr: (1968) Secondary epileptogenesis in rats. *Electroencephalography and Clinical Neurophysiology,* **25,** 494–498.

Engel J: (1989) *Seizures and epilepsy.* Philadelphia: Davis.

Epictetus: (1948) *The Enchiridion.* Translated by TW Higginson. Upper Saddle River, NJ: Prentice-Hall.

Epstein R, Lanza R, Skinner BF: (1980) Symbolic communication between two pigeons. *Science,* **207,** 543–545.

Erdelyi MH: (1992) Psychodynamics and the unconscious. *American Psychologist,* **47,** 784–787.

Essock-Vitale S, Seyfarth RM: (1987) Intelligence and social cognition. In BB Smuts, DL Cheney, RM Seyfarth, RW Wrangham, & TT Struhsaker (eds.), *Primate societies.* Chicago: University of Chicago Press.

Fahrenbach WH: (1985) Anatomical circuitry of lateral inhibition in the eye of the horseshoe crab. *Proceedings of the Royal Society of London B,* 225, 219–249.

Fairbank JA, Keane TM: (1982) Flooding for combat-related stress disorders: Assessment of anxiety reduction across traumatic memories. *Behavior Therapy,* 13, 499–510.

Falconer MA: (1954) Clinical manifestations of temporal lobe epilepsy and their recognition in relation to surgical treatment. *British Medical Journal,* 2, 939.

Farah MJ: (1989) The neural basis of mental imagery. *Trends in Neurosciences,* 12, 395–399.

Farah MJ: (1990) *Visual agnosia: Disorders of object recognition and what they tell us about normal vision.* Cambridge, MA: MIT Press.

Farah MJ, Perronet F: (1989) Event-related potentials in the study of mental imagery. *Journal of Psychophysics,* 3, 99–109.

Farah MJ, Weisberg LL, Monheit M, Peronnet F: (1989) Brain activity underlying mental imagery: Event-related potentials during mental image generation. *Journal of Cognitive Neuroscience,* 1, 302–316.

Feinberg I: (1974) Changes in sleep cycle patterns with age. *Journal of Psychiatric Research,* 10, 283.

Felleman DJ, Van Essen DC: (1991) Distributed hierarchical processing in the primate cerebral cortex. *Cerebral Cortex,* 1, 1–47.

Fenichel O: (1945) *The psychoanalytic theory of neurosis.* New York: Norton.

Ferenczi S: (1919/1980) Technical difficulties in the analysis of a case of hysteria. In S Ferenczi, *Further contributions to the theory and technique of psycho-analysis.* New York: Brunner/Mazel.

Ferenczi S: (1920/1980) The further development of an active therapy in psychoanalysis. In S Ferenczi, *Further contributions to the theory and technique of psycho-analysis.* New York: Brunner/Mazel.

Ferenczi S: (1923/1980) On forced phantasies. In S Ferenczi, *Further contributions to the theory and technique of psycho-analysis.* New York: Brunner/Mazel.

Ferenczi S: (1925a/1980) Psycho-analysis of sexual habits. In S Ferenczi, *Further contributions to the theory and technique of psycho-analysis.* New York: Brunner/Mazel.

Ferenczi S: (1925b/1980) Contra-indications to the "active" psycho-analytical technique. In S Ferenczi, *Further contributions to the theory and technique of psycho-analysis.* New York: Brunner/Mazel.

Ferenczi S: (1927/1955) The adaptation of the family to the child. In S Ferenczi, *Problems and methods of psychoanalysis.* New York: Basic Books.

Festinger L: (1957) *A theory of cognitive dissonance.* Evanston, IL: Row, Peterson.

Festinger L, Carlsmith JM: (1959) Cognitive consequences of forced compliance. *Journal of Abnormal and Social Psychology,* 58, 203–210.

Field T: (1996) Attachment and separation in young children. *Annual Review of Psychology,* 47, 541–561.

Fischer KW, Rose SP: (1994) Dynamic development of coordination of components in brain and behavior. In G Dawson & KW Fischer (eds.), *Human behavior and the developing brain.* New York: Guilford Press.

Fisher SA, Fischer TM, Carew TJ: (1997) Multiple overlapping processes underlying short-term synaptic enhancement. *Trends in Neurosciences,* 20, 170–177.

Flynn J: (1967) The neural basis of aggression in cats. In DH Glass (ed.), *Neurophysiology and emotion.* New York: Rockefeller University Press.

Flynn JP: (1976) Neural basis of threat and attack. In RG Grenell & S Gabey (eds.), *Biological foundations of psychiatry.* New York: Raven Press.

Fodor JA: (1983) The modularity of mind: An essay on faculty psychology. Cambridge, MA: MIT Press.

Folkard S: (1975) Diurnal variation in logical reasoning. *British Journal of Psychology,* 66, 1–8.

Folkard S: (1982) Circadian rhythms and human memory. In FM Brown & RC Graebner (eds.), *Rhythmic aspects of behavior.* Hillsdale, NJ: Erlbaum.

Fonagy P: (1991) Thinking about thinking: Some clinical observations in the treatment of a borderline patient. *International Journal of Psycho-Analysis,* 72, 639–656.

Fonberg E: (1973) The normalizing effect of lateral amygdalar lesions upon the dorsomedial amygdalar syndrome in dogs. *Acta Neurobiologiae Experimentalis,* 33, 449–466.

Forster FN, Liske EE: (1963) Role of environmental cues in temporal lobe epilepsy. *Neurology,* 13, 301.

Fouts R: (1997) *Next of kin: What chimpanzees have taught me about who we are.* New York: Morrow.

Fouts R, Fouts DH, van Cantfort TE: (1989) The infant Loulis learns signs from cross-fostered chimpanzees. In RA Gardner, BT Gardner, & TE van Cantfort (eds.), *Teaching sign language to chimpanzees.* Albany: State University of New York Press.

Fox PT, Ingham RJ, Ingham JC, Hirsch TB, Downs JH, Martin C, Jerabek P, Glass T, Lancaster JL: (1996) A PET study of the neural systems of stuttering. *Nature,* 382, 158–162.

Frank KA: (1992) Combining action techniques with psychoanalytic therapy. *International Review of Psycho-Analysis,* 19, 57–77.

Frank RA, Stutz RM: (1984) Self-deprivation: A review. *Psychological Bulletin,* 96, 384–393.

Freeman WJ: (1975) Mass action in the nervous system. New York: Academic Press.

Freeman W: (1987) Simulation of chaotic EEG patterns with a dynamic model of the olfactory system. *Biological Cybernetics,* 56, 139–150.

Freeman WJ: (1992) Tutorial in neurobiology. *International Journal of Bifurcation and Chaos,* 2, 451–482.

Freeman W: (1995) *Societies of brains: A study in the neuroscience of love and hate.* Hillsdale, NJ: Erlbaum.

Freeman W, Watts J: (1946) Pain of organic disease relieved by prefrontal lobotomy. *Lancet,* i, 29 June, 953–955.

Freud A: (1966) *The ego and the mechanisms of defense.* New York: International Universities Press.

Freud S: (1895/1966) Project for a scientific psychology. *Standard edition,* Vol. 1. London: Hogarth Press.

Freud S: (1900) The interpretation of dreams. *Standard edition,* Vol. 5. London: Hogarth Press.

Freud S: (1901/1966) The psychopathology of everyday life. *Standard edition*, Vol. 6. London: Hogarth Press.

Freud S: (1911/1957) Formulations regarding the two principles of mental functioning. *Collected Papers*, Vol. 4. London: Hogarth Press.

Freud S: (1913/1958) On beginning the treatment. *Standard edition*, Vol. 12. London: Hogarth Press.

Freud S: (1923) The ego and the id. *Standard edition*, Vol. 19. London: Hogarth Press.

Freud S: (1937) Analysis, terminable and interminable. *Collected papers*, Vol. 5. London: Hogarth Press.

Freud S: (1940) An outline of psycho-analysis. *Standard edition*, Vol. 23. London: Hogarth Press.

Friedman HR, Janas JD, Goldman-Rakic PS: (1990) Enhancement of metabolic activity in the diencephalon of monkeys performing working memory tasks: A 2-deoxyglucose study in behaving rhesus monkeys. *Journal of Cognitive Neuroscience*, 2, 18–31.

Frith U: (1989) *Autism: Explaining the enigma*. London: Blackwell.

Fuller JL, Rosvold HE, Pribram KH: (1957) The effect on affective and cognitive behavior in the dog of lesions of the pyriform–amygdala–hippocampal complex. *Journal of Comparative and Physiological Psychology*, 50, 89–96.

Fulton JF, Bailey P: (1929) Tumors in the region of the third ventricle: Their diagnosis and relation to pathological sleep. *Journal of Nervous and Mental Disease*, 69, 1–25, 145–164, 261.

Fuster JM: (1980) *The prefrontal cortex*. 1st ed. New York: Raven Press.

Fuster JM: (1989) *The prefrontal cortex*. 2nd ed. New York: Raven Press.

Fuster JM: (1997) *The prefrontal cortex*. 3rd ed. New York: Raven Press.

Gabbay FH: (1992) Behavior–genetic strategies in the study of emotion. *Psychological Science*, 3, 50–55.

Gaffan D: (1992) The role of the hippocampus–fornix–mammillary system in episodic memory. In LR Squire & N Butters (eds.), *Neuropsychology of memory*. 2nd ed. New York: Guilford Press.

Gaffan D, Murray EA: (1990) Amygdalar interaction with the mediodorsal nucleus of the thalamus and the ventromedial prefrontal cortex in stimulus–reward associative learning in the monkey. *Journal of Neuroscience*, 10, 3479–3493.

Gage FH, Olton DS, Bolanowski D: (1978) Activity, reactivity, and dominance following septal lesions in rats. *Behavioral Biology*, 22, 203–210.

Gallup GG: (1970) Chimpanzees: Self-recognition. *Science*, 167, 86–87.

Gallup G[G]: (1982) Self-awareness and the emergence of mind in primates. *American Journal of Primatology*, 2, 237–248.

Gallup GG: (1994a) Monkeys, mirrors, and minds. *Behavioral and Brain Sciences*, 17, 572–573.

Gallup GG: (1994b) Self-recognition: Research strategies and experimental design. In ST Parker, RW Mitchell, & ML Boccia (eds.), *Self-awareness in animals and humans: Developmental perspectives*. Cambridge, UK: Cambridge University Press.

Gardner BT, Gardner RA: (1971) Two-way communication with an infant chimpanzee. In AM Schrier & F Stollnitz (eds.), *Behavior of nonhuman primates*, Vol. 4. New York: Academic Press.

Gardner D, Lucas PB, Cowdry RW: (1987) Soft sign neurological abnormalities in borderline personality disorder and normal control subjects. *Journal of Nervous and Mental Disease,* 175, 177–180.

Gardner RA, Gardner BT, van Cantfort TE (eds.): (1989) *Teaching sign language to chimpanzees.* Albany: State University of New York Press.

Gascon GG, Lombroso CT: (1971) Epileptic (gelastic) laughter. *Epilepsia,* 12, 63–76.

Gastaut H, Colomb H: (1954) Étude du comportement sexuel chez les épileptiques psychomoteurs. *Annales Médico-Psychologiques (Paris),* 112, 659–696.

Gazzaniga MS: (1985) *The social brain.* New York: Basic Books.

Gazzaniga MS: (1995) Consciousness and the cerebral hemispheres. In MS Gazzaniga (ed.), *The cognitive neurosciences.* Cambridge, MA: MIT Press.

Gazzaniga MS, Bogen JE, Sperry RW: (1962) Some functional effects of sectioning the cerebral commissures in man. *Proceedings of the National Academy of Sciences USA,* 48, 1765–1769.

Gazzaniga MS, Fendrich R, Wessinger CM: (1994) Blindsight reconsidered. *Current Directions in Psychological Science,* 3, 93–96.

Gazzaniga MS, LeDoux JE: (1978) *The integrated mind.* New York: Plenum Press.

Gazzaniga MS, Wilson DH, LeDoux JE: (1977) Language, praxis, and the right hemisphere: Clues to some mechanisms of consciousness. *Neurology,* 27, 1144–1147.

Geschwind N: (1981) The perverseness of the right hemisphere. *Behavioral and Brain Sciences,* 4, 106–107.

Geschwind N, Galaburda AM: (1987) *Cerebral lateralization: Biological mechanisms, associations, and pathology.* Cambridge, MA: MIT Press.

Gilden L, Vaughan HG Jr., Costa LD: (1966) Summated human EEG potentials with voluntary movement. *Electroencephalography and Clinical Neurophysiology,* 20, 433–438.

Gill MM: (1982) *Analysis of transference, Vol. 1: Theory and technique.* New York: International Universities Press.

Gilman S, Bloedel JR, Lechtenberg R: (1981) *Disorders of the cerebellum.* Philadelphia: Davis.

Gittelman R, Mannuzza S, Shenker R, Bonagura N: (1985) Hyperactive boys almost grown up: I. Psychiatric status. *Archives of General Psychiatry,* 42, 937–947.

Gladue BA: (1994) The biopsychology of sexual orientation. *Current Directions in Psychological Science,* 3, 150–154.

Gladue BA, Green R, Hellman RE: (1984) Neuroendocrine response to estrogen and sexual orientation. *Science,* 225, 1496–1499.

Glass L, Mackey MC: (1979) Pathological conditions resulting from instabilities in physiological control systems. *Annals of the New York Academy of Science,* 316, 214–235.

Glass L, Mackey MC: (1988) *From clocks to chaos: The rhythms of life.* Princeton, NJ: Princeton University Press.

Glickstein M: (1993) Motor skills but not cognitive tasks. *Trends in Neurosciences,* 16, 450–451.

Glickstein M, Yeo C: (1990) The cerebellum and motor learning. *Journal of Cognitive Neuroscience,* 2, 69–80.

Globus A, Scheibel AB: (1967) Pattern and field in cortical structure: The rabbit. *Journal of Comparative Neurology,* **131,** 155–172.

Globus GG: (1992) Toward a noncomputational cognitive neuroscience. *Journal of Cognitive Neuroscience,* **4,** 299–310.

Goldberg E, Barr WB: (1991) Three possible mechanisms of unawareness of deficit. In GP Prigatano & DL Schachter (eds.), *Awareness of deficit after brain injury.* New York: Oxford University Press.

Goldberg E, Bilder RM: (1987) The frontal lobes and hierarchical organization of cognitive control. In E Perecman (ed.), *The frontal lobes revisited.* New York: IRBN Press.

Goldberg G, Mayer NH, Toglia JU: (1981) Medial frontal cortex infarction and the alien hand sign. *Archives of Neurology,* **38,** 683–686.

Goldberger L, Holt RR: (1958) Experimental interference with reality contact (perceptual isolation): Method and group results. *Journal of Nervous and Mental Disease,* **127,** 99.

Goldenberg G, Podreka I, Steiner M, Willmes K, Suess E, Deecke L: (1989) Regional cerebral blood flow patterns in visual imagery. *Neuropsychologia,* **27,** 641–664.

Goldfarb W: (1943) Infant rearing and problem behavior. *American Journal of Orthopsychiatry,* **13,** 249–265.

Goldiamond I: (1958) Indicators of perception: I. Subliminal perception, subception, unconscious perception—An analysis in terms of psychophysical indicator methodology. *Psychological Bulletin,* **55,** 373–411.

Goldman PS: (1976) Maturation of the mammalian nervous system and the ontogeny of behavior. In JS Rosenblatt, RA Hinde, E Shaw, & C Beer (eds.), *Advances in the study of behavior,* Vol. 7. New York: Academic Press.

Goldman PS, Nauta WJH: (1977) Columnar distribution of cortico-cortical fibers in the frontal association, limbic, and motor cortex of the developing rhesus monkey. *Brain Research,* **122,** 393–413.

Goldman-Rakic PS: (1984) Modular organization of prefrontal cortex. *Trends in Neurosciences,* **7,** 419–424.

Goldman-Rakic PS, Porrino LJ: (1985) The primate mediodorsal (MD) nucleus and its projection to the frontal lobe. *Journal of Comparative Neurology,* **242,** 535–560.

Goldman-Rakic PS, Schwartz ML: (1982) Interdigitation of contralateral and ipsilateral columnar projections to frontal association cortex in primates. *Science,* **216,** 755–757.

Goldstein K: (1908) Zur Lehre der motorischen Apraxis. *Zeitschrift für Psychologie und Neurologie,* **11,** 169–187, 270–283.

Goldstein K: (1939) *The organism: A holistic approach to biology derived from pathological data in man.* New York: American Book Co.

Goldstein K: (1942) *Aftereffects of brain injuries in war: Their evaluation and treatment.* New York: Grune & Stratton.

Gollin ES: (1966) An organism-oriented concept of development. Paper presented at the annual meeting of the American Psychological Association, New York.

Gollin ES: (1981) Development and plasticity. In ES Gollin (ed.), *Developmental plasticity: Behavioral and biological aspects of variations in development.* New York: Academic Press.

Gollin ES: (1984a) Developmental malfunctions: Issues and problems. In ES Gollin (ed.), *Malformations of development.* New York: Academic Press.

Gollin ES: (1984b) Early experience and developmental plasticity. *Annals of Child Development,* 1, 239–261.

Gollin ES, Stahl G, Morgan E: (1988) On the uses of the concept of normality in developmental biology and psychology. In HW Reese (ed.), *Advances in child development and behavior.* New York: Academic Press.

Goodall J: (1971) *In the shadow of man.* London: Collins.

Goodall J: (1990) *Through a window.* Boston: Houghton Mifflin.

Goodglass H, Kaplan E: (1972) *The assessment of aphasia and related disorders.* Philadelphia: Lea & Febiger.

Gottesman II: (1991) *Schzophrenia genetics: The origins of madness.* New York: Freeman.

Graf P, Squire LR, Mandler G: (1984) The information that amnesic patients do not forget. *Journal of Experimental Psychology: Learning, Memory and Cognition,* 10, 164–178.

Green CE: (1968) *Lucid dreams.* London: Hamish Hamilton.

Green C, McCreery C: (1994) *Lucid dreaming: The paradox of consciousness during sleep.* London: Routledge.

Greenough WT: (1986) What's special about development? Thoughts on the bases of experience-sensitive synaptic plasticity. In WT Greenough & JM Juraska (eds.), *Developmental neuropsychobiology.* New York: Academic Press.

Greenwald AG: (1992) New Look 3. *American Psychologist,* 47, 766–779.

Grigsby JP: (1987) The use of imagery in the treatment of posttraumatic stress disorder. *Journal of Nervous and Mental Disease,* 175, 55–59.

Grigsby J, Hartlaub G: (1994) Procedural learning and the development and stability of character. *Perceptual and Motor Skills,* 79, 355–370.

Grigsby J, Johnston CL: (1989) Depersonalization, vertigo and Ménière's disease. *Psychological Reports,* 64, 527–534.

Grigsby J, Kaye K: (1991) Chaos theory, circadian dysregulation and disorders characterized by disturbances of integration. In J Kotásková (ed.), *Proceedings of the 6th Prague International Conference on Psychological Development and Personality Formative Processes.* Prague: Czechoslovak Academy of Sciences.

Grigsby J, Kaye K: (1993) Incidence and correlates of depersonalization following head trauma. *Brain Injury,* 7, 507–513.

Grigsby J, Kaye K: (1995) Many neurologic and psychiatric disorders may reflect deterministic chaos. *Brain and Cognition,* 28, 103.

Grigsby J, Kaye K, Baxter J, Shetterly SM, Hamman RF: (1998) Executive cognitive abilities and functional status among community-dwelling older persons in the San Luis Valley Health and Aging Study. *Journal of the American Geriatrics Society,* 46, 590–596.

Grigsby J, Kaye K, Eilertsen TB, Kramer AM: (2000) The Behavioral Dyscontrol Scale and functional status among elderly medical and surgical rehab patients. *Journal of Clinical Geropsychology,* in press.

Grigsby J, Kaye K, Robbins LJ: (1992) Reliabilities, norms and factor structure of the Behavioral Dyscontrol Scale. *Perceptual and Motor Skills,* 74, 883–892.

Grigsby J, Kaye K, Robbins LJ: (1995) Behavioral disturbance and impairment of executive functions among the elderly. *Archives of Gerontology and Geriatrics*, 21, 167–177.

Grigsby J, Rosenberg NL, Busenbark D: (1995) Chronic pain is associated with deficits in information processing. *Perceptual and Motor Skills*, 81, 403–410.

Grigsby J, Schneiders JL: (1991) Neuroscience, modularity and personality theory: Conceptual foundations of a model of complex human functioning. *Psychiatry*, 54, 21–38.

Grigsby J, Schneiders JL, Kaye K: (1991) Reality testing, the self and the brain as modular distributed systems. *Psychiatry*, 54, 39–54.

Grigsby J, Stevens D: (2000) The role of multiple memory systems in the development of relationships. (Unpublished mansucript).

Grinder RE: (1964) Relations between behavioral and cognitive dimensions of conscience in middle childhood. *Child Development*, 35, 881–891.

Grinspoon L, Bakalar JB: (1979) *Psychedelic drugs reconsidered.* New York: Basic Books.

Gross CG, Sergent J: (1992) Face recognition. *Current Opinion in Neurobiology*, 2, 156–61.

Gur RC, Gur RE, Obrist WD, Skolnick BE, Reivich M: (1987) Age and regional cerebral blood flow at rest and during cognitive activity. *Archives of General Psychiatry*, 44, 617–621.

Hagerman RJ: (1996) Physical and behavioral phenotype. In RJ Hagerman & A Cronister (eds.), *Fragile X syndrome: Diagnosis, treatment, and research.* 2nd ed. Baltimore: Johns Hopkins University Press.

Halberg F: (1968) Physiologic considerations underlying rhythmometry, with special reference to emotional illness. In J de Ajuriaguerra (ed.), *Cycles biologiques et psychiatrie* (Symposium Bel Air III, Geneva, September 1967). Geneva: Masson.

Halberg F, Johnson EAA, Brown BW, Bittner JJ: (1960) Susceptibility rhythm to *E. coli* endotoxin and bioassay. *Proceedings of the Society for Experimental Biology and Medicine*, 103, 142–144.

Halgren E, Marinkovic K: (1995) Neurophysiological networks integrating human emotions. In MS Gazzaniga (ed.), *The cognitive neurosciences.* Cambridge, MA: MIT Press.

Hampson E: (1990) Estrogen-related variations in human spatial and articulatory-motor skills. *Psychoneuroendocrinology*, 15, 97–111.

Hampson E, Kimura D: (1988) Reciprocal effects of hormonal fluctuations on human motor and perceptual–spatial skills. *Behavioral Neuroscience*, 102, 456–459.

Happé F, Frith U: (1992) How autistics see the world. *Behavioral and Brain Sciences*, 15, 159–160.

Happé F, Ehlers S, Fletcher P, Frith U, Johansson M, Gillberg C, Dolan R, Frackowiak R, Frith C: (1996) "Theory of mind" in the brain. Evidence from a PET scan study of Asperger syndrome. *Neuroreport*, 8, 197–201.

Hare RD: (1978) Electrodermal and cardiovascular correlates of psychopathy. In RD Hare & D Schalling (eds.), *Psychopathic behavior.* New York: Wiley.

Harlow HF: (1958) The nature of love. *American Psychologist*, 13, 673–685.

Harlow HF, Harlow MK: (1973) Social deprivation in monkeys. In *Readings from Scientific American: The nature and nurture of behavior.* San Francisco: Freeman.

Harlow JM: (1868) Recovery from the passage of an iron bar through the head. *Massachusetts Medical Society Publication, 2,* 327–346.

Hartmann H: (1950) *Ego psychology and the problem of adaptation.* New York: International Universities Press.

Harwerth RS, Smith ELI, Duncan GC, Crawford MLJ, von Noorden GK: (1986) Multiple sensitive periods in the development of the primate visual system. *Science, 232,* 235–238.

Haug H, Barmwater U, Eggers R, Fischer D, Kuhl S, Sass NL: (1983) Anatomical changes in aging brain: Morphometric analysis of the human prosencephalon. In J Cervos-Navarro & HI Sarkander (eds.), *Neuropharmacology (Aging, Vol. 21).* New York: Raven Press.

Hayes C: (1951) *The ape in our house.* New York: Harper.

Hayes KJ, Nissen CH: (1971) Higher mental functions of a home-raised chimpanzee. In AM Schrier & F Stollnitz (eds.), *Behavior of nonhuman primates,* Vol. 4. New York: Academic Press.

Head H: (1920) *Studies in neurology.* London: Oxford University Press.

Head H, Holmes G: (1911) Sensory disturbances from cerebral lesions. *Brain, 34,* 102–254.

Heath RG: (1964) Pleasure response of human subjects to direct stimulation of the brain: Physiologic and psychodynamic consideration. In RG Heath (ed.), *The role of pleasure in behavior.* New York: Harper & Row.

Heatherington AW, Ranson SW: (1942) Hypothalamic lesions and adiposity in the rat. *Anatomical Record, 78,* 149–172.

Hebb DO: (1949) *The organization of behavior: A neuropsychological theory.* New York: Wiley.

Hécaen H, Albert ML: (1978) *Human neuropsychology.* New York: Wiley.

Hécaen H, Angelergues R: (1962) Agnosia for faces (prosopagnosia). *Archives of Neurology, 7,* 24–32.

Heilman KM: (1979) Neglect and related disorders. In KM Heilman & E Valenstein (eds.), *Clinical neuropsychology.* New York: Oxford University Press.

Heilman KM, Rothi LJ: (1985) Apraxia. In KM Heilman & E Valenstein (eds.), *Clinical neuropsychology.* 1st ed. New York: Oxford University Press.

Henriques JB, Davidson RJ: (1991) Left frontal hypoactivation in depression. *Journal of Abnormal Psychology, 100,* 535–545.

Herrnstein RJ: (1979) Acquisition, generalization, and discrimination reversal of a natural concept. *Journal of Experimental Psychology: Animal Behavior, 5,* 116–129.

Herrnstein RJ: (1985) Riddles of natural categorisation. In L Weiskrantz (ed.), *Animal intelligence.* Oxford, UK: Clarendon Press.

Herrnstein RJ, Loveland D: (1964) Complex visual concepts in the pigeon. *Science, 146,* 549–551.

Herskowitz J, Rosman NP, Geschwind N: (1984) Seizures induces by singing and recitation: A unique form of reflex epilepsy in childhood. *Archives of Neurology, 41,* 1102–1103.

Heston LL: (1966) Psychiatric disorders in foster home reared children of schizophrenic mothers. *British Journal of Psychiatry, 112,* 819–825.

Heyes CM: (1993) Reflections on self-recognition in primates. *Animal Behaviour, 47,* 909–919.

Hirsch HVB, Spinelli DN: (1971) Modification of the distribution of receptive field orientation in cats by selective visual exposure during development. *Experimental Brain Research*, 13, 509–527.

Hoebel BG, Teitelbaum P: (1962) Hypothalamic control of feeding and self-stimulation. *Science*, 135, 375–377.

Hoebel BG, Thompson RD: (1969) Aversion to lateral hypothalamic stimulation caused by intragastric feeding or obesity. *Journal of Comparative and Physiological Psychology*, 68, 536–543.

Houk JC: (1991) Red nucleus: Role in motor control. *Current Opinion in Neurobiology*, 1, 610–615.

Hubel DH: (1988) *Eye, brain, and vision*. New York: Scientific American Library.

Hubel DH, Wiesel T: (1959) Receptive fields of single neurones in the cat's striate cortex. *Journal of Physiology (London)*, 148, 574–491.

Hubel DH, Wiesel T: (1962) Receptive fields, binocular interaction and functional architecture in the cat's visual cortex. *Journal of Physiology (London)*, 160, 106–154.

Hubel DH, Wiesel T: (1963) Receptive fields of cells in striate cortex of very young, visually inexperienced kittens. *Journal of Neurophysiology*, 26, 994–1002.

Hubel DH, Wiesel TN, LeVay S: (1977) Plasticity of ocular dominance columns in monkey striate cortex. *Philosophical Transactions of the Royal Society of London, Series B: Biological Sciences* 278, 377–409.

Huffman MA, Wrangham RW: (1994) Diversity of medicinal plant use by chimpanzees in the wild. In RW Wrangham, WC McGrew, FBM de Waal, & PG Heltne (eds.), *Chimpanzee cultures*. Cambridge, MA: Harvard University Press.

Hull CL: (1943) *Principles of behavior*. New York: Appleton-Century-Crofts.

Ikeda A, Lüders HO, Burgess RC, Shibasaki H: (1992) Movement-related potentials recorded from supplementary motor area and primary motor area. *Brain*, 115, 1017–1043.

Irwin OC: (1942) Can infants have IQs? *Psychological Review*, 49, 69.

Isaacson RL: (1982) *The limbic system*. 2nd ed. New York: Plenum Press.

Ison JR, McAdam DW, Hammond GR: (1973) Latency and amplitude changes in the acoustic startle reflex of the rat produced by variation in auditory prestimulation. *Physiology and Behavior*, 10, 1035–1039.

Ivry RB, Keele SW: (1989) Timing functions of the cerebellum. *Journal of Cognitive Neuroscience*, 1, 136–152.

Iwai E, Yukie M: (1987) Amygdalofugal and amygdalopetal connections with modality-specific visual cortical areas in macaques (*Macaca fuscata, M. mulatta*, and *M. fascicularis*). *Journal of Comparative Neurology*, 261, 362–387.

Jacewicz MM, Hartley AA: (1987) Age differences in the speed of cognitive operations: Resolution of inconsistent findings. *Journal of Gerontology*, 42, 88–96.

Jacobs L, Grossman L: (1980) Three primitive reflexes in normal adults. *Neurology*, 30, 184–192.

Jacobs WJ, Nadel L: (1985) Stress-induced recovery of fears and phobias. *Psychological Review*, 92, 512–531.

James W: (1890) *The principles of psychology*. New York: Holt.

Jantsch E: (1980) *The self-organizing universe*. Oxford, UK: Pergamon Press.

Jeannerod M: (1994) The representing brain: Neural correlates of motor intention and imagery. *Behavioral and Brain Sciences*, 17, 187–245.

Jeavons PM, Harding GFA: (1975) Photosensitive epilepsy: A review of the literature and a study of 460 patients. In *Clinics in Developmental Medicine, No. 561*. Philadelphia: Lippincott.

Jenkins WM, Merzenich MM, Ochs MT, Allard T, Guic-Robles E: (1990) Functional reorganization of primary somatosensory cortex in adult owl monkeys after behaviorally controlled tactile stimulation. *Journal of Neurophysiology,* 63, 82–104.

Jenkins WM, Merzenich MM, Recanzone G: (1990) Neocortical representational dynamics in adult primates: Implications for neuropsychology. *Neuropsychologia,* 28, 573–584.

Jentsch JD, Redmond DE Jr, Elsworth JD, Taylor JR, Youngren KD, Roth RH: (1997) Enduring cognitive deficits and cortical dopamine dysfunction in monkeys after long-term administration of phencyclidine. *Science,* 277, 953–955.

Johnson MH, Magaro PA: (1987) Effects of mood and severity on memory processes in depression and mania. *Psychological Bulletin,* 101, 28–40.

Johnson MK, Raye CL: (1981) Reality monitoring. *Psychological Review,* 88, 67–85.

Johnson-Laird P: (1987) How could consciousness arise from the computations of the brain? In C Blakemore & S Greenfield (eds.), *Mindwaves: Thoughts on intelligence, identity and consciousness*. London: Blackwell.

Jones EE, Kanouse DE, Kelley HH, Nisbett RE, Valins S, Weiner B: (1972) *Attribution: Perceiving the causes of behavior*. Morristown, NJ: General Learning Press.

Jones RK: (1966) Observations on stammering after localized cerebral injury. *Journal of Neurology, Neurosurgery, and Psychiatry,* 29, 192–195.

Joyce J: (1934/1946) *Ulysses*. New York: Random House. (First published in Paris, 1922).

Joynt RJ: (1981) Are two heads better than one? *Behavioral and Brain Sciences,* 4, 108–109.

Jung CG: (1928/1959) *The archetypes and the collective unconscious*. New York: Pantheon.

Kaas JH: (1987) The organization of the neocortex in mammals: Implications for theories of brain function. *Annual Review of Psychology,* 38, 129–151.

Kaas JH: (1989) Why does the brain have so many visual areas? *Journal of Cognitive Neuroscience,* 1, 121–135.

Kaas JH: (1991) Plasticity of sensory and motor maps in adult mammals. *Annual Review of Neuroscience,* 14, 137–167.

Kaas JH: (1992) Do humans see what monkeys see? *Trends in Neurosciences,* 15, 1–3

Kaas JH: (1995) The evolution of isocortex. *Brain, Behavior, and Evolution,* 46, 187–196.

Kaas JH, Huerta MF: (1988) Subcortical visual system of primates. In HP Steklis (ed.), *Comparative primitive biology, Vol. 4, Neuroscience*. New York: Liss.

Kagan J: (1989) Temperamental contributions to social behavior. *American Psychologist,* 44, 668–674.

Kagan J, Reznick JS, Snidman N: (1988) Biological bases of childhood shyness. *Science,* 240, 167–171.

Kagan J, Snidman N: (1991) Infant predictors of inhibited and uninhibited profiles. *Psychological Science,* 2, 40–44.

Kagan J, Snidman N, Arcus DM: (1992) Initial reactions to unfamiliarity. *Current Directions in Psychological Science,* 1, 171–174.

Kandel ER: (1984) Steps toward a molecular grammar for learning: Explorations into the nature of memory. In KJ Isselbacher (ed.), *Medicine, science and society* (Symposia celebrating the Harvard Medical School bicentennial). New York: Wiley.

Kandel ER: (1991a) Nerve cells and behavior. In ER Kandel, JH Schwartz, & TM Jessell (eds.), *Principles of neural science.* 3rd ed. New York: Elsevier.

Kandel ER: (1991b) Cellular mechanisms of learning and the biological basis of individuality. In ER Kandel, JH Schwartz, & TM Jessell (eds.), *Principles of neural science.* 3rd ed. New York: Elsevier.

Kandel ER, Abrams T, Bernier L, Carew TJ, Hawkins RD, Schwartz JH: (1983) Classical conditioning and sensitization share aspects of the same molecular cascade in *Aplysia. Cold Spring Harbor Symposium in Quantitative Biology,* 48, 821–830.

Kaplan E: (1983) Process and achievement revisited. In S Wapner & B Kaplan (eds.), *Toward holistic developmental psychology.* Hillsdale, NJ: Erlbaum.

Kapp BS, Pascoe JP, Bixler MA: (1984) The amygdala: A neuroanatomical systems approach to its contributions to aversive conditioning. In N Butters & LR Squire (eds.), *Neuropsychology of memory.* New York: Guilford Press.

Kapp BS, Wilson A, Pascoe J, Supple W, Whalen PJ: (1990) A neuroanatomical systems analysis of conditioned bradycardia in the rabbit. In M Gabriel & J Moore (eds.), *Learning and computational neuroscience: Foundations of adaptive networks.* Cambridge, MA: MIT Press.

Kapur N, Scholey K, Moore E, Barker S, Brice J, Thompson S, Shiel A, Carn R, Abbot P, Fleming J: (1996) Long-term retention deficits in two cases of disproportionate retrograde amnesia. *Journal of Cognitive Neuroscience,* 8, 416–434.

Karni A, Sagi D: (1995) A memory system in the adult visual cortex. In B Julesz & I Kovács (eds.), *Maturational windows and adult cortical plasticity.* (Santa Fe Institute Studies in the Sciences of Complexity, Proceedings, Vol. 23). Reading, MA: Addison-Wesley.

Kauer JA, Malenka RC, Nicoll RA: (1988) A persistent postsynaptic modification mediates long-term potentiation in the hippocampus. *Neuron,* 1, 911–917.

Kaye K: (1996) [Paraphrenic patients with significant sensory deficits.] Unpublished raw data.

Kaye K, Grigsby J: (1991) Frontal lobe dysfunction and decreased activity associated with normal aging. In J Kotásková (ed.), *Proceedings of the 6th Prague International Conference on Psychological Development and Personality Formative Processes.* Prague: Czechoslovak Academy of Sciences.

Kaye K, Grigsby J, Robbins LJ, Korzun B: (1990) Prediction of independent functioning and behavior problems in geriatric patients. *Journal of the American Geriatrics Society,* 38, 1304–1310.

Keane TM, Kaloupek DG: (1982) Imaginal flooding in the treatment of a posttraumatic stress disorder. *Journal of Consulting and Clinical Psychology,* 50, 138–140.

Kelley AE, Stinus L: (1984) Neuroanatomical and neurochemical substrates of affective behavior. In NA Fox & RJ Davidson (eds.), *The psychobiology of affective development.* Hillsdale, NJ: Erlbaum.

Kelso JAS: (1981) On the oscillatory basis of movement. *Bulletin of the Psychonomic Society,* **18,** 63.

Kelso JAS: (1984) Phase transitions and critical behavior in human bimanual coordination. *American Journal of Physiology: Regulatory, Integrative and Comparative Physiology,* **15,** R1000-R1004.

Kelso JAS: (1995) *Dynamic patterns: The self-organization of brain and behavior.* Cambridge, MA: MIT Press.

Kelso JAS, Ding M, Schöner G: (1992) Dynamic pattern formation: A primer. In J Mittenthal & A Baskin (eds.), *Principles of organization in organisms* (Santa Fe Institute Studies in the Sciences of Complexity, Proceedings, Vol. 13). Reading, MA: Addison-Wesley.

Kemper MB, Hagerman RJ, Ahmad RS, Mariner R: (1986) cognitive profiles in the spectrum of clinical manifestations in heterozygous fra(X) females. *American Journal of Medical Genetics,* **23,** 139–156.

Kentridge RW, Heywood CA, Weiskrantz L: (1997) Residual vision in multiple retinal locations within a scotoma: Implications for blindsight. *Journal of Cognitive Neuroscience,* **9,** 191–202.

Kierkegaard S: (1849/1954) *The sickness unto death.* In S Kierkegaard, *Fear and trembling and The sickness unto death.* Translated by W Lowrie. Princeton, NJ: Princeton University Press.

Kihlstrom JF: (1987) The cognitive unconscious. *Science,* **237,** 1445–1452.

Kihlstrom JF, Barnhardt TM, Tataryn DJ: (1992) The psychological unconscious: Found, lost, and regained. *American Psychologist,* **47,** 788–791.

Kihlstrom JF, Klein SB: (1994) The self as a knowledge structure. In RS Wyer & TK Srull (eds.), *Handbook of social cognition,* Vol. 1. Hillsdale, NJ: Erlbaum.

Kilgard MP, Merzenich MM: (1998) Cortical map reorganization enabled by nucleus basalis activity. *Science,* **279,** 1714–1718.

Kim JJ, Fanselow MS: (1992) Modality-specific retrograde amnesia of fear. *Science,* **256,** 675–677.

Kim JJ, Thompson RF: (1997) Cerebellar circuits and synaptic mechanisms involved in classical eyeblink conditioning. *Trends in Neurosciences,* **20,** 177–181.

King AJ, Moore DR: (1991) Plasticity of auditory maps in the brain. *Trends in Neurosciences,* **14,** 31–37.

Kinney HC, Korein J, Panigrahy A, Dikkes P, Goode R: (1994) Neuropathological findings in the brain of Karen Ann Quinlan: The role of the thalamus in the persistent vegetative state. *New England Journal of Medicine,* **330,** 1469–1475.

Kinsbourne M: (1988) Integrated field theory of consciousness. In AJ Marcel & E Bisiach (eds.), *Consciousness in contemporary science.* New York: Oxford University Press, 239–256.

Kinsbourne M: (1995) Models of consciousness: Serial or parallel in the brain? In MS Gazzaniga (ed.), *The cognitive neurosciences.* Cambridge, MA: MIT Press.

Kinsbourne M, Warrington EK: (1962) A study of finger agnosia. *Brain,* **85,** 47–66.

Kiser RS, German DC: (1978) Opiate effects on aversive midbrain stimulation in rats. *Neuroscience Letters,* **10,** 197–202.

Kling A, Brothers L: (1992) The amygdala and social behavior. In JP Aggleton (ed.), *The amygdala: Neurobiological aspects of emotion, memory, and mental dysfunction.* New York: Wiley.

Knowlton BJ, Mangels JA, Squire LR: (1996) A neostriatal habit learning system in humans. *Science, 273,* 1399–402.

Kohlberg L: (1976) Moral stages and moralization. In T Lickona (ed.), *Moral development and behavior.* New York: Holt, Rinehart & Winston.

Kolb LC: (1984) The post-traumatic stress disorders of combat: A subgroup with a conditioned emotional response. *Military Medicine, 149,* 237–243.

Kolb LC, Mutalipassi LR: (1982) The conditioned emotional response: A sub-class of the chronic and delayed post-traumatic stress disorder. *Psychiatric Annals, 12,* 979–987.

Kosslyn SM: (1980) *Image and mind.* Cambridge, MA: Harvard University Press.

Kosslyn SM: (1994) *Image and brain.* Cambridge, MA: MIT Press.

Kosslyn SM, Alpert NM, Thompson WL, Maljkovic V, Weise SB, Chabris CF, Hamilton SE, Rauch SL, Buonanno FS: (1993) Visual mental imagery activates topographically organized visual cortex. *Journal of Cognitive Neuroscience, 5,* 263–287.

Kripke DF, Mullaney DJ, Atkinson M, Wolf S: (1978) Circadian rhythm disorders in manic depressives. *Biological Psychiatry, 13,* 335–351.

Krubitzer L: (1995) The organization of neocortex in mammals: Are species differences really so different? *Trends in Neurosciences, 18,* 408–417.

Kunst-Wilson WR, Zajonc RB: (1980) Affective discrimination of stimuli that cannot be recognized. *Science, 207,* 557–558.

LaBerge S, Levitan L, Dement W: (1986) Lucid dreaming: physiological correlates of consciousness during REM sleep. *Journal of Mind and Behaviour, 7,* 251–258.

LaBerge S, Nagel L, Dement W, Zarcone V: (1981) Lucid dreaming verified by volitional communication during REM sleep. *Perceptual and Motor Skills, 52,* 727–732.

Lackner JR: (1988) Some propriocieptive influences on the perceptual representation of body shape and orientation. *Brain, 111,* 281–297.

Laing RD: (1960) *The divided self.* London: Tavistock.

Lambert NM, Hartsough CS, Sassone D, Sandoval J: (1987) Persistence of hyperactivity symptoms from childhood to adolescence and associated outcomes. *American Journal of Orthopsychiatry, 57,* 22–32.

Landis T, Graves R, Benson F, Hebben N: (1982) Visual recognition through kinaesthetic mediation. *Psychological Medicine, 12,* 515–531.

Langer EJ, Imber LG: (1979) When practice makes imperfect: Debilitating effects of overlearning. *Journal of Personality and Social Psychology, 37,* 2014–2024.

Langton CG: (1988) Artificial life. In C Langton (ed.), *Artificial life: Santa Fe Institute studies in the sciences of complexity.* Reading, MA: Addison-Wesley.

Langton CG: (1991) Life at the edge of chaos. In CG Langton, C Taylor, JD Farmer, & S Rasmussen (eds.), *Artificial Life II (Santa Fe Institute Studies in the Sciences of Complexity, Proceedings, Vol. 10).* Reading, MA: Addison-Wesley.

LaRue A: (1992) *Aging and neuropsychological assessment.* New York: Plenum Press.

Lawes INC: (1988) The central connections of area postrema define the paraventricular system involved in antinoxious behaviours. In J Kucharczyk, D Stewart, & A Miller (eds.), *Nausea and vomiting: Recent research and clinical advances.* Boca Raton, FL: CRC Press.

Lazarus A: (1981) *The practice of multimodal therapy.* New York: McGraw-Hill.

Lazarus RS: (1984) On the primacy of cognition. *American Psychologist,* 39, 124–129.

Lazarus RS, McCleary RA: (1951) Autonomic discrimination without awareness: A study of subception. *Psychological Review,* 58, 113–122.

LeDoux JE: (1995) Emotion: Clues from the brain. *Annual Review of Psychology,* 46, 209–235.

LeDoux J: (1996) *The emotional brain.* New York: Simon & Schuster.

LeDoux JE, Gazzaniga MS: (1981) The split brain: A duel with duality as a model of mind. *Behavioral and Brain Sciences,* 4, 109–110.

LeDoux JE, Iwata J, Cicchetti P, Reis DJ: (1988) Different projections of the central amygdaloid nucleus mediate autonomic and behavioral correlates of conditioned fear. *Journal of Neuroscience,* 8, 2517–2529.

LeDoux JE, Romanski L, Xagoraris A: (1989) Indelibility of subcortical emotional memories. *Journal of Cognitive Neuroscience,* 1, 238–243.

LeDoux JE, Sakaguchi A, Reis DJ: (1984) Subcortical efferent projections of the medial geniculate nucleus mediate emotional responses conditioned to acoustic stimuli. *Journal of Neuroscience,* 4, 683–698.

LeDoux JE, Sakaguchi A, Iwata J, Reis DJ: (1986) Interruptions of projections from the medial geniculate body to an archi-neostriatal field disrupts the classical conditioning of emotional responses to acoustic stimuli in the rat. *Neuroscience,* 17, 615–627.

Leiner HC, Leiner AL, Dow RS: (1986) Does the cerebellum contribute to mental skills? *Behavioral Neuroscience,* 100, 443–454.

Leiner HC, Leiner AL, Dow RS: (1989) Reappraising the cerebellum: What does the hindbrain contribute to the forebrain? *Behavioral Neuroscience,* 103, 998–1008.

Lenz FA, Gracely RH, Hope EJ, Baker FH, Rowland LH, Dougherty PM, Richardson RT: (1994) The sensation of angina can be evoked by stimulation of the human thalamus. *Pain,* 59, 119–125.

Lenz FA, Gracely RH, Romanoski AJ, Hope EJ, Rowland LH, Dougherty PM: (1995) Stimulation in the human somatosensory thalamus can reproduce both the affective and sensory dimensions of previously experienced pain. *Nature Medicine,* 1, 910–913.

Lenz FA, Seike M, Lin YC, Baker FH, Rowland LH, Gracely RH, Richardson RT: (1993a) Neurons in the area of human thalamic nucleus ventralis caudalis respond to painful heat stimuli. *Brain Research,* 623, 235–240.

Lenz FA, Seike M, Richardson RT, Lin YC, Baker FH, Khoja I, Jaeger CJ, Gracely RH: (1993b) Thermal and pain sensations evoked by microstimulation in the area of the human ventrocaudal nucleus (Vc). *Journal of Neurophysiology,* 70, 200–212.

Lethmate J, Dücker G: (1973) Untersuchungen zum Selbsterkennen im Spiegel bei Orang-utans und einigen anderen Affenarten. *Zeitschrift für Tierpsychologie,* 33, 248–269.

Leuner H: (1969) Guided affective imagery (GAI): A method of intensive psychotherapy. *American Journal of Psychotherapy,* 34, 4–11.

LeVay S: (1991) A difference in hypothalamic structure between heterosexual and homosexual men. *Science,* 253, 1034–1037.

Levenson RW: (1992) Autonomic nervous system differences among emotions. *Psychological Science,* 3, 23–27.

Levin HS, Culhane KA, Hartmann J, Evankovich K, Mattson AJ, Harward H, Ringholz G, Ewing-Cobbs L, Fletcher JM: (1991) Developmental changes in performance on tests of purported frontal lobe functioning. *Developmental Neuropsychology,* 7, 377–395.

Levine PA, Frederick A: (1997) *Waking the tiger: Healing trauma.* Berkeley, CA: North Atlantic Books.

Lewicki P, Hill T, Czyzewska M: (1992) Nonconscious acquisition of information. *American Psychologist,* 47, 796–801.

Lewis M: (1990) The development of intentionality and the role of consciousness. *Psychological Inquiry,* 1, 231–248.

Lewis M: (1994) Myself and me. In ST Parker, RW Mitchell, ML Boccia (eds.), *Self-awareness in animals and humans: Developmental perspectives.* New York: Cambridge University Press.

Lewis M, Brooks-Gunn J: (1979) *Social cognition and the acquisition of self.* New York: Plenum Press.

Lewy AJ, Sack RL: (1987) Phase typing and bright light therapy of chronobiologic sleep and mood disorders. In A Halaris (ed.), *Chronobiology and psychiatric disorders.* New York: Elsevier.

Lezak MD: (1983) *Neuropsychological assessment.* 2nd ed. New York: Oxford University Press.

Lhermitte F: (1983) "Utilization behavior" and its relation to lesions of the frontal lobes. *Brain,* 106, 237–255.

Lhermitte F: (1951) Visual hallucinations of the self. *British Medical Journal,* i, 431–439.

Liang KC, Juler R, McGaugh JL: (1986) Modulating effects of posttraining epinephrine on memory: Involvement of the amygdala noradrenergic system. *Brain Research,* 368, 125–133.

Libet B: (1964) Brain stimulation and the threshold of conscious experience. In JC Eccles (ed.), *Brain and conscious experience.* New York: Springer-Verlag.

Libet B: (1973) Electrical stimulation of cortex in human subjects, and conscious sensory aspects. In A Iggo (ed.), *Handbook of sensory physiology, Vol. 2, Somatosensory system.* New York: Springer-Verlag.

Libet B: (1985) Unconscious cerebral initiative and the role of conscious will in voluntary action. *Behavioral and Brain Sciences,* 10, 529–566.

Libet B: (1989) Conscious subjective experience vs. unconscious mental functions: A theory of the cerebral processes involved. In RMJ Cotterill (ed.), *Models of brain function.* Cambridge, UK: Cambridge University Press.

Libet B: (1992) The neural time-factor in perception, volition and free will. *Revue de Métaphysique et de Morale,* 97, 255–272

Libet B, Alberts WW, Wright EW, Delattre LD, Levin G, Feinstein B: (1964) Production of threshold levels of conscious sensation by electrical stimulation of human somatosensory cortex. *Journal of Neurophysiology,* 27, 546–578.

Libet B, Pearl DK, Morledge DE, Gleason CA, Hosobuchi Y, Barbaro NM: (1991) Control of the transition from sensory detection to sensory awareness in man by the duration of a thalamic stimulus. *Brain,* 114, 1731–1757.

Libon D, Goldberg E: (1990) The effect of age on frontal systems and visuospatial functioning. Paper presented at the 18th annual meeting of the International Neuropsychological Society, Orlando, FL, February.

Lichtenberg JD: (1975) The development of the sense of self. *Journal of the American Psychoanalytic Association,* 23, 453–484.

Linden DJ, Connor JA: (1995) Long-term synaptic depression. *Annual Review of Neuroscience,* 18, 319–357.

Lindsay J, Ounsted C, Richards P: (1979) Long-term outcome in children with temporal lobe seizures: II. Marriage, parenthood, and sexual indifference. *Developmental Medicine and Child Neurology,* 21, 433–440.

Lissauer H: (1890) Ein Fall von Seelenblindheit nebst einen Beitrag zur Theorie der selben. *Archiv für Psychiatrie,* 21, 222–270.

Llinás R, Paré D: (1996) The brain as a closed system modulated by the senses. In R Llinás & PS Churchland (eds.), *The mind–brain continuum: Sensory processes.* Cambridge, MA: MIT Press.

Loeber R: (1982) The stability of antisocial and delinquent behavior: A review. *Child Development,* 53, 1431–1446.

Loeber R, Stouthamer-Loeber M, Green SM: (1987) Age of onset of conduct problems, different developmental trajectories, and unique contributing factors. Paper presented at meeting of the Society for Research in Child Development, Baltimore, MD, April.

Lorenz EN: (1963) Deterministic nonperiodic flow. *Journal of Atmospheric Science,* 20, 282–293.

Lukianowicz, N: (1958) Autoscopic phenomena. *Archives of Neurology and Psychiatry,* 80, 199–207.

Luria AR: (1961) *The role of speech in the regulation of normal and abnormal behavior.* New York: Irvington.

Luria AR: (1965) Two kinds of motor perseveration in massive injury of the frontal lobes. *Brain,* 88, 1–10.

Luria AR: (1966) *Human brain and psychological processes.* New York: Harper & Row.

Luria AR: (1969) Frontal lobe syndromes. In PJ Vinken & GW Bruyn (eds.), *Handbook of clinical neurology,* Vol. 2. Amsterdam: North-Holland.

Luria AR: (1973) *The working brain.* New York: Basic Books.

Luria AR: (1976) *The nature of human conflicts.* New York: Liveright.

Luria AR: (1979) *The making of mind.* M Cole & S Cole (eds.). Cambridge, MA: Harvard University Press.

Luria AR: (1980) *Higher cortical functions in man.* 2nd ed. New York: Basic Books.

Luria AR, Pravdina-Vinarskaya EN, Yarbuss AL: (1963) Disorders of ocular movement in a case of simultanagnosia. *Brain,* 86, 219–228.

Lykken DT: (1957) A study of anxiety in the sociopathic personality. *Journal of Abnormal and Social Psychology,* 55, 6–10.

Lynch G: (1986) *Synapses, circuits, and the beginnings of memory.* Cambridge, MA: MIT Press.

Lytton H: (1990) Child and parent effects in boys' conduct disorder: A reinterpretation. *Developmental Psychology,* 26, 683–697.

Mackey MC, Glass L: (1977) Oscillation and chaos in physiological control systems. *Science,* 197, 287–289.

Mackey MC, Milton JG: (1987) Dynamical diseases. *Annals of the New York Academy of Science*, **504**, 16–32.

Mandelbrot BB: (1982) *The fractal geometry of nature*. New York: Freeman.

Manger P, Sum M, Szymanski M, Ridgway S, Krubitzer L: (1998) Modular subdivisions of dolphin insular cortex: Does evolutionary history repeat itself? *Journal of Cognitive Neuroscience*, **10**, 153–166.

Marcus Aurelius: (1991) *Meditations*. Translated by G Long. Amherst, NY: Prometheus Books.

Margules DL, Lewis MJ, Dragovich JA, Margules AS: (1972) Hypothalamic norepinephrine: Circadian rhythms and the control of feeding behavior. *Science*, **178**, 640–643.

Markowitsch HJ: (1995) Which brain regions are critically involved in the retrieval of old episodic memory? *Brain Research Reviews*, **21**, 117–127.

Markowitsch HJ, Calabrese P, Liess J, Haupts M, Durwen HF, Gelhen W: (1993) Retrograde amnesia after traumatic injury of the temporo-frontal cortex. *Journal of Neurology, Neurosurgery and Psychiatry*, **56**, 988–992.

Markram H, Lübke J, Frotscher M, Sakmann B: (1997) Regulation of synaptic efficacy by coincidence of postsynaptic APs and EPSPs. *Science*, **275**, 213–215.

Marshal CR, Maynard RM: (1983) Vestibular stimulation for supranuclear gaze palsy: Case report. *Archives of Physical Medicine and Rehabilitation*, **64**, 134–146.

Marshall J, Halligan P: (1988) Blindsight and insight in visuo-spatial neglect. *Nature, London*, **336**, 766–777.

Marshall JF, Turner BH, Teitelbaum P: (1971) Sensory neglect produced by lateral hypothalamic damage. *Science*, **174**, 523–525.

Martin JH: (1991) The collective electrical behavior of cortical neurons: The electroencephalogram and the mechanisms of epilepsy. In ER Kandel, JH Schwartz, & TM Jessell (eds.), *Principles of neural science*, 3rd ed. New York: Elsevier.

Martin RS: (1991) Apathy: A neuropsychiatric syndrome. *Journal of Neuropsychiatry and Clinical Neurosciences*, **3**, 243–254.

Matsuzawa T: (1994) Field experiments on use of stone tools by chimpanzees in the wild. In RW Wrangham, WC McGrew, FBM de Waal, & PG Heltne (eds.), *Chimpanzee cultures*. Cambridge, MA: Harvard University Press.

Matthies H: (1982) Plasticity in the nervous system: An approach to memory research. In CA Marsan & H Matthies (eds.), *Neuronal plasticity and memory formation*. New York: Raven Press.

Mayer-Gross W: (1935) On depersonalization. *British Journal of Medical Psychology*, **15**, 103–122.

Maynard Smith J: (1978) Optimization theory in evolution. *Annual Review of Ecology and Systematics*, **9**, 31–56.

McCarthy RA, Warrington EK: (1990) *Cognitive neuropsychology: A clinical introduction*. San Diego, CA: Academic Press.

McClearn GE, Boo Johansson, Berg S, Pedersen NL, Ahern F, Petrill SA, Plomin R: (1997) Substantial genetic influence on cognitive abilities in twins 80 or more years old. *Science*, **276**, 1560–1563.

McClelland JL, Rumelhart DE, Hinton GE: (1986) The appeal of parallel distributed processing. In DE Rumelhart & JL McClelland (eds.), *Parallel distributed processing: Explorations in the microstructure of cognition*, Vol. 1, *Foundations*. Cambridge, MA: MIT Press.

McCrae RR, Costa PT: (1994) The stability of personality: Observations and evaluations. *Current Directions in Psychological Science*, 3, 173–175.

McCulloch WS: (1945) A heterarchy of values determined by the topology of nervous nets. *Bulletin of Mathematics and Biophysics*, 7, 89–93.

McFall M, Veith R, Murburg M: (1992) Basal sympathoadrenal function in post-traumatic stress disorder. *Biological Psychiatry*, 31, 1050–1056.

McGaugh JL: (1990) Significance and remembrance: The role of neuromodulatory systems. *Psychological Science*, 1, 15–25.

McGaugh JL, Introini-Collison IB, Cahill LF, Castellano C, Dalmaz C, Parent MB, Williams CL: (1993) Neuromodulatory systems and memory storage: Role of the amygdala. *Behavioural Brain Research*, 58, 81–90.

McGrew WC: (1992) *Chimpanzee material culture: Implications for human evolution*. Cambridge, UK: Cambridge University Press.

McGrew WC: (1994) Tools compared: The material of culture. In RW Wrangham, WC McGrew, FBM de Waal, & PG Heltne (eds.), *Chimpanzee cultures*. Cambridge, MA: Harvard University Press.

McKenna JJ, Mosko S, Dungy C, McAninch J: (1990) Sleep and arousal patterns of co-sleeping human mother/infant pairs: A preliminary physiological study with implications for the study of sudden infant death syndrome (SIDS). *American Journal of Physical Anthropology*, 83, 331–347.

McNamara JO: (1986) Kindling model of epilepsy. In AV Delgado-Escueta, AA Ward Jr., DM Woodbury, & RJ Porter (eds.), *Basic mechanisms of the epilepsies: Molecular and cellular approaches* (Advances in neurology, Vol. 44). New York: Raven Press.

Mead GH: (1934/1974) *Mind, self and society*. Chicago: University of Chicago Press.

Mecklinger A, Müller N: (1996) Dissociations in the processing of "what" and "where" information in working memory: An event-related potential analysis. *Journal of Cognitive Neuroscience*, 8, 453–473.

Mednick SA: (1977) A bio-social theory of the learning of law-abiding behavior. In SA Mednick & KO Christiansen (eds.), *Biosocial bases of criminal behavior*. New York: Gardner Press.

Meguro K, Ueda M, Yamaguchi T, Sekita Y, Yamazaki H, Oikawa Y, Kikuchi Y, Matsuzawa T: (1990) Disturbance in daily sleep/wake patterns in patients with cognitive impairment and decreased daily activity. *Journal of the American Geriatrics Society*, 38, 1176–1182.

Meijer JH, Rietveld WJ: (1989) Neurophysiology of the suprachiasmatic circadian pacemaker in rodents. *Physiology Review*, 69, 671–707.

Mendelson J: (1972) Ecological modulation of brain stimulation effects. *International Journal of Psychobiology*, 2, 285–304.

Merikle PM: (1992) Perception without awareness: Critical issues. *American Psychologist*, 47, 792–795.

Merzenich MM, Kaas JH, Wall J, Nelson RJ, Sur M, Felleman D: (1983a) Topographic reorganization of somatosensory cortical areas 3b and 1 in adult monkeys following restricted deafferentation. *Neuroscience*, 8, 33–55.

Merzenich MM, Kaas JH, Wall JT, Sur M, Nelson RJ, Felleman DJ: (1983b) Progression of change following median nerve section in the cortical representation of the hand in areas 3b and 1 in adult owl and squirrel monkeys. *Neuroscience,* 10, 639–65.

Merzenich MM, Recanzone GH, Jenkins WM, Grajski KA: (1990) Adaptive mechanisms in cortical networks underlying cortical contributions to learning and nondeclarative memory. *Cold Spring Harbor Symposium in Quantitative Biology,* 55, 873–87.

Mesulam M-M: (1982) A cortical network for directed attention and unilateral neglect. *Annals of Neurology,* 10, 309–325.

Michel F, Peronnet F: (1980) A case of cortical deafness: Clinical and electrophysiological data. *Brain and Language,* 10, 367–377.

Michel S, Geusz ME, Zaritsky JJ, Block GD: (1993) Circadian rhythm in membrane conductance expressed in isolated neurons. *Science,* 178, 640–643.

Middleton FA, Strick PL: (1994) Anatomical evidence for cerebellar and basal ganglia involvement in higher cognitive function. *Science,* 266, 458–461.

Miles HLW: (1986) How can I tell a lie? Apes, language and the problem of deception. In RW Mitchell & NS Thompson (eds.), *Deception: Perspectives on human and nonhuman deceit.* Albany: State University of New York Press.

Miles HLW: (1994) Me Chantek: The development of self-awareness in a signing orangutan. In ST Parker, RW Mitchell, ML Boccia (eds.), *Self-awareness in animals and humans: Developmental perspectives.* New York: Cambridge University Press.

Mill JS: (1861/1993) Utilitarianism. In *Utilitarianism, On liberty, Considerations on representative government, Remarks on Bentham's philosophy.* G Williams (ed.). London: Everyman.

Miller GA: (1956) The magical number seven, plus or minus two: Some limits on our capacity for processing information. *Psychological Review,* 63, 81–97.

Miller GA: (1962) *Psychology: The science of mental life.* New York: Harper & Row.

Milner B: (1962) Les troubles de la mémoire accompagnant des lésions hippocampiques bilatérales. In P Passouant (ed.), *Physiologie de l'hippocampe.* Paris: Centre National de la Recherche Scientifique.

Milner B: (1965) Memory disturbances after bilateral hippocampal lesions in man. In PM Milner & SE Glickman (eds.), *Cognitive processes and brain.* Princeton, NJ: Van Nostrand.

Milner B, Petrides M: (1984) Behavioural effects of frontal-lobe lesions in man. *Trends in Neurosciences,* 7, 403–407.

Milner P: (1974) A model for visual shape recognition. *Psychological Review,* 81, 521–535.

Milner PM: (1989) A cell assembly theory of hippocampal amnesia. *Neuropsychologia,* 27, 23–30.

Mishkin M, Malamut B, Bachevalier J: (1984) Memories and habits: Two neural systems. In G Lynch, JL McGaugh, & NM Weinberger (eds.), *Neurobiology of learning and memory.* New York: Guilford Press.

Mitchell SA: (1993) *Hope and dread in psychoanalysis.* New York: Basic Books.

Mittenberg W, Seidenberg M, O'Leary DS, DiGiulio DV: (1989) Changes in cerebral functioning associated with normal aging. *Journal of Clinical and Experimental Neuropsychology,* 11, 918–932.

Money J, Ehrhardt AA: (1972) *Man & woman boy & girl*. Baltimore: Johns Hopkins University Press.

Moniz E: (1936) Essai d'un traitement chirurgical de certaines psychoses. *Bulletin de l'Académie de Médicine*, 115, 385–392.

Monk TH, Gillin JC: (1984) Circadian lability and shift work intolerance. *Trends in Neurosciences*, 7, 459–460.

Mora F, Avrith DB, Phillips AG, Rolls ET: (1979) Effects of satiety on self-stimulation of the orbitofrontal cortex in the monkey. *Neuroscience Letters*, 13, 141–145.

Moreland RL, Zajonc RB: (1977) Is stimulus recognition a necessary condition for the occurrence of exposure effects? *Journal of Personality and Social Psychology*, 35, 191–199.

Moreland RL, Zajonc RB: (1979) Exposure effects may not depend on stimulus recognition. *Journal of Personality and Social Psychology*, 37, 1085–1089.

Morris RGM, Davis S, Butcher SP: (1990) Hippocampal synaptic plasticity and NMDA receptors: A role in information storage? *Philosophical Transactions of the Royal Society of London, Series B: Biological Sciences*, 329, 187–204.

Moscovitch M, Winocur G, Behrmann M: (1997) What is special about face recognition? Nineteen experiments on a person with visual object agnosia and dyslexia but normal face recognition. *Journal of Cognitive Neuroscience*, 9, 555–604.

Mountcastle VB: (1979) An organizing principle for cerebral function: The unit module and the distributed system. In FO Schmitt & FG Worden (eds.), *The neurosciences: Fourth study program*. Cambridge, MA: MIT Press.

Mountcastle VB: (1997) The columnar organization of the neocortex. *Brain*, 120, 707–722.

Muller D, Joly M, Lynch G: (1988) Contributions of quisqualate and NMDA receptors to the induction and expression of LTP. *Science*, 242, 1694–1697.

Multi-Society Task Force on Persistent Vegetative State (MSTFPVS): (1994) Medical aspects of the persistent vegetative state. (First of two parts.) *New England Journal of Medicine*, 330, 1499–1508.

Murphy GG, Glanzman DL: (1997) Mediation of classical conditioning in *Aplysia californica* by long-term potentiation of sensorimotor synapses. *Science*, 278, 467–471.

Nadel L: (1992) Multiple memory systems: What and why? *Journal of Cognitive Neuroscience*, 4, 179–188.

Nathanson M, Bergman PS, Gordon GG: (1952) Denial of illness. *Archives of Neurology and Psychiatry*, 68, 380–387.

Nauta WJH: (1964) Some efferent connections of the prefrontal cortex in the monkey. In JM Warren & K Akert (eds.), *The frontal granular cortex and behavior*. New York: McGraw-Hill.

Newman J, Baars BJ, Cho S-B: (1997) A neural Global Workspace model for conscious attention. *Neural Networks*, 10, 1195–1206.

Nilsson D-E, Pelger S: (1994) A pessimistic estimate of the time required for an eye to evolve. *Proceedings of the Royal Society of London, Series B: Biological Sciences*, 256, 53–58.

Nisbett RE, Ross L: (1980) *Human inference: Strategies and shortcomings of social judgment*. Englewood Cliffs, NJ: Prentice-Hall.

Nisbett RE, Wilson TD: (1977) Telling more than we can know: Verbal reports on mental processes. *Psychological Review,* **84,** 231–259.

Norman DA: (1981) Categorization of action slips. *Psychological Review,* **88,** 1–15.

Norman DA: (1986) Reflections on cognition and parallel distributed processing. In JL McClelland & DE Rumelhart (eds.), *Parallel distributed processing: Explorations in the microstructure of cognition,* Vol. 2. Cambridge, MA: MIT Press.

Norman DA, Shallice T: (1986) Attention to action: Willed and automatic control of behavior. In RJ Davidson, GE Schwartz, & D Shapiro (eds.), *Consciousness and self-regulation,* Vol. 4. New York: Plenum Press.

Noyes R, Kletti R: (1976) Depersonalization in the face of life-threatening danger: A description. *Psychiatry,* **39,** 19–27.

Ogden T: (1994) *Subjects of analysis.* Northvale, NJ: Aronson.

Olds J: (1958) Self-stimulation of the brain. *Science,* **127,** 315–324.

Olds J, Milner PM: (1954) Positive reinforcement produced by electrical stimulation of septal area and other regions of rat brain. *Journal of Comparative and Physiological Psychology,* **47,** 419–427.

Olds J, Olds ME: (1965) Drives, rewards, and the brain. In TM Newcombe (ed.), *New directions in psychology.* New York: Holt, Rinehart & Winston.

Olds ME, Olds J: (1963) Approach-avoidance analysis of rat diencephalon. *Journal of Comparative Neurology,* **120,** 259–295.

Olsen CW, Ruby C: (1941) Anosognosia and autotopognosia. *Archives of Neurology and Psychiatry,* **46,** 340–345.

Orton ST: (1925) "Word-blindness" in school children. *Archives of Neurology and Psychiatry,* **14,** 581–615.

Orton ST: (1937) *Reading, writing, and speech problems in children.* New York: Norton.

Overton DA: (1984) State dependent learning and drug discriminations. In LL Iverson, SD Iverson, & SH Snyder (eds.), *Handbook of psychopharmacology,* Vol. 18. New York: Plenum Press.

Paillard J, Michel F, Stelmach G: (1983) Localization without content: A tactile analogue of "blind sight." *Archives of Neurology,* **40,** 548–551.

Panksepp J, Siviy SM, Normansell LA: (1985) Brain opioids and social emotions. In M Reite & T Field (eds.), *The psychobiology of attachment and separation.* Orlando, FL: Academic Press.

Pardo JV, Pardo PJ, Raichle ME: (1993) Neural correlates of self-induced dysphoria. *American Journal of Psychiatry,* **150,** 713–719.

Parker ST, Mitchell RW, Boccia ML: (1994) *Self-awareness in animals and humans: Developmental perspectives.* Cambridge, UK: Cambridge University Press.

Passingham R: (1993) *The frontal lobes and voluntary action.* Oxford, UK: Oxford University Press.

Patterson FG, Cohn RH: (1994) Self-recognition and self-awareness in lowland gorillas. In ST Parker, RW Mitchell, ML Boccia (eds.), *Self-awareness in animals and humans: Developmental perspectives.* New York: Cambridge University Press.

Patterson F, Linden E: (1981) *The education of Koko.* New York: Holt, Rinehart and Winston.

Pavlov IP: (1927) *Conditioned reflexes: An investigation of the physiological activ-*

ity of the cerebral cortex. Translated by GV Anrep. London: Oxford University Press.

Pearlson GD, Kreger L, Rabins PV, Chase GA, Cohen B, Wirth JB, Schlaepfer TB, Tune LE: (1989) A chart review study of late-onset and early-onset schizophrenia. *American Journal of Psychiatry,* **146,** 1568–1574.

Pearlson GD, Petty RG: (1994) Late-life-onset psychoses. In CE Coffey & JL Cummings (eds.), *Textbook of geriatric neuropsychiatry.* Washington, DC: American Psychiatric Press.

Pedersen NL, Plomin R, Nesselroade JR, McClearn GE: (1992) A quantitative genetic analysis of cognitive abilities during the second half of the life span. *Psychological Science,* **3,** 346–353.

Penfield W, Rasmussen T: (1955) *The cerebral cortex of man.* New York: Macmillan.

Perry BD: (1994) Neurobiological sequelae of childhood trauma: Post-traumatic stress disorders in children. In M Murberg (ed.), *Catecholamines in post-traumatic stress disorder: Emerging concepts.* Washington, DC: American Psychiatric Press.

Perry BD, Pate JE: (1994) Neurodevelopment and the psychobiological roots of post-traumatic stress disorders. In LF Koziol & CE Stout (eds.), *The neuropsychology of mental illness: A practical guide.* Springfield, IL: Thomas.

Perry BD, Pollard RA, Blakley TL, Baker WL, Vigilante D: (1995) Childhood trauma, the neurobiology of adaptation, and "use-dependent" development of the brain: How "states" become "traits." *Infant Mental Health Journal,* **16,** 271–291.

Pettigrew JD, Garey LJ: (1974) Selective modification of single neuron properties in the visual cortex of kittens. *Brain Research,* **66,** 160–164.

Phillips RG, LeDoux JE: (1992) Differential contribution of amygdala and hippocampus to cued and contextual fear conditioning. *Behavioral Neuroscience,* **106,** 274–285.

Pick A: (1903) On reduplicative paramnesia. *Brain,* **26,** 260–267.

Pick A: (1908) *Über Storungen der Orientierung am eigenen Körper* (Arbeiten aus der deutschen psychiatrischen Universität-klinik in Prag). Berlin: Karger.

Pietrini P, Horwitz B, Grady CL: (1992) A positron emission tomography study of cerebral glucose metabolism (rCMRglc) and blood flow (rCBF) in normal human aging. *Gerontologist (special issue),* **32_** 242.

Pine F: (1985) *Developmental theory and clinical process.* New Haven, CT: Yale University Press.

Pinel JPJ, Rovner LI: (1978) Experimental epileptogenesis: Kindling-induced epilepsy in rats. *Experimental Neurology,* **58,** 190–202.

Pitkänen A, Savander V, LeDoux JE: (1997) Organization of intra-amygdaloid circuitries in the rat: An emerging framework for understanding functions of the amygdala. *Trends in Neurosciences,* **20,** 517–523.

Planck M: (1925) The unity of the physical universe. In *A survey of physics: Collection of lectures and essays.* New York: Dutton.

Plomin R, Daniels D: (1987) Why are children in the same family so different from one another? *Behavioral and Brain Sciences,* **10,** 1–60.

Plomin R, Owen MJ, McGuffin P: (1994) The genetic basis of complex human behaviors. *Science,* **264,** 1733–1739.

Plomin R, Rowe DC: (1977) A twin study of temperament in young children. *Journal of Psychology,* **97,** 107–113.

Poincaré H: (1905/1952) *Science and hypothesis.* New York: Dover.

Poirel C: (1982) Circadian rhythms in behavior and experimental psychopathology. In FM Brown & RC Graebner (eds.), *Rhythmic aspects of behavior.* Hillsdale, NJ: Erlbaum.

Poppen JL: (1946) Prefrontal lobotomy for intractable pain: Case report. *Lahey Clinic Bulletin,* **4,** 205–207.

Posner MI, DiGirolamo GJ, Fernandez-Duque D: (1997) Brain mechanisms of cognitive skills. *Consciousness and Cognition,* **6,** 267–290.

Posner MI, Peterson SE: (1990) The attention system of the human brain. *Annual Review of Neuroscience,* **13,** 25–42.

Posner MI, Raichle ME: (1994) *Images of mind.* New York: Scientific American Library.

Post RM: (1992) Transduction of psychosocial stress into the neurobiology of recurrent affective disorder. *American Journal of Psychiatry,* **149,** 999–1010.

Povinelli DJ: (1994) What chimpanzees (might) know about the mind. In RW Wrangham, WC McGrew, FBM de Waal, & PG Heltne (eds.), *Chimpanzee cultures.* Cambridge, MA: Harvard University Press.

Povinelli DJ, deBlois S: (1992) Young children's *(Homo sapiens)* understanding of knowledge formation in themselves and others. *Journal of Comparative Psychology,* **106,** 228–238.

Povinelli DJ, Nelson KE, Boysen ST: (1990) Inferences about guessing and knowing by chimpanzees *(Pan troglodytes).* *Journal of Comparative Psychology,* **104,** 203–210.

Povinelli DJ, Nelson KE, Boysen ST: (1992) Comprehension of social role reversal by chimpanzees: Evidence of empathy? *Animal Behavior,* **43,** 633–640.

Povinelli DJ, Parks KA, Novak MA: (1991) Do rhesus monkeys *(Macaca mulatta)* attribute knowledge and ignorance to others? *Journal of Comparative Psychology,* **105,** 318–325.

Povinelli DJ, Parks KA, Novak MA: (1992) Role reversal by rhesus monkeys, but no evidence of empathy. *Animal Behavior,* **44,** 269–281.

Powley TL, Keesey RE: (1970) Relationship of body weight to the lateral hypothalamic feeding syndrome. *Journal of Comparative and Physiological Psychology,* **70,** 25–36.

Pratt CL, Sackett GP: (1967) Selection of social partners as a function of peer contact during rearing. *Science,* **155,** 1133–1135.

Press F, Siever R: (1978) *Earth.* 2nd ed. San Francisco: Freeman.

Prigogine I: (1980) *From being to becoming: Time and complexity in the physical sciences.* New York: Freeman.

Prigogine I, Stengers I: (1984) *Order out of chaos: Man's new dialogue with nature.* Toronto: Bantam.

Puccetti R: (1981) The case for mental duality: Evidence from split-brain data and other considerations. *Behavioral and Brain Sciences,* **4,** 93–123.

Pylyshyn ZW: (1981) The imagery debate: Analogue media versus tacit knowledge. *Psychological Review,* **86,** 16–45.

Quay HC, Routh DK, Shapiro SK: (1987) Psychopathology of childhood: From description to validation. *Annual Review of Psychology,* **38,** 491–532.

Quitkin F, Rifkin A, Klein DF: (1976) Neurologic soft signs in schizophrenia and character disorders. *Archives of General Psychiatry,* 33, 845–853.

Raichle ME, Fiez JA, Videen TO, MacLeod AMK, Pardo JV, Fox PT, Petersen SE: (1994) Practice-related changes in human brain functional anatomy during nonmotor learning. *Cerebral Cortex,* 4, 8–26.

Raine A, Venables PH: (1981) Classical conditioning and socialization: A biosocial interaction. *Personality and Individual Differences,* 2, 273–283.

Ralph MR, Foster RG, Davis FC, Menaker M: (1990) Transplanted suprachiasmatic nucleus determines circadian period. *Science,* 247, 975–978.

Ramachandran VS, Levi L, Stone L, Rogers-Ramachandran D, McKinney R, Stalcup M, Arcilla G, Zweifler R, Schatz A, Flippin A: (1996) Illusions of body image: What they reveal about human nature. In R Llinás & PS Churchland (eds.), *The mind–brain continuum: Sensory processes.* Cambridge, MA: MIT Press.

Rapaport D: (1951) *Organization and pathology of thought.* New York: Columbia University Press.

Reeves AG, Plum F: (1969) Hyperphagia, rage, and dementia accompanying a ventromedial hypothalamic neoplasm. *Archives of Neurology,* 20, 616–624.

Reich W: (1949) *Character analysis.* 3rd ed. New York: Orgone Institute Press.

Reimann HA: (1963) *Periodic diseases.* Philadelphia: Davis.

Reimann HA: (1974) Clinical importance of biorhythms longer than the circadian. In LE Schering, F Halberg, & JE Pauly (eds.), *Chronobiology.* Tokyo: Igaku-Shoin.

Rescorla RA, Heth CD: (1975) Reinstatement of fear to an extinguished conditioned stimulus. *Journal of Experimental Psychology: Animal Behavior Processes,* 104, 88–96.

Rescorla RA, Wagner AR: (1972) A theory of Pavlovian conditioning: Variations in the effectiveness of reinforcement and nonreinforcement. In AH Black & WF Prokasy (eds.), *Classical conditioning II: Current research and theory.* New York: Appleton-Century-Crofts.

Richardson DE, Akil H: (1977) Pain reduction by electrical brain stimulation in man: I. Acute administration in periaqueductal and periventricular sites. *Journal of Neurosurgery,* 47, 184–194.

Ridley M: (1996) *Evolution.* 2nd ed. Cambridge, MA: Blackwell.

Rizzolatti G: (1994) Nonconscious motor images. *Behavioral and Brain Sciences,* 17, 220.

Rizzolatti G, Carmada R, Fogassi L, Gentilucci M, Luppino G, Matelli M: (1988) Functional organization of area 6 in the macaque monkey: II. Area F5 and the control of distal movements. *Experimental Brain Research,* 71, 491–507.

Roberts DW: (1991) Corpus callosum section. In SS Spencer & DD Spencer (eds.), *Surgery for epilepsy.* Boston: Blackwell.

Roberts W: (1960) Normal and abnormal depersonalization. *Journal of Mental Science,* 106, 478–493.

Roberts WW: (1958) Both rewarding and punishing effects from stimulation of posterior hypothalamus of cat with same electrode at same intensity. *Journal of Comparative and Physiological Psychology,* 51, 400–407.

Robinson RG, Kubos KL, Starr LB, Rao K, Price TR: (1984) Mood disorders in stroke patients: Importance of location of lesion. *Brain,* 107, 81–93.

Rodman HT, Gross CG, Albright TD: (1989) Afferent basis of visual response properties in area MT of the macaque: I. Effects of striate cortex removal. *Journal of Neuroscience,* 9, 2033–2050.

Roland PE: (1984) Metabolic measurements of the working frontal cortex in man. *Trends in Neurosciences,* 7, 430–435.

Roland PE, Friberg L: (1985) Localization of cortical areas activated by thinking. *Journal of Neurophysiology,* 53, 1219–1243.

Rolls ET: (1995) A theory of emotion and consciousness, and its application to understanding the neural basis of emotion. In MS Gazzaniga (ed.), *The cognitive neurosciences.* Cambridge, MA: MIT Press.

Rolls ET: (1999) *The brain and emotion.* Oxford, UK: Oxford University Press.

Rolls ET, Cooper SJ: (1974) Anesthetization and stimulation of the sulcal prefrontal cortex and brain-stimulation reward. *Physiology and Behavior,* 12, 563–571.

Rose SPR: (1993) Synaptic plasticity, learning, and memory. In M Baudry, RF Thompson, & JL Davis (eds.), *Synaptic plasticity: Molecular, cellular, and functional aspects.* Cambridge, MA: MIT Press.

Rössler OE, Hudson JL: (1990) Self-similarity in hyperchaotic data. In E Basar (ed.), *Chaos in brain function.* Berlin: Springer-Verlag.

Roth M: (1959) The phobic anxiety–depersonalization syndrome. *Proceedings of the Royal Society of Medicine,* 52, 587–595.

Rothman GR: (1980) The relationship between moral judgment and moral behavior. In M Windmiller, N Lambert, & E Turiel (eds.), *Moral development and socialization.* Boston: Allyn & Bacon.

Rubens AB: (1985) Caloric stimulation and unilateral visual neglect. *Neurology,* 35, 1019–1024.

Rudy JW, Morledge P: (1994) Ontogeny of contextual fear conditioning in rats: Implications for consolidation, infantile amnesia, and hippocampal system function. *Behavioral Neuroscience,* 108, 227–234.

Ruff GE, Levy EZ, Thaler VH: (1961) Factors influencing reactions to reduced sensory input. In P Solomon, PE Kubzansky, PH Leiderman, JH Mendelson, R Trumbull, & D Wexler (eds.), *Sensory deprivation.* Cambridge, MA: Harvard University Press.

Rumelhart DE, McClelland JL: (1986) PDP models and general issues in cognitive science. In DE Rumelhart & JL McClelland (eds.), *Parallel distributed processing: Explorations in the microstructure of cognition, Vol. 1, Foundations.* Cambridge, MA: MIT Press.

Rusak B, Zucker I: (1974) Fluid intake of rats in constant light and during feeding restricted to the light or dark portion of the illumination cycle. *Physiology and Behavior,* 13, 91–100.

Russo EB: (1992) Headache treatments by native peoples of the Ecuadorian Amazon: A preliminary cross-disciplinary assessment. *Journal of Ethnopharmacology,* 36, 193–206.

Saint-Cyr JA, Taylor AE: (1992) The mobilization of procedural learning: The "key signature" of the basal ganglia. In LR Squire & N Butters (eds.), *Neuropsychology of memory.* 2nd ed. New York: Guilford Press.

Salthouse T: (1985) Speed of behavior and its implications for cognition. In JE Birren & KW.Schaie (eds.), *Handbook of the psychology of aging.* 2nd ed. New York: Van Nostrand Reinhold.

Sarich V, Wilson AC: (1967) Immunological time scale for human evolution. *Science, 158,* 1200–1203.

Savage-Rumbaugh S, Lewin R: (1994) *Kanzi: The ape at the brink of the human mind.* New York: Wiley.

Savage-Rumbaugh ES, Pate JL, Lawson J, Smith ST, Rosenbaum S: (1983) Can a chimpanzee make a statement? *Journal of Experimental Psychology: General, 112,* 457–492.

Savage-Rumbaugh ES, Rumbaugh EM, Boysen S: (1978a) Symbolic communication between two chimpanzees *(Pan troglodytes). Science, 201,* 641–644.

Savage-Rumbaugh ES, Rumbaugh EM, Boysen S: (1978b) Linguistically mediated tool use and exchange by chimpanzees *(Pan troglodytes). Behavioral and Brain Sciences, 4,* 539–554.

Schachter DL: (1987) Implicit memory: History and current status. *Journal of Experimental Psychology: Learning, Memory and Cognition, 13,* 501–518.

Schachter DL: (1992) Priming and multiple memory systems: Perceptual mechanisms of implicit memory. *Journal of Cognitive Neuroscience, 4,* 244–256.

Schachter DL, Harbluk JL, McLachlan DR: (1984) Retrieval without recollection: An experimental analysis of source amnesia. *Journal of Verbal Learning and Verbal Behavior, 23,* 593–611.

Schachter S, Singer JE: (1962) Cognitive, social, and physiological determinants of emotional state. *Psychological Review, 69,* 379–399.

Schadé JP, Van Groenigen WB: (1961) Structural organization of the human cerebral cortex. *Acta Anatomica, 47,* 74–111.

Schafer R: (1976) *A new language for psychoanalysis.* New Haven, CT: Yale University Press.

Schaffer CE, Davidson RJ, Saron C: (1983) Frontal and parietal EEG asymmetries in depressed and nondepressed subjects. *Biological Psychiatry, 18,* 753–762.

Schaie KW, Parham IA: (1977) Cohort-sequential analysis of adult intellectual development. *Developmental Psychology, 13,* 649–653.

Schank RC: (1982) *Dynamic memory.* Cambridge, UK: Cambridge University Press.

Schank RC, Abelson R: (1977) *Scripts, plans, goals, and understanding.* Hillsdale, NJ: Erlbaum.

Scheibel AB: (1979) Development of axonal and dendritic neuropil as a function of evolving behavior. In FO Schmitt & FG Worden (eds.), *The neurosciences: Fourth study program.* Cambridge, MA: MIT Press.

Scheibel ME, Scheibel AB: (1958) Structural substrates for integrative patterns in the brainstem reticular core. In HH Jasper, LD Proctor, RS Knighton, WC Noshay, & RT Ostello (eds.), *Reticular formation of the brain.* Boston: Little, Brown.

Schell TL, Klein SB, Babey SH: (1996) Testing a hierarchical model of self-knowledge. *Psychological Science, 7,* 170–173.

Schilder P: (1935) *The image and appearance of the human body.* London: Routledge & Kegan Paul.

Schiller PH, True SD, Conway JL: (1980) Deficits in eye movements following frontal eye-field and superior colliculus ablations. *Journal of Neurophysiology, 44,* 1175–1189.

Schmidt K, Solant MV, Bridger WH: (1985) Electrodermal activity of undersocialized aggressive children: A pilot study. *Journal of Child Psychology and Psychiatry,* **26,** 653–660.

Schore AN: (1994) *Affect regulation and the origin of the self: The neurobiology of emotional development.* Hillsdale, NJ: Erlbaum.

Schore AN: (1996) The experience-dependent maturation of a regulatory system in the orbital prefrontal cortex and the origin of developmental psychopathology. *Development and Psychopathology,* **8,** 59–87.

Schultz JH, Luthe W: (1959) *Autogenic training.* New York: Grune & Stratton.

Schwartz SH, Feldman KA, Brown ME, Heingartner A: (1969) Some personality correlates of conduct in two situations of moral conflict. *Journal of Personality,* **37,** 41–57.

Scott TR, Giza BK: (1992) Gustatory control of ingestion. In DA Booth (ed.), *The neurophysiology of ingestion.* Manchester, UK: Manchester University Press.

Scoville WB, Milner B: (1957) Loss of recent memory after bilateral hippocampal lesions. *Journal of Neurology, Neurosurgery and Psychiatry,* **20,** 11–21.

Seay BM, Alexander BK, Harlow HF: (1964) Maternal behavior of socially deprived rhesus monkeys. *Journal of Abnormal and Social Psychology,* **69,** 345–354.

Seitz RJ, Roland PE, Bohm C, Greitz T, Stone-Elander S: (1990) Motor learning in man: A positron emission tomographic study. *NeuroReport,* **1,** 17–20.

Sem-Jacobsen CW: (1968) *Depth-electrographic stimulation of the human brain and behavior.* Springfield, IL: Thomas.

Seneca: (1958) On tranquility. In *The Stoic philosophy of Seneca: Essays and letters.* Translated by M Hadas. New York: Norton.

Serway RA, Faughn JS: (1989) *College physics.* 2nd ed. Philadelphia: Saunders.

Seyfarth RM: (1981) Do monkeys rank each other? *Behavioral and Brain Sciences,* **4,** 447–448.

Shaffer D, Schonfeld I, O'Connor PA, Stokman C, Trautman P, Shafer S, Ng S: (1985) Neurological soft signs: Their relationship to psychiatric disorder and intelligence in childhood and intelligence. *Archives of General Psychiatry,* **42,** 342–351.

Shallice T: (1988) *From neuropsychology to mental structure.* Cambridge, UK: Cambridge University Press.

Shallice T, Fletcher P, Frith CD, Grasby P, Frackowiak RSJ, Dolan RJ: (1994) Brain regions associated with acquisition and retrieval of verbal episodic memory. *Nature,* **368,** 633–635.

Shapiro MF, Fink M, Bender MB: (1952) Exosomesthesia or displacement of cutaneous sensation into extrapersonal space. *Archives of Neurology and Psychiatry,* **68,** 481–490.

Sherwin BB: (1988) Estrogen and/or androgen replacement therapy and cognitive functioning in surgically menopausal women. *Psychoneuroendocrinology,* **13,** 345–357.

Shorvon H: (1945/46) The depersonalization syndrome. *Proceedings of the Royal Society of Medicine,* **39,** 779–792.

Shrager J, Johnson MH: (1995) Waves of growth in the development of cortical function: A computational model. In B Julesz & I Kovács, *Maturational windows and adult cortical plasticity.* Reading, MA: Addison-Wesley.

Sibley CG, Ahlquist JE: (1987) DNA hybridization evidence of hominoid phylogeny: Results from an expanded data set. *Journal of Molecular Evolution,* 26, 99–121.

Siegel J, Wang RY: (1974) Electroencephalographic, behavioral, and single-unit effects produced by stimulation of forebrain inhibitory structures in cats. *Experimental Neurology,* 42, 28–50.

Siegel M, Kurzrok N, Barr WB, Rowan AJ: (1992) Game-playing epilepsy. *Epilepsia,* 33, 93–97.

Siegelbaum SA, Kandel ER: (1991) Learning-related synaptic plasticity: LTP and LTD. *Current Opinion in Neurobiology,* 1, 113–120.

Silberpfennig J: (1941) Contributions to the problem of eye movements. *Confinia Neurologica,* 4, 1–13.

Simon H, LeMoal M, Cardo B: (1975) Self-stimulation in the dorsal pontine tegmentum in the rat. *Behavioral Biology,* 13, 339–347.

Singer JL: (1974) *Imagery and daydreaming methods in psychotherapy and behavior modification.* New York: Academic Press.

Singer W: (1996) Neuronal synchronization: A solution to the binding problem? In R Llinás & PS Churchland (eds.), *The mind–brain continuum: Sensory processes.* Cambridge, MA: MIT Press.

Singer W, Engel AK, Kreiter AK, Munk MHJ: (1997) Neuronal asemblies: Necessity, signature, detectability. *Trends in Cognitive Science,* 1, 252–261.

Singer W, Gray CM: (1995) Visual feature integration and the temporal correlation hypothesis. *Annual Review of Neuroscience,* 18, 555–586.

Skarda CA, Freeman WJ: (1987) How brains make chaos in order to make sense of the world. *Behavioral and Brain Sciences,* 10, 161–195.

Smith DD: (1991) Indeterminacy in psychology. *Psychological Reports,* 69, 771–777.

Smith DD: (1992) Longitudinal stability of personality. *Psychological Reports,* 70, 483–498.

Smith DD: (1993) Brain, environment, heredity, and personality. *Psychological Reports,* 72, 3–13.

Smith KU, Akelaitis AJ: (1942) Studies on the corpus callosum: I. Laterality in behavior and bilateral motor organization in man before and after section of the corpus callosum. *Archives of Neurology and Psychiatry,* 47, 519–543.

Snapir N, Yaakobi M, Robinson B, Ravona H, Perek M: (1976) Involvement of the medial hypothalamus and the septal area in the control of food intake and body weight in geese. *Pharmacology, Biochemistry and Behavior,* 5, 609–615.

Sobesky WE, Hull CE, Hagerman RJ: (1994) Symptoms of schizotypal personality disorder in fragile X females. *Journal of the American Academy of Child and Adolescent Psychiatry,* 33, 247–255.

Sobesky WE, Porter D, Pennington BF, Hagerman RJ: (1995) Dimensions of shyness in fragile X females. *Developmental Brain Dysfunction,* 8, 280–292.

Spencer WA, Thompson RF, Neilson DR Jr: (1966) Response decrement of the flexion reflex in the acute spinal cat and transient restoration by strong stimuli. *Journal of Neurophysiology,* 29, 221–239.

Spencer-Booth Y, Hinde RA: (1971) Effects of 6 days separation from mother on 18- to 32-week-old rhesus monkeys. *Animal Behavior,* 19, 174–191.

Sperry RW: (1966) Brain bisection and mechanisms of consciousness. In JC Eccles (ed.), *Brain and conscious experience.* New York: Springer-Verlag.

Sperry R[W]: (1982) Some effects of disconnecting the cerebral hemispheres. *Science*, **217**, 1223–1226.

Spezzano C: (1993) *Affect in psychoanalysis: A clinical synthesis.* Hillsdale, NJ: Analytic Press.

Spitz RA: (1945) Hospitalism: An inquiry into the genesis of psychiatric conditions in early childhood. *Psychoanalytic Study of the Child*, **1**, 53–74.

Spitz RA: (1946) Anaclitic depression. *Psychoanalytic Study of the Child*, **2**, 313–342.

Spitz RA, Wolf KM: (1946) Hospitalism: A follow-up report on investigation described in Volume 1, 1945. *Psychoanalytic Study of the Child*, **2**, 313–342.

Springer SP, Deutsch G: (1981) *Left brain, right brain.* San Francisco: Freeman.

Squire LR: (1987) *Memory and brain.* New York: Oxford University Press.

Squire LR: (1992) Declarative and nondeclarative memory: Multiple brain systems supporting learning and memory. *Journal of Cognitive Neuroscience*, **4**, 232–243.

Squire LR, Zola-Morgan S: (1988) Memory: Brain systems and behavior. *Trends in Neurosciences*, **11**, 170–175.

Stampfl TG, Levis DJ: (1967) Essentials of implosive therapy: A learning theory based on psychodynamic behavioral therapy. *Journal of Abnormal Psychology*, **72**, 496–507.

Steegman AT, Winer B: (1961) Temporal lobe epilepsy resulting from ganglioglioma. *Neurology*, **11**, 406.

Stellar E: (1954) The physiology of motivation. *Psychological Review*, **61**, 5–22.

Steriade M, McCormick DA, Sejnowski TJ: (1993) Thalamocortical oscillations in the sleeping and aroused brain. *Science*, **262**, 679–685.

Stern DN: (1985) *The interpersonal world of the infant: A view from psychoanalytic developmental psychology.* New York: Basic Books.

Storrie-Baker HJ, Segalowitz SJ, Black SE, McLean JAG, Sullivan N: (1997) Improvement of hemispatial neglect with cold-water calorics: An electrophysiological test of the arousal hypothesis of neglect. *Journal of the International Neuropsychological Society*, **3**, 394–402.

Streifler M, Hofman S: (1976) Sinistrad mirror writing and reading after brain concussion in a bi-systemic (Oriento–Occidental) polyglot. *Cortex*, **12**, 356–364.

Stuss DT: (1991) Disturbance of self-awareness after frontal system damage. In GP Prigatano & DL Schachter (eds.), *Awareness of deficit after brain injury.* New York: Oxford University Press.

Stuss DT: (1992) Biological and psychological development of executive functions. *Brain and Cognition*, **20**, 8–23.

Stuss DT, Benson DF: (1986) *The frontal lobes.* New York: Raven Press.

Stuss DT, Benson DF: (1987) The frontal lobes and the control of cognition and memory. In E Perecman (ed.), *The frontal lobes revisited.* New York: IRBN Press.

Stuss DT, Benson DF, Kaplan EF, Weir WS, Naeser MA, Lieberman I, Ferrill D: (1983) The involvement of orbitofrontal cerebrum in cognitive tasks. *Neuropsychologia*, **21**, 235–248.

Suchy Y, Blint A, Osmon DC: (1997) Behavioral Dyscontrol Scale: Criterion and predictive validity in an inpatient rehabilitation unit population. *The Clinical Neuropsychologist*, **11**, 258–265.

Suzuki S: (1970) *Zen mind, beginner's mind.* New York: Weatherhill.

Swaab DF, Hofman MA: (1990) An enlarged suprachiasmatic nucleus in homosexual men. *Brain Research,* 537, 141–148.

Szentágothai J: (1967) The anatomy of complex integrative units in the nervous system. In K Lissak (ed.), *Recent developments of neurobiology in Hungary, Vol. 1, Results in neuroanatomy, neurochemistry, neuropharmacology, and neurophysiology.* Budapest: Akadémiai Kiadó.

Szentágothai J: (1975) The "module-concept" in cerebral cortex architecture. *Brain Research,* 95, 475–498.

Szentágothai J: (1979) Local neuron circuits of the neocortex. In FO Schmitt & FG Worden (eds.), *The neurosciences: Fourth study program.* Cambridge, MA: MIT Press.

Szentágothai J: (1980) Principles of neural organization. In J Szentágothai, M Palkovits, & J Hamori (eds.), *Advances in physiological sciences, Vol. 1, Regulatory functions of the CNS: Principles of motion and organization.* Budapest: Akadémiai Kiadó, 1–16.

Szentágothai J: (1983) The modular architectonic principle of neural centers. *Review of Physiology, Biochemistry, and Pharmacology,* 98, 11–61.

Szentágothai J: (1987) The "brain–mind" relation: A pseudoproblem? In C Blakemore & S Greenfield (eds.), *Mindwaves: Thoughts on intelligence, identity and consciousness.* Oxford, UK: Blackwell.

Szentágothai J, Arbib MA: (1974) Conceptual models of neural organization. *Neurosciences Research Program Bulletin,* 12, 307–510.

Takahashi JS: (1991) Circadian rhythms: From gene expression to behavior. *Current Opinion in Neurobiology,* 1, 556–561.

Talairach J, Bancaud J, Geier S, Bordas-Ferrer M, Bonis A, Szikla G, Rusu M: (1973) The cingulate gyrus and human behaviour. *Electroencephalography and Clinical Neurophysiology,* 34, 45–52.

Target M, Fonagy P: (1996) Playing with reality: II. The development of psychic reality from a theoretical perspective. *International Journal of Psycho-Analysis,* 77, 459–479.

Teasdale JD, Fogarty SJ: (1979) Differential effects of induced mood on retrieval of pleasant and unpleasant events from episodic memory. *Journal of Abnormal Psychology,* 88, 248–257.

Teasdale JD, Russell ML: (1983) Differential effects of induced mood on the recall of positive, negative and neutral words. *British Journal of Clinical Psychology,* 22, 163–172.

Teitelbaum P: (1955) Sensory control of hypothalamic hyperphagia. *Journal of Comparative and Physiological Psychology,* 48, 158–163.

Teitelbaum P, Epstein AN: (1962) The lateral hypothalamic syndrome: Recovery of feeding and drinking after lateral hypothalamic lesions. *Psychological Review,* 69, 74–90.

Tellegen A, Lykken DT, Bouchard TJ Jr, Wilcox K, Segal NS, Rich S: (1988) Personality similarity in twins reared apart and together. *Journal of Personality and Social Psychology,* 54, 1031–1039.

Tempkins O: (1945) *The falling sickness: A history of epilepsy from the Greeks to the beginnings of modern neurology.* Baltimore: Johns Hopkins University Press.

Terry RD, DeTeresa R, Hansen LA: (1987) Neocortical cell counts in normal human adult aging. *Annals of Neurology,* **21,** 530–539.

Thelen E, Kelso JAS, Fogel A: (1987) Self-organizing systems and infant motor development. *Developmental Review,* **7,** 39065.

Thelen E, Smith LB: (1994) *A dynamic systems approach to the development of cognition and action.* Cambridge, MA: MIT Press.

Thierry AM, Tassin JP, Blanc G, Glowinski J: (1978) Studies on mesocortical dopamine systems. *Advances in Biochemical Psychopharmacology,* **17,** 205–216.

Thomas A, Chess S: (1977) *Temperament and development.* New York: Brunner/Mazel.

Thomas A, Chess S: (1980) *The dynamics of psychological development.* New York: Brunner/Mazel.

Thompson RF: (1986) The neurobiology of learning and memory. *Science,* **233,** 941–947.

Thompson RF: (1988) The neural basis of basic associative learning of discrete behavioral responses. *Trends in Neurosciences,* **11,** 152–155.

Thorndike EL: (1911) *Animal intelligence: Experimental studies.* New York: Macmillan.

Tomasello M: (1994) The question of chimpanzee culture. In RW Wrangham, WC McGrew, FBM de Waal, & PG Heltne (eds.), *Chimpanzee cultures.* Cambridge, MA: Harvard University Press.

Tootell RBH, Dale AM, Sereno MI, Malach R: (1996) New images from human visual cortex. *Trends in Neurosciences,* **19,** 481–489.

Tootell RBH, Silverman MS, Switkes E, DeValois RL: (1982) Deoxyglucose analysis of retinotopic organization in primate striate cortex. *Science,* **218,** 902–904.

Tranel D, Damasio AR: (1985) Knowledge without awareness: An autonomic index of facial recognition by prosopagnosics. *Science,* **228,** 1453–1455.

Tranel D, Damasio A[R]: (1988) Nonconscious face recognition in patients with face agnosia. *Behavioural Brain Research,* **30,** 235–249.

Tranel D, Damasio A[R], Damasio H: (1988) Intact recognition of facial expression, gender, and age in patients with impaired recognition of face identity. *Neurology,* **38,** 680–696.

Traub RD, Miles R, Wong RKS: (1989) Model of the origin of rhythmic population oscillations in the hippocampal slice. *Science,* **243,** 1319–1325.

Travis J: (1994) Glia: The brain's other cells. *Science,* **266,** 970–972.

Trueman RH: (1965) Mirror writing. *Postgraduate Medicine,* **38,** 469–476.

Ts'o DY, Gilbert CD, Wiesel TN: (1986) Relationships between horizontal interactions and functional architecture in cat striate cortex as revealed by cross-correlation analysis. *Journal of Neuroscience,* **6,** 1160–1170.

Tuller B, Kelso JAS: (1989) Environmentally specified patterns of movement coordination in normal and split-brain subjects. *Experimental Brain Research,* **74,** 306–316.

Tulving E: (1985) On the classification problem in learning and memory. In L Nilsson & T Archer (eds.), *Perspectives on learning and memory.* Hillsdale NJ: Erlbaum.

Tulving E: (1987) Multiple memory systems and consciousness. *Human Neurobiology,* **6,** 67–80.

Tulving E, Kapur S, Craik FIM, Moscovitch M, Houle S: (1994a) Hemispheric encoding/retrieval asymmetry in episodic memory: Positron emission tomography findings. *Proceedings of the National Academy of Sciences USA*, **91**, 2016–2020.

Tulving E, Kapur S, Markowitsch HJ, Craik FIM, Habib R, Houle S: (1994b) Neuroanatomical correlates of retrieval in episodic memory: Auditory sentence recognition. *Proceedings of the National Academy of Sciences USA*, **91**, 2012–2015.

Tulving E, Markowitsch HJ, Kapur S, Habib R, Houle S: (1994c) Novelty encoding networks in the human brain: Data from positron emission tomography studies. *NeuroReport*, **5**, 2525–2528.

Ungerleider LG: (1995) Functional brain imaging studies of cortical mechanisms for memory. *Science,* **270**, 769–775.

Ursin H, Kaada BR: (1960) Functional localization within the amygdaloid complex in the cat. *Electroencephalography and Clinical Neurophysiology*, **12**, 1–20.

Valenstein ES: (1973) *Brain control: A critical examination of brain stimulation and psychosurgery.* New York: Wiley.

Vallar G, Sterzi R, Bottini G, Cappa S, Rusconi ML: (1990) Temporary remission of left hemianesthesia after vestibular stimulation: A sensory neglect phenomenon. *Cortex,* **26**, 123–131.

Vallar G, Bottini G, Rusconi ML, Sterzi R: (1993) Exploring somatosensory hemineglect by vestibular stimulation. *Brain,* **116**, 71–86.

van Eeden F: (1913) A study of dreams. *Proceedings of the Society for Psychical Research,* **26**(Pt. 47), 431–461.

Van Essen DC, Maunsell JHR: (1983) Hierarchical organization and functional streams in the visual cortex. *Trends in Neurosciences,* **6**, 370–375.

van Hooff JARAM: (1994) Understanding chimpanzee understanding. In RW Wrangham, WC McGrew, FBM deWaal, & PG Heltne (eds.), *Chimpanzee cultures.* Cambridge, MA: Harvard University Press.

Vauclair J: (1996) *Animal cognition: An introduction to modern comparative psychology.* Cambridge, MA: Harvard University Press.

Victor M, Agamanolis D: (1990) Amnesia due to lesions confined to the hippocampus: A clinical-pathologic study. *Journal of Cognitive Neuroscience,* **2**, 246–257.

von der Malsburg C: (1981) *The correlation theory of brain function.* Internal report, Max Planck Institute for Biophysical Chemistry, Göttingen, Germany.

von der Malsburg C: (1996) The binding problem of neural networks. In R Llinás & PS Churchland (eds.), *The mind–brain continuum: Sensory processes.* Cambridge, MA: MIT Press.

von der Malsburg C, Schneider W: (1986) A neural cocktail-party processor. *Biological Cybernetics,* **54**, 29–40.

von Senden M: (1932/1960) *Space and sight: The perception of space and shape in the congenitally blind before and after operation.* Glencoe, IL: Free Press.

Vygotsky L: (1934/1986) *Thought and language.* A Kozulin (ed.). Cambridge, MA: MIT Press.

Wada JA (ed.): (1976) *Kindling.* New York: Raven Press.

Wada JA, Osawa T: (1976) Spontaneous recurrent seizure state induced by daily electrical amygdaloid stimulation in Senegalese baboons, *Papio papio. Neurology,* **26**, 273–286.

Wada JA, Sato M, Corcoran ME: (1974) Persistent seizure susceptibility and recurrent spontaneous seizures in kindled cats. *Epilepsia,* **15,** 465–478.

Walsh AC, Brown BB, Kaye K, Grigsby J: (1994) *Mental capacity: Legal and medical aspects of assessment and treatment.* 2nd ed. Colorado Springs, CO, & New York: Shepherd's/McGraw-Hill.

Walters JR, Seyfarth RM: (1987) Conflict and cooperation. In BB Smuts, DL Cheney, RM Seyfarth, RW Wrangham, & TT Struhsaker (eds.), *Primate societies.* Chicago: University of Chicago Press.

Warrington EK, Shallice T: (1984) Category specific semantic impairments. *Brain,* **107,** 829–854.

Warrington E[K], Weiskrantz L: (1973) The effect of prior learning on subsequent retention in amnesic patients. *Neuropsychologia,* **20,** 233–248.

Wehr TA, Goodwin FK: (1983) Biological rhythms in manic-depressive illness. In Wehr TA, Goodwin FK (eds.), *Circadian rhythms in psychiatry.* Pacific Grove, CA: Boxwood Press.

Weingartner H, Miller H, Murphy DL: (1977) Mood-state-dependent retrieval of verbal associations. *Journal of Abnormal Psychology,* **86,** 276–284.

Weinstein EA: (1981) *Woodrow Wilson: A medical and psychological biography.* Princeton, NJ: Princeton University Press.

Weinstein EA, Kahn RL: (1950) Syndrome of anosognosia. *Archives of Neurology and Psychiatry,* **64,** 772–791.

Weinstein EA, Kahn RL: (1955) *Denial of illness: Symbolic and physiological aspects.* Springfield, IL: Thomas.

Weiskrantz L: (1986) *Blindsight: A case study and implications.* Oxford, UK: Clarendon Press.

Weiskrantz L: (1995) Blindsight—not an island unto itself. *Current Directions in Psychological Science,* **4,** 146–151.

Weiskrantz L: (1997) *Consciousness lost and found: A neuropsychological exploration.* Oxford, UK: Oxford University Press.

Weiskrantz L, Warrington E: (1979) Conditioning in amnesic patients. *Neuropsychologia,* **17,** 187–194.

Weiskrantz L, Warrington E, Sanders MD, Marshall J: (1974) Visual capacity in the hemianopic field following a restricted occipital ablation. *Brain,* **97,** 709–728.

Weiss G, Hechtman L, Milroy T, Perlman T: (1985) Psychiatric status of hyperactives as adults: A controlled prospective 15-year follow-up of 63 hyperactive children. *Journal of the American Academy of Child Psychiatry,* **24,** 211–220.

Weiss J, Sampson H: (1986) *The psychoanalytic process.* New York: Guilford Press.

Weiss PA: (1967) 1 + 1 ≠ 2 (One plus one does not equal two). In GC Quarton, T Melnechuk, & FO Schmitt (eds.), *The neurosciences: A study program.* New York: Rockefeller University Press.

Weiss PA: (1969) The living system: Determinism stratified. In A Koestler & JR Smythies (eds.), *Beyond reductionism.* Boston: Beacon Press.

Weiss PA: (1971) The basic concept of hierarchic systems. In PA Weiss (ed.), *Hierarchically organized systems in theory and practice.* New York: Hafner.

Welsh MC, Pennington BF, Groisser DB: (1991) A normative-developmental study of executive function: A window on prefrontal function in children. *Developmental Neuropsychology,* **7,** 131–149.

Werner H: (1937) Process and achievement: A basic problem of education and developmental psychology. *Harvard Educational Review,* **7,** 353–368.

Wessinger CM, Fendrich R, Gazzaniga MS: (1997) Islands of residual vision in hemianopic patients. *Journal of Cognitive Neuroscience, 9,* 203–221.

Weyandt LL, Willis WG: (1994) Executive functions in school-aged children: Potential efficacy of tasks in discriminating clinical groups. *Developmental Neuropsychology, 10,* 27–38.

Whelihan WM, Lescher EL: (1985) Neuropsychological changes in frontal functions with aging. *Developmental Neuropsychology, 1,* 371–380.

Whitehead AN, Russell B: (1910–1913) *Principia mathematica.* 2nd ed. Cambridge, UK: Cambridge University Press.

Whiten A, Byrne RW: (1988) Tactical deception in primates. *Behavioral and Brain Sciences, 11,* 233–273.

Wiesel TN, Hubel DH: (1963) Single-cell responses in striate cortex of kittens deprived of vision in one eye. *Journal of Neurophysiology, 26,* 1003–1017.

Wiesel TN, Hubel DH: (1965) Comparison of the effects of unilateral and bilateral eye closure on cortical unit responses in kittens. *Journal of Neurophysiology, 28,* 1029–1040.

Wilson S, Barber T: (1983) The fantasy-prone personality: Implications for understanding imagery, hypnosis, and parapsychological phenomena. In A Sheikh (ed.), *Imagery: Current theory, research, and applications.* New York: Wiley.

Wilson TD: (1985) Strangers to ourselves: The origins and accuracy of beliefs about one's own mental states. In JH Harvey & G Weary (eds.), *Attribution: Basic issues and applications.* New York: Academic Press.

Winn P: (1995) The lateral hypothalamus and motivated behavior: An old syndrome reassessed and a new perspective gained. *Current Directions in Psychological Science, 4,* 182–187.

Winn P, Tarbuck A, Dunnett SB: (1984) Ibotenic acid lesions of the lateral hypothalamus: Comparison with the electrolytic lesion syndrome. *Neuroscience, 12,* 225–240.

Winnicott DW: (1960) The theory of the parent–infant relationship. *International Journal of Psycho-Analysis, 41,* 585–595.

Winnicott DW: (1960/1965) Ego distortion in terms of true and false self. In DW Winnicott, *The maturational processes and the facilitating environment.* London: Hogarth Press.

Wise RA: (1980) The dopamine synapse and the notion of "pleasure centers" in the brain. *Trends in Neurosciences, 3,* 91–94.

Wise RA: (1996) Addictive drugs and brain stimulation reward. *Annual Review of Neuroscience, 19,* 319–340.

Wolpe J: (1958) *Psychotherapy by reciprocal inhibition.* Palo Alto, CA: Stanford University Press.

Yakovlev PI, Lecours A-R: (1967) The myelogenetic cycles of regional maturation of the brain. In A Minkowski (ed.), *Regional development of the brain in early life.* Oxford, UK: Blackwell.

Yamadori A, Albert ML: (1973) Word category aphasia. *Cortex, 9,* 83–89.

Yamamoto J, Egawa I, Yamamoto S, Shimizu A: (1991) Reflex epilepsy induced by calculation using a "soroban," a Japanese traditional calculator. *Epilepsia, 32,* 39–43.

Yeo CH, Hardiman MJ, Glickstein M: (1984) Discrete lesions of the cerebellar cortex abolish the classically conditioned nictitating membrane response of the rabbit. *Behavioural Brain Research, 13,* 261–266.

Yeomans JS: (1982) The cells and axons mediating medial forebrain bundle reward. In BG Hoebel & D Novin (eds.), *The neural basis of feeding and reward.* Brunswick, ME: Haer Institute.

Yeterian EH, Pandya DN: (1985) Corticothalamic connections of the posterior parietal cortex in the rhesus monkey. *Journal of Comparative Neurology,* 237, 408–426.

Zajonc RB: (1968) Attitudinal effects of mere exposure. *Journal of Personality and Social Psychology Monograph,* 9(2, Pt. 2), 1–28.

Zajonc R: (1980) Feeling and thinking: Preferences need no inferences. *American Psychologist,* 35, 151–175.

Zajonc RB: (1982) Affective and cognitive factors in preferences. *Journal of Consumer Research,* 9, 123–131.

Zajonc RB: (1984) On the primacy of affect. *American Psychologist,* 39, 117–123.

Zajonc RB, McIntosh DN: (1992) Emotions research: Some promising questions and some questionable promises. *Psychological Science,* 4, 70–74.

Zatz LM, Jernigan TL, Ahumada AJ: (1982) White matter changes in cerebral computed tomography relating to aging. *Journal of Computer Assisted Tomography,* 6, 19–23.

Zimbardo P, Ebbesen E: (1969) *Influencing attitudes and changing behavior.* Reading, MA: Addison-Wesley.

Zola-Morgan S, Squire LR: (1986) Memory impairment in monkeys following lesions of the hippocampus. *Behavioral Neuroscience,* 100, 165–170.

Zola-Morgan S, Squire LR: (1990) The neuropsychology of memory: Parallel findings from humans and nonhuman primates. *Annals of the New York Academy of Sciences,* 608, 434–456.

Zola-Morgan S, Squire LR, Amaral DG: (1989) Lesions of the hippocampal formation but not lesions of the fornix or the mammillary nuclei produce long-lasting memory impairment in monkeys. *Journal of Neuroscience,* 9, 897–912.

Zuckerman M: (1995) Good and bad humors: Biochemical basis of personality and its disorders. *Psychological Science,* 6, 325–332.

INDEX

A

Abstract ideas, 231
Acid-base reaction, 113
Action potential
  description of, 41, 42–43, 44
  myelinization of neurons and, 46
  neuronal firing and, 133–134
  synaptic efficacy and, 44
Action slips, 284–285
Active approach (Ferenczi), 309, 322
Adaptation
  conscious functioning and, 258–260
  efficiency and, 32
  evolutionary compared to psychological, 32
  experience-dependent type of, 27
  of neural plasticity, 16
  recurrence of behavior and, 51
  self-organizing capacity and, 131
ADHD (attention-deficit/hyperactivity disorder)
  character and, 321
  control parameters and, 123–124
  executive functioning and, 291
  as heritable, 30
  temperament and, 196, 197
Adynamia, 76
Affect and self-representations, 333–334
Affective disorders
  as dynamic disorders, 156–157
  See also Depression
Aggression in primate groups, 206–207

Aging brain
  frontal lobes and, 291–292
  neural networks and, 141–142
Agnosia, 70–72, 341–342
  apperceptive, 70–71, 72
  finger, 341
  visual, 70–72, 269–270
Allesthesia, 341
Ambiguity and conscious functioning, 223–224, 241–244
Ambivalence, 159
Amnesia, 89–91, 271–272
  anterograde, 89–91
  infantile, 318, 369–370
  post-traumatic, 1
  retrograde, 89–91
  source, 88
Amygdala
  cortical and subcortical connections of, 186
  emotional learning and, 96, 98, 187
  emotion regulation and, 185–186
  excitability and, 195
  fear conditioning and, 176
  memory and, 85, 88–89
  startle behavior and, 98
Angle of repose, 115
Anosognosia, 250–251, 274, 345–346
Anterior commissure, 242
Anthropoidea, 33
Apathy, 297
Aphasic disorder, 345

Apoptosis, 46, 290
Apparent randomness, 114
Appetite regulation, 181–183
Apraxia, 285–286
    ideational, 285–286
ideomotor, 285
Architecture of brain, 54–55
Arousal and learning, 98, 365–367
Articulatory loop, 101
Asomatognosia, 337, 341
Assessment and modular hypothesis, 80–
    81
Associative agnosia, 71–72
Asymbolia for pain, 342
Attachment
    critical periods and, 48, 360
    primates and, 205–206
    procedural learning and, 315
Attention, 232–233, 234
Attention-deficit/hyperactivity disorder.
    See ADHD (attention-deficit/hy-
    peractivity disorder)
Attractors
    chemical equilibrium as, 114
    compared to repellors, 111–112
    levels of analysis and, 280–281
    in nervous system, 143
    overview of, 108
    states as, 168
Attributions, 7–8, 273
Austin (chimpanzee), 215–216, 219
Autism, 192, 201, 340
Automaticity of character, 311–312
Autoscopic phenomena, 343–344
Autosomal dominant transmission, 30
Autotopagnosia, 341

B
Baars, B.J.
    conscious and nonconscious function-
        ing and, 234–235
    global workspace metaphor of, 235–236
    model of voluntary activity of, 258
Baboons
    dominance in, 206–207
    tactical deception by, 214
Background activity, 134, 142, 145
Basal ganglia
    anatomy of, 74, 288
    excitation and inhibition in, 135–136

habit memory and, 92
    injury to, 76
    schemas and, 283
Basal nucleus, 52
Basin of attraction
    ambivalence and paranoia and, 159–
        160
    broad type, 144, 160
    depression and, 169
    description of, 112, 124
    perseveration and, 158
Behavior
    attributions about, 241–244
    change in with language in nonhuman
        primates, 218–219
    classes of, 222–223
    delay between initiation of and aware-
        ness of, 235–236, 253–255
    elicited type, 183–184
    as emergent process, 302–303
    genetic influence on, 192–194
    levels of analysis of, 280–281
    as paradoxical, 102
    probabilistic basis of, 130
    rationality and, 303
    reconciliatory type, 208
    self-destructive type, 261
    state influence on, 171–172
    strategies to change, 355–356
    superstitious type, 25–26
    voluntary control of, 257–258
    See also Regulation of behavior
Behavioral control. *See* Regulation of
    behavior
Behavioral Dyscontrol Scale, 292
Behaviorism, 6, 225
Bifurcation
    description of, 113, 117–118
    examples of, 118–119
Binding problem, 55, 77–79
Biological model
    bifurcation in, 118
    dynamics and, 105
    energy conservation and, 106–107
    hierarchical organization and, 55–56
    relationship to psychological model, 8–
        9, 13–15
    structure and function, relationship be-
        tween, 58
    temperament and, 189

Blindsight, 248–249
Blobs, 69
Body schema
   as basic level of self, 329–330, 332–333
   disturbances of, 344–346
   overview of, 340–344
   in unilateral spatial neglect, 337–339
Borderline personality disorder
   modularity of self and, 352–353, 354
   mood disturbance in, 321
   temperament and, 201, 362
Boutons, 42
Brain
   aging of, 141–142, 291–292
   architecture of, 54–55
   chaotic activity in, 142–143
   development of, 40, 46
   as emergent property, 13
   euphoria with injury to, 184–185,
      274–275
   focal injury to, 251–252
   intracranial electrical stimulation of,
      178–180
   maturation of memory systems and,
      94–95
   modular architecture of, 4, 58–60,
      242–244
   pattern recognition and generation in,
      229–230
   sense of agency and, 255–257
   theories of function of, 56–58
   See also Conscious functioning (or
      processing); Nonconscious func-
      tioning (or processing); *specific
      brain structures* (i.e., Amygdala)
Brainstem, 69–70
Buffers, 101, 239–240

C
Calcarine cortex, 66
Callosotomy, 242–244, 272–273, 346–
   350
Caloric testing, 250–251
Caregivers
   ego functions and, 266–267
   relationships with, 315–316
   self-representations and, 335
   separation from, 205–206
   temperament of infant and, 198–199
   See also Attachment

Cartesian interactionism, 15–16
Categorization capacity of chimpanzees,
   216
Caudate nucleus, 123–124, 135, 288
Cellular map of visual world, 61
Central executive (Baddeley), 233
Central nervous system (CNS)
   body schema and, 340
   development of, 40
   external stimulation and, 147–148
   neural plasticity and, 45–46
   sensitivity to changes in activity of,
      160–162
   structural-functional organization of,
      56–58
Cerebellum, 75
Cerebral time-on theory, 253
Change
   arousal level and, 365–367
   in character, 319–320, 370–372
   critical period and, 359–360
   dynamics of, 358–359
   in hierarchical system, 358
   insight and, 372
   learning and, 325, 367–369
   in state, 362–365
   synaptic plasticity and, 360–361
   temperament and, 361–362
Chaos, system on the edge of, 110
Chaotic activity in brain, 142–143
Chaotic or strange attractor, 108
Chaotic systems, 108, 110, 114
Character
   automaticity of, 311–312
   change in, 319–320, 370–372
   compared to self, 332
   definition of, 310–311
   dissociability of self and, 318–319
   dynamics and, 317–318
   history of concept of, 308–310
   nonconscious quality of, 318
   overview of, 305–306
   pathology in, 320–321
   procedural learning and, 18, 91, 310–
      311, 316–317, 325
   representations of and reactions to
      others', 324
   repression and, 321–322
   sensitive periods in development of,
      313–314

Character (*cont.*)
  temperament and development of, 314–315
  theory of, 23
  therapeutic approach to, 102, 322–323
  variability in, 319–320
Chemical equilibrium, 113–114, 121–122
Chemical synapse, 42, 43
Chemical systems, 14–15
Chimpanzee cultures
  cooperative behavior in, 219
  dominance in, 207–208
  procedural learning in, 35–37
  reconciliation in, 208
  reflective self-awareness and, 210, 211
  symbolic language and, 215–216
  tactical deception in, 214
  theory of mind and, 212–213
Cingulate gyrus, 255–257
Cingulate gyrus, anterior, 76
Circadian pacemaker, 61
Circadian rhythm, 152
Classical conditioning, 99, 368–369
CNS. *See* Central nervous system (CNS)
Cognition
  influence of state on, 171–172
  rhythmic variation in, 153–154
Cognition in nonhuman primates
  attachment and separation, 205–206
  attribution and theory of mind, 212–218
  dominance and social hierarchies, 206–208
  learning language and, 218–219
  overview of, 22, 203–205
  reconciliation after conflict, 208
  reflective self-awareness, 209–212
  self-representations, 211–212
Cognitive ability, conservation of across order Primates, 35
Cognitive appraisal theory, 177–178
Cognitive therapy, 364
Coma, 229
Commissurotomy. *See* Callosotomy
Complex cells, 69
Complex partial seizure, 228, 276
Concretization of perceptions of world, 316–317
Conditioned fear, 96–98, 176, 186

Conditioned stimulus, 99, 368
Conduct disorder, 196
Confabulation, 158–159, 271
Conscious functioning (or processing)
  ambiguity and, 223–224, 241–244
  basic aspects of, 227–229
  compared to nonconscious functioning, 234–235
  conditioned fear and, 97
  description of, 22, 222–224, 226
  as emergent process, 225–226
  Freud on, 224–225
  as global workspace, 235–236
  limitations of, 233–234, 351
  manifestations of, 227
  representational activity and, 230–232
  value of, 258–260
  working memory, attention, and, 232–233
Conservation of traits across evolution, 33
Contention scheduling system (Shallice), 282–283, 284
Control of information processing, 234
Control parameter, 122–124, 147
Cooperative activity of primates, 207, 219
Corpus callosum, 241–244
Cortex
  association, 288
  basal prefrontal, 184–185
  declarative memory and, 88
  dorsolateral prefrontal (DLPC)
    compared to OMPC, 288–290
    inhibition of habitual behavior and, 295–296
    voluntary behavior and, 257
  emotion and, 176–177
  habit memory and, 92
  inferior temporal, 252
  left temporal and amnesia, 89–90
  orbitofrontal, 184–185
  orbitomedial prefrontal (OMPC), 288–290, 296
  primary motor, 72–74
  primary somatosensory, 74
  somatosensory, plasticity of, 51–52
  superior posterior temporal, 276–277
Cortical module, 58
Coupled systems, 136

Critical period
  for attachment, 48, 360
  brain development and, 47
  definition of, 46
  in development of character, 313–314
  for language, 360
  neural plasticity and, 45–46
  personality change and, 359–360
  visual system development and, 46–48
Critical state
  chaotic activity and, 142–143
  description of, 115
  in organisms, 116–117
  psychotherapy and, 130
  See also Self-organized criticality
Crossover and DNA, 31
Culture
  evolution and, 35–37
  See also Chimpanzee cultures

D
Darwin, Charles, 28
Decerebrate rigidity, 1
Declarative memory
  dissociability of, 87–89
  flexibility of, 176
  infantile amnesia and, 369
  modularity of, 84
  procedural learning and, 93
  reactivation of, 90
  timing of development of, 94–95
Déjà vu, 275
Delay between initiation of and aware-
    ness of action, 235–236, 253–255
Dendrites, 41, 46
Dendritic spines, 41, 46
Depersonalization, 275–276
Depolarization, 133, 135–136
Depression
  compared to apathy, 297
  as disturbance of periodic functioning,
    156–157
  lateralization of affect in, 174–175
  neural networks and, 143–144
  neurochemical tuning and, 363
  phase space and, 125–126
  processing speed and, 233
  self-representations and, 334
  state and, 169
Derealization, 275–276

Descartes, René, 15–16, 226
Diagnosis and modular hypothesis, 80–
    81
Dishabituation, 367
Disinhibition, 76
Dissipative structure, 121
Dissociability
  of anterograde and retrograde amne-
    sia, 89–91
  of awareness and perception, 247–252
  of character and self, 318–319
  of declarative memory, 87–89
  of memory systems, 85–86
  of moral judgment and moral behav-
    ior, 300–302
  of procedural learning, 86–87
  of self-representation and awareness of
    self, 327–328, 330–331
Dissociative state, 354
Distractibility, 158, 198
DNA, 31, 35
Dominance, social
  in humans, 208–209
  in nonhuman primates, 206–208
Dopamine, 180, 181
Dostoevsky, Fyodor, 343–344
Double dissociation, 87, 88, 228–229
Dreams, 228
Drive reduction theory of motivation,
    179
DSM-IV, 80–81
Dualism, 15–16, 226
Dynamic disorders
  cause of, 160
  disturbances of periodic functioning
    and affective disorders, 156–157
  overview of, 21
  perseveration, distractibility, and con-
    fabulation, 157–159
  rhythmic process in, 155
  types of, 155–156
Dynamic equilibrium, 113–114
Dynamics, science of
  attractors, 108
  change and, 358–359
  chaotic systems, 108, 110, 114
  character and, 317–318
  chemical equilibrium, 113–114
  energy expenditure, 119–121
  fluctuations and bifurcations, 117–119

Dynamics, science of (*cont.*)
  nonlinear systems and unpredictability,
    112–113
  overview of, 20–21, 104–107
  periodicity, 107–108
  quasi-periodicity and apparent ran-
    domness, 114
  repellors, 110–112
  self-organized criticality, 114–116
  temperament and, 190–191
Dyscalculia, 30
Dysexecutive syndrome
  case examples of, 298–300
  failure to initiate and inhibit behavior
    in, 294–297
  impairment of insight in, 293–294
  overview of, 293
Dyskinesia, 136
Dyslexia, 30

E
Earthquake example, 115–116
Ecological niche
  adaptation and, 32
  evolution and, 26–27
  organism and, 16
Efficiency of conscious and nonconscious
    functioning, 223
Ego, Freud on, 263–264
Ego functions
  description of, 263
  as emergent processes, 264–265
  examples of, 264
  as modular, 267
  relationships with caregivers and, 266–
    267
Electroconvulsive therapy (ECT), 157
Electroencephalogram (EEG), 114
Elicited behavior, 183–184
Emergent materialism, 16
Emotion
  amygdala and, 185–186
  biology of, 173–174
  lateralization of depressive affect, 174–
    175
  LeDoux neuropsychological theory of,
    176–178
  seizure activity and, 175
  state and, 169–170
Emotional attachment. *See* Attachment

Emotional learning, 96, 98, 187
Emotional memory, 84–85, 96–99
Energy conservation, 106–107, 119–
    121
Energy of activation, 127, 128
Entropy, 106, 121–122
Environment
  relationship of organism to, 16
  state and, 363–364
  temperament and, 196–200
  transactions of brain with, 147–148
Epilepsy. *See* Seizure
Episodic memory
  description of, 87
  early childhood and, 370
  lateralization in, 90–91
Epistemological solipsism, 267
Equilibrium, 113–114, 116–117
Estrogen, 154, 193
Euphoria and brain injury, 184–185,
    274–275
Evolutionary biology
  cognition in humans compared to that
    in great apes, 203–205
  conservation of traits, 33
  genetic mutations and, 29–31
  importance of, 25
  overview of, 20, 25–26
  See also Adaptation; Primates
Excitatory postsynaptic potential, 43,
    44
Excitatory stimulation, 133, 135–136
Executive cognitive functions
  dysexecutive syndrome and, 293–297
  movement and, 77
  neuroanatomy of, 287–293
  overview of, 286–287
Exosomesthesia, 270–271, 342
Experience
  acquisition of behavioral control and,
    297–298
  activation of neural networks and,
    126–127
  changes in functioning as result of,
    83–84
  in development of character, 314
  synaptic modification by, 45, 49–50,
    51
  temperament and, 189–190
Explicit memory, 85, 92, 246

Extinction
    of fear response, 97
    of learned behavior, 368–369
Eyes and natural selection, 33

F
Fantasy play by nonhuman primates, 217
Fantasy-prone individual, 240
Fear conditioning. *See* Conditioned fear
Fear-potentiated startle paradigm, 97
Feedforward and feedback activity
    amygdala and cortex and, 176
    overview of, 137–139
    perception and movement and, 75, 76–77
Fenichel, Otto, on character, 306–308
Ferenczi, Sándor, on character, 308–309, 322
Fitness, 26–27
Flaccidity, 74
Focal injury to brain, 251–252
Fornix, 89
Fovea, 237
Fragile X syndrome, 192
Freud, Sigmund
    on character pathology, 307
    on ego, 263–264
    on parapraxes, 283–284
    on unconscious, 224–225, 260
Frontal lobes
    in aging brain, 141–142, 291–292
    anatomy of, 290
Function, relationship to structure, 58
Functional systems, 4, 19, 55

G
Gage, Phineas, 5–6
Gender identity, 360
Generalizability of learning, 88
Genetic influence on behavior, 38, 192–194
Genetic mutations, 29–31
Genotype, 33, 35, 38
Glia, 41
Global workspace metaphor of conscious functioning (Baars), 235–236
"Good enough" fit, 199–200, 315
"Goodness of fit," 190, 198

Gorillas, self-awareness in, 210–211
Greely, A.W., 172

H
Habit memory, 92
Habitual behavior
    activation of, 371–372
    changing, 312
    consciousness and, 259
    inhibition or override of, 295–296, 303
    as nonconscious, 279–280
    overview of, 22
    procedural learning and, 99
    volition and, 255
    See also Nonconscious functioning (or processing)
Habituation, 367–368
Harlow, Harry F., 48, 206
Head trauma, effects of on personality, 3–6
Hebb, D.O., model of synaptic modification, 45, 334
Hemianopia, 70
Hemiautotopagnosia, 274, 341–342
Hemiplegia, 73
Hemispatial neglect, 249–251, 337–339
Hemispheric dominance, disruptions of, 160–161
Heritability
    of attention-deficit and learning disorders, 30
    of intelligence, 28, 192–193
    of temperament, 190–191
Heterarchy, 57, 58
Heterozygosity, 29
Hierarchical organization
    of biological systems, 55–58, 72–77
    change in, 358
    of schemas, 282
    of self-representation, 327–328, 332–333
Hippocampus
    memory and, 85, 88, 90, 105
    oscillatory dynamics and, 136
Hominoids, 33, 35
Homozygosity, 29
Hormone replacement therapy, 154
Hunger example of state influence, 171–172

Huntington's disease, 30, 74
Hypercolumns, 69
Hyperpolarization, 133, 135–136
Hypomania, 233
Hypothalamus
    appetite and, 181–183
    stimulation of and elicited behavior,
        183–184

I
Ideomotor theory (James), 258
Illusions and hallucinations, paroxysmal,
    343–344
Imagery and perception, 236–237, 239–
    241
Imperfect fit, 199
Implicit memory, 85, 92, 95–96, 246–
    247
Impulsivity, 296
Infradian rhythm, 152, 154
Inhibited children, 195–196, 197
Inhibition, disorders of, 294–297
Inhibitory postsynaptic potential, 43,
    44
Inhibitory stimulation, 133, 135–136
Initiation, disorders of, 294–296
Inner speech, 101
Insight
    change and, 372
    consciousness and, 260
    dysexecutive syndrome and, 293–294
    impairments of, 274, 344–346
Instantaneous physiological state. See
    State
Intelligence, 28, 192–193
Interictal period, 175
Interneuron, 43
Intracranial electrical stimulation of
    brain, 178–180

J
Jamais vu, 275
James, William, 225, 258, 259, 328
Jet lag, 123, 157

K
Kierkegaard, Søren, 328
Kindling, 112, 151–152
Kinesthetic sense, 74
Koko (gorilla), 210–211, 216–217

L
Labyrinths, 76
Language
    behavior change in nonhuman pri-
        mates with, 218–219
    conscious functioning and, 235
    critical periods and, 360
    mediation of in brain, 59
    unitary sense of self and, 352
    See also Symbolic language
Lateral geniculate nucleus (LGN), 61, 66
Lateral hypothalamus (LH), 182–184
Lateral inhibition, 135
Lateralization
    of depressive affect, 174–175
    of episodic memory, 90–91
Law of cosmic laziness, 119–121
Learning
    arousal and, 98, 365–367
    change and, 367–369
    culture and, 35–37
    from experience, 20
    generalizability of, 88
    neural basis of, 45
    as physiological process, 14–15
    regulation of behavior and, 297–298
    speed of, 93
    See also Procedural learning
Learning disabilities, 30–31
LeDoux, J.E., 176–178
Left hemisphere
    callosotomy and, 348
    mnestic deficits and, 90–91
    rationalization and, 255
Levels of analysis, 13–15, 18, 280–281
Libet, Benjamin, 253–255
Local relaxation time, 117
Locked-in syndrome, 229
Lockwood, James B., 172
Long-term depression, 50
Long-term memory, 49–50, 51
Long-term potentiation, 50, 151
Lucid dreaming, 228
Luria, A.R., 4, 56
Lying by nonhuman primates, 217–218

M
Macaque monkeys, 66, 208
Macropsia, 343
Macrosomatagnosia, 343

Magnocellular tract, 288, 290
Mammillary bodies, 89
Mania, 233, 317–318
Medial forebrain bundle, 180–181
Medicinal plants, 37
Melatonin, 152
Membrane potential, 134
Memory
    amygdala and, 85, 88–89
    brain development and, 94–95
    context-dependent type, 170–171
    dissociability of, 85–89
    emotional memory, 84–85, 96–99
    episodic type, 87, 90–91, 370
    examples of, 83–84
    explicit type, 85, 92, 246
    hippocampus and, 85, 88, 90, 105
    implicit type, 85, 92, 95–96, 246–247
    long-term, 49–50, 51
    modularity of, 20
    of pain, 99–100
    primacy and recency effects in, 101
    PTSD and, 103
    self-representations and, 335–337
    semantic, 87, 90–91
    treatment of psychological conditions
        and, 81, 85
    working memory, 101–102
    See also Declarative memory; Proce-
        dural learning; Working memory
Ménière's disease, 276
Menstrual cycle, 154
Mental duality, 346–347, 350
Mere exposure effect, 246
Micropsia, 343
Microsomatagnosia, 343
Migraine headache, 343
Mill, John Stuart, on moral philosophy, 7
Mind, 17, 226, 229
Minnesota Multiphasic Personality In-
    ventory (MMPI), 81
Mirror focus, 151–152
Mirror self-recognition, 210
Mirror writing, 161
Mnestic process, types of, 84–85
Model
    clinical implications of, 23–24, 375–
        376
    development of, 11–12
    philosophical basis of, 13–15

Modular systems
    assessment and diagnosis and, 80–81
    binding problem and, 77–79
    ego functions as, 267
    motor functioning as, 72–77
    neural systems evolution toward, 57
    overview of, 4–5
    personality and, 79
    psychopathology and, 79–80
    reality testing as, 269–275
    regulation of appetite as, 181–183
    self as, 333–334, 346–350
    states as, 168–170
    treatment and, 81
    visual system as, 60–61, 66, 68–69,
        72
Modulatory input, 133–134
Modules, 58–60
Monism, 16
Mood and state, 169
Mood-congruent memory, 170
Moral judgment and moral behavior,
    300–302
Motivation, 178–181
Motor functioning, 72–77
Multistability, 124
Mutations, 29–31
Myelinization of neurons, 46

N
Natural selection
    conditions of, 28
    manipulation of others and, 214
    overview of, 20, 38
    survival of the fittest, 26–27
    variation and, 28–29
Nature-nurture debate, 191–192
Nerve impulse. See Action potential
Nervous system. See Central nervous sys-
    tem (CNS)
Neural dynamics. See Dynamics, science
    of
Neural network
    activation of, 126–127
    description of, 50, 131–132
    dynamics of, 142–144
    levels of analysis of, 280–281
    processing in, 139–142
    synaptic plasticity and, 50–51
Neural plasticity. See Synaptic plasticity

Neural processing
    computational aspect of, 57
    energy expenditure and, 120
Neurobiology of learning, 15
Neurochemical tuning, 363
Neuromodulators, 98, 133–134
Neuron
    cortical, 134
    firing of, 133–134
    myelinization of, 46
    number and kinds of, 132
    structure and function of, 40–43
Neuronal synchronization, 78
Neuronal units, 60
Neurosis, 307, 309–310
Neurotransmitter, 43, 44
Neurotrophic factors, 46
Nonconscious functioning (or processing)
    character and, 318
    compared to conscious functioning,
        234–235
    description of, 22, 222–224, 226, 245
    emotional processing and, 178
    experimental psychology and, 245–246
    Freud on, 224–225
    self-organizing activity and, 231
    as unconscious in psychodynamics,
        260–262
Nonequilibrium phase transition. See Bi-
        furcation
Nonlinear systems
    neuronal activity as, 133–134
    state as, 168–170, 187
    unpredictability in, 112–113
Norepinephrine, 98
Novelty
    conscious functioning and, 259
    nonconscious functioning and, 247–
        248
Nucleotide, 31

O
Ocular dominance columns, 69
Odor stimulus, 141
Old World monkeys, 33, 35
Olfactory bulb, 141, 142, 183
Opiods, 98
Organism
    relationship to environment, 16
    self-organized criticality in, 116–117

Oscillatory activity, 78, 136–137
Others' reactions and self, 332

P
Pain
    asymbolia for pain, 342
    brain and, 148
    memories of, 84–85, 99–100
    seizure and, 151
Paradoxical human behavior, 102
Parallel processing, 139–140
Paranoia, 159–160
Paraphrenia, 148–149
Parapraxes, 283–284
Parasitic infections and medicinal plants,
        37
Paresthesia, 341
Parietal lobe, 344
Parkinson's disease, 74, 87, 136
Parvocellular fibers, 288, 290
Passive-aggressive personality, 319, 321
Pattern recognition and generation, 229–
        230
Pavy, Octave, 172
Perception
    concretization of, 316–317
    disorders of, 269–271
    imagery and, 236–237, 239–241
    reality testing and, 267–269
Perceptual ability. See Visual system
Perceptual quantum, 78
Periodic attractor, 108, 109
Periodicity
    overview of, 107–108
    regulation of, 152
    state and, 168
Perseveration, 157–158, 295
Persistent vegetative state, 228–229
Personality
    conservative energy expenditure and,
        120
    definition of, 19
    effects of head trauma on, 3–6
    as emergent property of brain pro-
        cesses, 13, 17, 105
    fluctuations in, 356–358
    as modular system, 4, 79
    self-organized criticality and, 127–129
    stability of, 356
    synaptic plasticity and, 360–361

Pharmacological means of changing state, 363
Phase portrait, 124, 125, 166–168
Phase space
  attractors and repellors and, 112
  overview of, 124–126
  self-representations and, 352
Phencyclidine (PCP), 363
Phonological loop, 239–240
Phonological short-term store, 101
Physiological state. *See* State
Plasma membrane, 42
Poincaré, Jules-Henri, 104
Point attractor, 108, 109
Postsynaptic neuron, 44
Posttraumatic stress disorder (PTSD), 103, 144, 365–366
Prefrontal cortex
  anatomy of, 287–290
  attention regulation and, 234
  development of, 40, 94, 290–293
  dysexecutive syndrome and, 270, 293–297
  euphoria after injury to, 274–275
  insight and, 345
  movement and, 76, 283
  novelty and, 247–248
Premotor area, medial, 76, 255–257. *See also* Supplementary motor area
Presynaptic neuron, 42–43
Pretectal area, 61
Pretectum, 61, 69
Primates
  categorization capacity of, 216
  cooperative activity of, 207, 219
  dominance in, 206–207
  lying by, 217–218
  overview of, 33–35
  self-awareness in, 210–211
  tactical deception by, 214
  visual system of, 60–61, 66, 68–69
  See also Chimpanzee cultures; Cognition in nonhuman primates
Priming, 95–96, 247
Probabilistic phenomena
  activation of neural networks as, 126–127
  behavior as, 51, 130, 371–372
  dynamics and, 106
  state as, 165–166

synaptic efficacy and, 44–45
synaptic plasticity and, 39
temperament and, 11
Procedural knowledge
  expressions of, 316
  nonconscious functioning and, 231, 247
  overview of, 92–94
Procedural learning
  character and, 18, 91, 310–311, 313–314, 316–317
  character change and, 325
  culture and, 36–37
  declarative memory and, 93
  definition of, 36
  dissociability of, 86–87
  inertial quality of, 356
  infantile amnesia and, 369
  as modular, 84
  in monkeys, 208
  overview of, 91–92
  relationships with caregivers and, 315–316
  timing of development of, 94–95
Projection neuron, 43
Propanolol, 98
Prosimii, 33
Prosopagnosia, 251–252
Psychodynamics, 105, 260–262
Psychological activity and rhythmic process, 155
Psychological adaptation, 32
Psychological model
  bifurcation in, 119
  relationship to biological model, 8–9, 13–15
Psychological theories of temperament, 189
Psychological treatment
  of character, 102, 320, 322–324, 370–372
  cognitive therapy, 364
  critical state and, 130
  infantile amnesia and, 369–370
  modular hypothesis and, 81, 85
  of PTSD, 365–366
  self-organized criticality and, 130
  self-representations and, 336–337
  temperament and, 200–202
  in terms of dynamics, 359

Psychopathology
    modular hypothesis and, 79–80
    modularity of self and, 352–353
    temperament and, 199–200, 362
Psychotherapy. *See* Psychological treat-
    ment
PTSD (posttraumatic stress disorder),
    103, 144, 365–366
Pupillary reflexes and brainstem, 69–70
Putamen, 135, 288

Q

Quadrantanopia, 70
Quasi-periodicity, 114
Quinlan, Karen Ann, 229

R

Rapid eye movement (REM) sleep
    consciousness and, 228
    learning and, 15
    oscillatory dynamics and, 136
Rationality and behavior, 303
Rationalization
    conscious functioning and, 224, 241–
        244
    left hemisphere and, 255
    reality testing and, 272–273
Reaction rate, 113
Readiness potential (RP), 253–255, 257
Reality monitoring, 267, 271–272
Reality testing
    description of, 263, 267
    disorders of complex somatesthetic
        perception and, 270–271
    disorders of perception and, 269–270
    euphoria after frontal lobe injury and,
        274–275
    factors in disorders of, 277–278
    mnestic disturbances and, 271–272
    rationalization and, 272–273
    reflective awareness and denial of ill-
        ness and, 274
    representations and, 267–269
    sense of reality and, 275–277
Receptors, 43
Reconciliation behavior, 208
Red nucleus, 74–75
Reduplicative paramnesia, 271
Reentrance or reentry, 58–59
Refractory period, absolute, 44, 133

Reflective self-awareness
    description of, 278
    evolutionary advantage of, 220
    in great apes, 209–211
    language and, 221
    reality testing and, 274
    self-representations and, 330–331
    temperament and, 199
Reflex epilepsy, 149–151
Refractory period, relative, 44, 133
Regulation of behavior
    caregivers and development of, 266–
        267
    determinants of, 302–303
    learning, development, and acquisition
        of skill of, 297–298
    moral judgment and moral behavior,
        300–302
    overview of, 22, 279–280
    schemas and, 281–283
    See also Executive cognitive functions
Reich, Wilhelm, on character, 309–310,
    322–323
REM sleep. *See* Rapid eye movement
    (REM) sleep
Repellors, 110–112, 168
Repetition of task, 93–94
Representational space, 334
Representations
    conscious functioning and, 230–232
    description of, 224
    depictitive, 231
    motor, 345–346
    neurobiology of, 236
    propositional, 231
    reality testing and, 267–269
    of self and world, 337–340
    self-organized criticality and personal-
        ity and, 127–129
    types of, 231–232
    See also Self-representations
Repression and development of character,
    321–322
Resistance, 260–262
Reticular system, 66
Retinohypothalamic tract, 61, 70
Rhesus monkeys, 206, 208
Rhythmic movement, 137
Rhythmic process, significance of, 154–
    155

Rhythmic variation in cognition, 153–154
Right hemisphere
    callosotomy and, 348
    mnestic deficits and, 90–91

S
Sandpile example, 115
Saturn, rings of, 110–111
Schemas
    activation of behavior and, 281–282
    disruption of, 283–286
    Ferenczi conceptualization compared
        to, 308
    hierarchical organization of, 282
    levels of analysis of, 280–281
    overview of, 286
    selection and activation of, 282–283
Schizophrenia
    diagnostic category of, 80
    genetic influence on, 192
    modularity of self and, 352–353
    rationalization and, 273
Seasonal affective disorder, 156
Seizure
    complex partial type, 228, 276
    corpus callosotomy in, 242–244
    emotional functioning and, 175
    kindling and, 112, 151–152
    learning and, 112
    paroxysmal illusions and hallucina-
        tions and, 343
    reflex epilepsy, 149–151
    tonic-clonic type, 135
    triggers for, 149–151
Self
    callosotomy and modularity of, 346–
        350
    description of, 23
    difficulty of defining, 328–329
    dissociability of character and, 318–
        319
    as modular functional system, 333–
        334
    organization of, 329
    psychopathology and, 352–353
    purposes of, 329–330
    unitary sense of, 350–352
    See also Self-representations
Self-awareness. See Reflective self-aware-
    ness

Self-destructive behavior, 261
Self-organization
    adaptation and, 131
    description of, 116
    as nonconscious functioning, 231
Self-organized criticality
    characteristics of, 116–117
    nervous system and, 142–143
    overview of, 114–116
    personality and, 127–129
    psychotherapy and, 130
Self-organizing system, 121–124
Self-representations
    description of, 232
    disorders of, 337–339
    in great apes, 211–212
    as hierarchically organized, 327–328,
        332–333
    limitations of, 331–332
    overview of, 23
    self-awareness and, 330–331
    sensory stimuli and, 339–340
    socialization and, 334
    stability and change of, 335–337
    See also Body schema
Self-stimulation, 179–181
Semantic memory, 87, 90–91
Sense of agency, 255–257
Sense of reality, 275–277
Sensitive period. See Critical period
Sensitization, 367–368
Sensory buffer, 240
Sensory deprivation and overload, 147–
    148
Sensory perception without awareness,
    248–249
Sensory stimuli
    neurodynamics and, 146–149
    primacy of over vision, 341–342
    self-representations and, 339–340
Separation from caregiver, 205–206
Separatrix, 111–112
Septum, 136
Sequential processing, 139
Sexual orientation, 193–194
Shallice, T., theory of behavioral self-reg-
    ulation, 281–283, 284
Shame, 334
Sherman (chimpanzee), 215–216, 219
Short-term memory. See Working memory

Short-term synaptic enhancement, 49
Shyness
    repellors and, 112
    temperament and, 197, 314
    types of in children, 195–196
Sickle cell trait, 29
Sign language. *See* Symbolic language
Simple cells, 68
Simultanagnosia, 71
Skin conductance, 252
Sleep
    consciousness and, 228
    oscillatory dynamics and, 136
    REM type, 15
Sleep-wake cycle, 152, 153
Social context
    for cognition, 204
    for self-representations, 334
Social hierarchies in nonhuman primates,
        206–208
Social learning, 36–37
Soma, 41
Somatic perception disorders, 270–271
Somototopical map, 73
Spandrels, 32, 258
Spasticity, 74
Speed
    of information processing, 233
    of learning process, 93
Split-brain syndrome, 234–235, 241–
        244, 272–273, 346–350
Splitting of self, 352–353
Stable attractor, 108
State
    alterations in, 362–364
    character and, 318
    context-dependent memory and, 170–
        171
    description of, 21–22, 126, 164–165
    as dynamic process, 165–168
    as global attractor, 143–144
    influence of on behavior and cogni-
        tion, 171–172
    as instantaneous, 164
    as modular, 168–170
    as nonlinear, 168–170, 187
    rhythmic process in, 154–155
    temperament and, 195
    transient change and, 365

State space. *See* Phase space
Stimulus generalization, 144
Striatum, 135
Structure, relationship to function, 58
Stuttering, 160–162
Subliminal perception, 246
Superior colliculus, 61, 70
Superstitious behavior, 25–26
Supplementary motor area (SMA), 76,
        255–257
Suprachiasmatic nucleus (SCN), 61, 70,
        153
Survival of the fittest, 26–27
Symbolic language
    acquisition of by apes, 22
    Austin and Sherman and, 215–216
    importance of great apes learning,
        220–221
    Koko and, 216–217
    Washoe and, 215
Synapse
    description of, 14, 41, 42, 132–133
    efficacy of, 44–45
    long-term memory and, 49–50, 51
    modification of by experience, 45
    structure and function of, 43–44
Synaptic cleft, 43
Synaptic plasticity
    in adults, 49–50
    changes in across lifespan, 360–361
    critical periods and, 45–48
    description of, 14, 20, 39
    neural networks and, 50–51
    personality change and, 359–360
    personality fluctuations and, 358
    short-term synaptic enhancement and,
        49
    somatosensory cortex and, 51–52
    theories of, 15
Synaptic strength, 134, 140
Synaptic vesicle, 43
Synergy, 77
Synthesis, 263, 350
Szentágothai, Janos, 4

T
Tactical deception, 213–215, 217–218
Taste, 183
Tectonic plate example, 115–116

Temperament
  change and, 361–362
  conduct disorder and hyperactivity,
    196
  development of character and, 314–
    315
  dimensions of, 194–195
  dynamics and, 190–191
  ego functions and, 265
  environment and, 196–200
  inhibited and uninhibited children,
    195–196, 197
  overview of, 10–11, 22, 189–190
  psychological treatment and, 200–
    202
  state and, 168–169
Temporal lobe epilepsy, 175
Temporal lobes
  amnesia and, 89–90
  memory and, 85–86
Temporal organization of processes, 21
Terminal arborizations, 41–42
Terminology in book, 10–11
Thalamotomy, stereotactic, 99
Thalamus
  dorsomedial, 76, 288
  and memory of pain, 99
Thalassemias, 29–30
Theories
  of behavioral self-regulation (Shallice),
    281–283, 284
  of brain function, 56–58
  of character, 23
  definition of, 9
  of emotion (LeDoux), 176–178
  of learning, 15
  of readers of book, 8
  of synaptic plasticity, 15
  of temperament, 189
Theory of mind
  autism and, 201
  caring for young and, 220
  great apes and, 205, 212–218
  overview of, 7–8
Thermodynamics, second law of, 119–
  120, 121
Time, patterns of activity across, 152–
  155
Time-locked, 78

Timing
  of development of procedural and de-
    clarative learning, 94–95
  evolutionary change and, 31
  modification of synapses by experience
    and, 45
Tool acquisition and use, 36–37
Topographical organization
  of brain modules, 59–60
  of somatosensory cortex, 52
Traits, conservation of across evolution,
  33
Trauma, 320, 335–336, 359, 362
  See also Posttraumatic stress disorder
    (PTSD)

U
Ultradian rhythm, 152
Unconditioned response, 368
Unconditioned stimulus, 99, 368
Unconscious in psychodynamics, 260–
  262
Unilateral spatial neglect, 249–251, 337–
  339
Uninhibited children, 195–196, 197
Unitary sense of self, 350–352
Unpredictability, 112–113
Utilization behavior (Lhermitte), 296–297

V
Variation and natural selection, 28–29
Vermis, 75
Vestibulo-oculomotor reflex, 76
Vibrissae, 33
Vicki (chimpanzee), 216, 217
Visual buffer, 239–240
Visual system
  architecture of, 54–55
  critical periods and development of,
    46–48
  effects of injury to regions of, 69–72
  imagery and perception in, 236–237,
    239–241
  as modular organization, 60–61, 66,
    68–69, 72
  neural networks and, 140–141
  overview of, 20
  primacy of somatesthetic sensation
    over, 341–342

Visuospatial sketchpad, 101
Volition, 253–255
Voluntary control of behavior, 257–258

W
Washoe (chimpanzee), 215
Wilderness encounters, 337, 366–367
Wilson, Woodrow, 249

Working memory
aging and, 292
capacity of, 103, 233–234
conscious functioning and, 232–233
as modular, 85
overview of, 101–102
short-term synaptic enhancement and,
  49